Darwin's Illness

UNIVERSITY PRESS OF FLORIDA

Florida A&M University, Tallahassee
Florida Atlantic University, Boca Raton
Florida Gulf Coast University, Ft. Myers
Florida International University, Miami
Florida State University, Tallahassee
New College of Florida, Sarasota
University of Central Florida, Orlando
University of Florida, Gainesville
University of North Florida, Jacksonville
University of South Florida, Tampa
University of West Florida, Pensacola

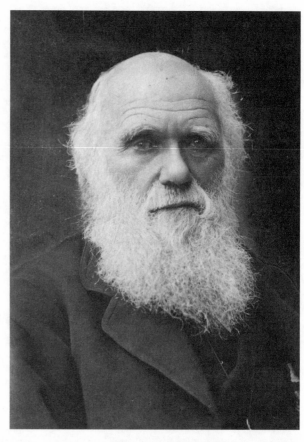

University Press of Florida
Gainesville · Tallahassee · Tampa · Boca Raton · Pensacola
Orlando · Miami · Jacksonville · Ft. Myers · Sarasota

DARWIN'S ILLNESS

Ralph Colp Jr., M.D.

Foreword by James Moore

12   11   10   09   08   6   5   4   3   2   1

Library of Congress Cataloging-in-Publication Data
Colp, Ralph, 1924–
Darwin's illness / Ralph Colp, Jr.
p. cm.
Includes bibliographical references.
ISBN 978–0–8130–3231–3 (alk. paper)
1. Darwin, Charles, 1809–1882. 2. Naturalists—Great Britain—Biography.
3. Chronic diseases—Case studies. I. Title.
QH31.D2C623 2008
576.8′20929–dc22
[B]
2007051226

The University Press of Florida is the scholarly publishing agency for the State
University System of Florida, comprising Florida A&M University, Florida Atlantic
University, Florida Gulf Coast University, Florida International University, Florida
State University, New College of Florida, University of Central Florida, University
of Florida, University of North Florida, University of South Florida, and University
of West Florida.

University Press of Florida
15 Northwest 15th Street
Gainesville, Fla. 32611-2079
www.upf.com

To the memory of my mother, who shared my interest in Darwin, and for my wife, who supported me throughout my work on Darwin.

Contents

Foreword

Charles Darwin is the patient, and his doctor is Ralph Colp Jr. For forty years, Dr. Colp has been examining the great naturalist; no one knows his corpus better. No one since the death of Darwin's wife in 1896 has possessed more intimate details of his daily existence. And no doctor, biographer, or historian is likely to surpass Colp's insights for a generation. *Darwin's Illness* may not be the end, but it is unquestionably the vital starting point for all future reflection on the health of history's most famous sick scientist.

Doctors know three things for sure about Darwin: he sailed around the world, he had a beard, and he was sick a lot. And they think they know why he was sick. Every consultant has a diagnosis; every GP has a hunch. A history of medical controversies since Darwin's day could be written around discussions of his disordered state. Darwin himself (with medical training) had theories, his doctors had theories, and for a century medical and psychiatric journals have published theories. Like a Victorian whodunit, with a plethora of lurid clues, the subject remains irresistible.

Dr. Colp starts with those clues. Chapter by painstaking chapter, he sets down Darwin's case history in chronological order. The evidence for every passing complaint and persistent condition has been ferreted out from every biographical byway, including Darwin's unpublished manuscripts and jottings, recollections of his relatives, friends, and physicians, *The Correspondence of Charles Darwin*, now half completed, and a host of revealing letters yet to be published in that great work. Over the years it has been my privilege and education to assist Dr. Colp with his research. From these rich sources, Darwin emerges reincarnate, presenting an array of symptoms in all their corporeal horror.

Have a man's intimate bodily functions ever been recorded in such detail? Still in his fifties, Darwin himself reported "25 years extreme spasmodic daily & nightly flatulence: occasional vomiting, on two occasions prolonged during months. Vomiting preceded by shivering, hysterical crying[,] dying sensations . . . & copious very palid [*sic*] urine. Now vomiting & every passage of flatulence preceded by ringing of ears." For much of his life, Darwin was (as Janet Browne frankly admits) a "noisy and smelly" presence, his wretched belly a barometer of an anxious or overwrought mind; and he sought to shield even his oldest friends from the effects. "I sh[oul]d not like to be in the House ... as my retching is apt to be extremely loud," he once warned a dying colleague.

Practically everything known about Darwin's illness is recorded in Colp's early chapters, and as the awful details emerge, he recounts an often desperate quest for remedies. Doctors came and went, shaking their heads and prescribing the latest nostrums. There was nothing Darwin wouldn't try (except mesmerism, clairvoyance, and prayer): acids and alkalis, ice and heat, emetics and purgatives, opium, arsenic, "electric chains," and "Condy's Ozonised Water." The treatment he stuck with longest was the fashionable "water cure." Depressed after his father's death and fearing that he himself was "rapidly going the way of all flesh," he spent four months under Dr. James Manby Gully at the hydropathic spa of Malvern. At home he kept up the aquatic ritual—heat lamp followed by icy showers and soaking sheets—recording the effects in a foolscap health diary.

This was Darwin's only extended experiment on a human subject. He observed himself obsessively, a believer in "survival of the fittest" struggling with his own mortality, an evolutionist jotting down the changes in his organism day and night for six agonizing years. The diary, kept from 1849 to 1855, testifies to Darwin's tenacious mental state on the eve of starting the *Origin of Species*, and in an appendix to *Darwin's Illness* this extraordinary document is fully transcribed for the first time. Dr. Colp spent many years deciphering the abysmal handwriting and cryptic abbreviations. His meticulously annotated text is a boon to Darwin scholars and will shed new light on the self-help culture of Victorian fringe medicine.

What was wrong with Darwin? Dr. Colp gives a judicious survey of the many theories put forward since his patient's death. Was the cause an overbearing father, himself a physician? Or was it the seasickness he suffered aboard the *Beagle*? Or was he afflicted by the absence of his mother, who died when he was eight? Was it arsenic poisoning? Adrenal malfunction is possible, but suppose Darwin had systemic lupus or lactose intolerance. Or did he suffer from Chagas' disease or Crohn's? Or was he just a hypochondriac? Dr. Colp ascribes Darwin's disordered state to arrested Chagas' plus fluctuating mental pressures from his taxing work on evolution and other personal stresses.

Darwin's Illness is much more than a persuasively intimate account of a Victorian invalid. It is also a history of ideas about that illusive illness or shifting set of symptoms and the diagnoses favoring either physical or psychosomatic causation chart controversies in medical knowledge. The subject of this book—illness and patient—will continue to fascinate doctors. And as long as creative genius is associated with mental and physical suffering, a much wider audience will be intrigued. Indeed, Dr. Colp's picture of Darwin jotting down the effects of amyl nitrate on his failing heart up to forty-eight hours before he died—"14 April: 1 attack slight pain 1 dose . . . 17 April: Only traces of pain no dose"—is strangely reminiscent of ourselves. We share his obsession with survival and fitness.

James Moore
Cambridge, England

Preface

In 1977 I published my first book, *To Be an Invalid: The Illness of Charles Darwin*. In it, based largely on Darwin's extant correspondence, I gave the history of an illness that Darwin once described as "my old enemy."[1] At the time Darwin made this comment, he had experienced twenty-three years of daily discomfort that sometimes increased in intensity and duration and was frequently associated with other kinds of symptoms. I evaluated a number of theories about the possible causes of the illness.

In the three decades that have followed the appearance of my book, knowledge of Darwin's correspondence has greatly increased. There has been the publication of a calendar of all his published and unpublished letters (first printed in 1985 and then updated in 1994) and the publication of fifteen volumes of his correspondence, 1821–67. I have also learned new facts about Darwin's personal life from his notebooks, his wife's diary, the recollections of his children and friends, and comprehensive biographies by Adrian Desmond and James Moore, *Darwin* (1991), and Janet Browne, *Charles Darwin: Voyaging* (1995) and *Charles Darwin: The Power of Place* (2002).

This increased knowledge showed me that many changes needed to be made in my book. These changes will be published by 2009, the bicentennial of Darwin's birth on 12 February and the 150th anniversary of the publication of *On the Origin of Species* on 26 November. This is the date of publication given in Morse Peckham's recently reissued variorum edition of *Origin*.

In the course of making these changes, although limitations of space have not made it possible to reprint my transcription of the Darwin family receipts and memoranda book, I have produced this new book, which is more informative than *To Be an Invalid*. Some of the additions I have made consist of new facets and insights on Darwin's pre-*Beagle* health, on the possibility he may have contracted Chagas' disease in South America, and on the occasional illnesses he had soon after he returned to England from the *Beagle*. I then discuss the onset of his lifelong adult illness and the possibility that Chagas' disease may have been one of the causes of this illness.

New information has enabled me to delineate several episodes of Darwin's illness that were hitherto unrecorded, to offer new explanations for some of his large and small increases of illness, to narrate a fuller and more detailed history of his symptoms and treatments, and to give a more intimate portrait of him as a scientist and man by depicting the manifold and complex ways that illness influenced his work and his relationships with family and friends.

As theories about the possible causes of the illness have continued to proliferate, I have evaluated each of these, showing how they were often stimulated not only by new information about Darwin but also by new expansions in medical and psychiatric knowledge.

In an appendix to *Darwin's Illness* I have added a complete transcription of Darwin's 1849–55 "diary of health," which I had previously only partly quoted. I believe that the diary is a remarkable personal and medical document, because it is the only time that Darwin gives a chronicle of his various daily symptoms over a period of several years, shows the different treatments he used, and shows many of the possible reasons for increases in severity of his symptoms.

As far as I can judge, this book may contain practically everything that is known about Darwin's illness.

Acknowledgments

My greatest debt is to Jim Moore for years of friendship and sharing with me his very great knowledge of Darwin, as well as for his unstinting aid in my work on Darwin. Without his presence, this book would not have been possible.

I am further indebted to Randal Keynes and David Kohn for discussing with me their areas of expertise on Darwin. Additionally, Richard Milner has informed me about advances in different areas of Darwin research.

I owe a special debt to my son-in-law, Professor Barry Rubin, who encouraged me to do a second edition of *To Be an Invalid* and who then found a publisher for this edition. Thanks also must go to my daughter, Judy Colp Rubin, for helping to edit this book.

Among the many individuals with whom I have had valuable talks about Darwin, I should like to mention Dr. Jeremiah Barondes, Frederick Burkhardt, Paul Elovitz, Howard Gruber, Edna Healey, Jeffery Kaye, Richard Darwin Keynes, Silvan Schweber, and Leonard Wilson.

I am also indebted to the Syndics of the Cambridge University Library for permission to publish Darwin documents in their possession; to Richard Darwin Keynes for permission to quote from Emma Darwin's diary; and to the College Archive, Imperial College London, for permission to quote from Darwin's letters to Huxley. Documents in the possession of the Wedgwood Museum are published by courtesy of the Wedgwood Museum Trust, Barlaston, Staffordshire. Darwin's health diary is transcribed with permission of English Heritage, Down House (Darwin Collection).

Finally, thanks to Karen Abraham for doing a superb job in typing successive versions of my manuscript.

The Illness

1

"Violent Fatigues," Bad Lips, and Unwell Hands

When Charles Darwin was between fifteen and twenty-two years old, he was omnivorous of life and eagerly participated in many activities with friends and relatives. He also suffered from three kinds of disturbances to his health.

The first kind happened when he sometimes reacted to certain events, pleasant or unpleasant, by experiencing episodes which his physician father, Dr. Robert Darwin, and younger sister, Catherine, called "violent fatigues" and which he later called "mental fatigue or rather excitement." Episodes consisted of trembling, chills, shivering, and a gastrointestinal disorder of an unspecified nature. These occurred in varying intensities, durations, and combinations, and they were followed by periods of fatigue, lasting for varying lengths of time, which Darwin referred to as being "knocked up."[1]

His siblings worried about how these episodes might disturb him and predicted that exposures to certain unpleasant events would cause him to have particular symptoms. Early in 1825, when he was sixteen, his older brother, Erasmus, who was then a medical student, wrote him a letter about dissecting a human cadaver and, referring to his strong negative feelings about this kind of dissecting, commented: "I don't fancy it w^ld. have suited you especially before breakfast." The following year, after becoming a medical student at the University of Edinburgh and listening to Professor Alexander Monro's lectures on human anatomy, Darwin was stimulated by feelings of revulsion (perhaps accompanied by unpleasant stomach sensations) to write to his family that Dr. Monro was "dirty in person & actions," and "I dislike him & his Lectures so much that I cannot speak with decency about them." He would recollect that the subject of anatomy "disgusted" him and that "it has proved one of the greatest evils in my life that I was not urged to practice dissection, for I should soon have got over my disgust; and the practice would have been invaluable for all my future work."

In addition to Monro's lectures, he "attended on two occasions the operating theatre in the hospital at Edinburgh, and saw two very bad operations, one on a child, but rushed away before they were completed. Nor did I ever attend again, for hardly any inducement would have been strong enough to make me do so; this being long before the blessed days of chloroform."[2]

He was horrified by the strapped screaming patients, the violence and cruelty of the surgeons as they hacked and cut at body parts, and by the sight of blood pouring into buckets and on the floor. He became "haunted" by what he had seen and would speak about it many years later. He would continue to be horrified at instances where individuals inflicted pain on each other, and he would always have (in the words of his son George) "a morbid horror of the sight or even of the word *blood*."[3]

Two events that stimulated his deep feelings were caused by dogs. When he was at Edinburgh, Catherine wrote him that his dog, Sparks, had been sent from the Darwin household to another household, and that the loss of Sparks would "be a shock to all your nerves, and will spoil a good many breakfasts."

Several years later, after Darwin had terminated medical studies at Edinburgh and become a pre-divinity student at Cambridge University, he and his Cambridge friend John Herbert attended an exhibition of "learned dogs." Herbert recollected how in the middle of the exhibition, "one of the dogs failed in performing the trick his master told him to do—on the man reproving, the dog put on the most piteous expression, as if in fear of the whip. Darwin seeing it, asked me to leave with him, saying, 'come along, I can't stand this any longer; how those poor dogs must have been licked.'" Darwin's reasons for suddenly leaving the exhibition were not only to avoid being knocked up by his painful perceptions of cruelties to dogs but to also avoid the possibility that these perceptions might then haunt him, as he had been haunted by the horrors of the Edinburgh operations. Throughout his life he would be sensitive to individuals maltreating dogs, horses, and other domestic animals.[4]

On two occasions, he had physical symptoms because of mental experiences that were unusually pleasant, the first when he was fifteen and successfully hunted birds, the second when he was twenty and developing "a strong taste for music." "How well I remember," he wrote in his autobiography, "killing my first snipe, and my excitement was so great that I had much difficulty in reloading my gun from the trembling of my hands." He soon learned to control his trembling, and was able to reload his gun rapidly so as to kill record numbers of birds. He also continued to experience feelings of excitement, so that he came to regard hunting as a "most holy cause."[5]

He recollected how listening to certain kinds of music when he was at Cambridge caused him to have "intense pleasure, so that my backbone would sometimes shiver." Herbert remembered how he frequently went to King's College Chapel to hear the Anthem in the afternoon service and that "what gave him the greatest delight was some grand symphony or overture, of Mozart's or Beethoven's, with their full harmonies. For a simple melody he cared little." Herbert adds that one afternoon, after he and Darwin had heard a "very beautiful anthem" at King's Chapel, Darwin commented on his shivering by saying to Herbert "with a deep sigh, 'How's your backbone?'"[6]

On 8 October 1829, Darwin attended two events at the Birmingham Musical Festival: a morning orchestral and choral performance of Handel's *Messiah* (which especially stirred him), and evening enactments from three Italian operas. In both the morning and evening, there was singing and acting by the beautiful and charismatic young soprano Maria Malibran. In a letter to his friend William Darwin Fox, Darwin commented that the festival was "the most glorious thing I ever experienced," "very superior" to any concerts he had "ever heard before," and that Malibran was "quite the most charming person I ever saw." He added: "It knocked me up most dreadfully, & I never will attempt again to go to two things the same day." This first statement meant that, whereas hearing an anthem for an afternoon at Cambridge stimulated him to sigh because of one occurrence of shivering, hearing a variety of "glorious" musical events in the morning and again in the evening at Birmingham overly stimulated him. His way of preventing being knocked up again was by planning to curtail the amount of time that he would spend listening to the music that made him shiver.[7]

Darwin's second kind of ill health was a recurring skin disorder on his lips and hands. Herbert described the first disorder, many years later, as "an eruption about the mouth." In letters to Fox in 1829, Darwin recounted the history of the eruption, along with the stresses that may have caused it.

"My life," he wrote Fox early in January, "is very quiet & uniform, & what makes it more so, my lips have lately taken to be bad, which will prevent my going to Edinburgh." He went on to write about studying for the Cambridge Little-Go examination, scheduled to take place the next term, and having "doubt & tribulation" over being able to pass it. At the suggestion of his Cambridge tutor, he postponed taking the examination for a year.

He then informed Fox how, when he had gone out hunting with one of the sons of his friend Squire Owen, the copper cap from the first shot that he fired had flown out of his gun and cut young Owen's "eye so badly. . . .that he has been in bed for a week. I think I never in my life time was half so much frightened." The wound may have produced much bleeding, thus immediately stimulating Darwin's feelings of horror over seeing blood, which may have been followed by guilt over having injured Owen.[8]

In two letters in April, Darwin expressed feelings of depression: "I find Cambridge rather stupid, & as I know scarcely any one that walks, & this joined with my lips not being quite well, has reduced me to sort of Hybernation," and "I have been in such perfect & absolute state of idleness, that it is enough to paralyze all one's faculties."

In July, after starting out from his home in Shrewsbury to collect beetles, accompanied by another beetle collector, Frederick Hope, he told Fox: "The first two days I went on pretty well, taking several good insects, but for the rest of that week, my lips became suddenly so bad, & I myself not very well, that I was unable to leave the room, & on the Monday I retreated with grief and sorrow back again to Shrewsbury. . . . But the days that I was unable to go out, M^r. Hope did wonders taking several rare species. . . . I am sure you will properly sympathise with my unfortunate situation; I am determined to go over the same ground that he does before Autumn comes, & if working hard will procure insects I will bring home a glorious stock." Darwin's rivalry over beetle collecting with Hope would change into his becoming "quite disgusted" with Hope's entomological activities. After July 1829, he resumed beetle collecting and for many years had no lip complaints in his extant letters. He may have had complaints that were undocumented, for in July 1833, when he was voyaging on the *Beagle*, his sister Susan wrote him: "I hope you keep quite well. . . . Do your lips plague you now?"[9]

Herbert later recollected that Darwin treated his lips by taking "small doses of arsenic" and that his father warned him of the possible toxic effects of arsenic. This is the only reference to Darwin's actually taking arsenic. Herbert does not tell the size and frequency of the "small doses" that Darwin used, whether he took them locally or internally, or whether he was medicated by a doctor, or by himself.[10]

Darwin's third disturbance of health was numbness of his hands (paresthesia), which in a 6 September 1831 letter to Susan he described as follows: "My hands are not quite well—& I have observed that if I once get them well & change my manner of living about the same time they will generally remain well." He gives no further information on the clinical nature of his hand condition or the ways he treated it. This was his earliest recorded mention of hand paresthesia, which would occur on several occasions in his later life.[11]

In his autobiography, looking back on the Cambridge University years of 1828–31, Darwin commented: "I was then in excellent health, and almost always in high spirits." He regarded his health as excellent because the interruptions resulting from his violent fatigue, lip eruption, and hand paresthesia were short and temporary. He was soon able to resume his patterns of beetle collecting and friendships with Cambridge men and his special friendship, which combined feelings of reverence with love, for Cambridge botany professor John Stevens Henslow. Being "*almost* always" in high spirits may refer to the depressions that were associated with the lip eruption. These depressions resulted not only from the mental stresses that caused the eruption but also from feelings of shame over its facial disfigurements and perhaps also from the toxic side effects of arsenic.[12]

2

The *Beagle* Illnesses

On 29 August 1831, through the influence of Professor Henslow, Darwin was offered the position of naturalist on the HMS *Beagle,* which was preparing to sail around the world. Stimulated by a recent reading of Alexander von Humboldt's *Personal Narrative* descriptions of travels in South America and the island of Teneriffe and by a passion to visit Teneriffe's tropical vegetation, he "immediately" accepted the offer.[1] The next day he refused it, mainly because of his father's objections. "Even if I was to go," he wrote, "my Father disliking would take away all energy, & I should want a good stock of that." After his uncle Josiah Wedgwood persuaded his father to give support, he again accepted the offer on 1 September.[2]

He recollected how from 30 August through 1 September, "My mind was like a swinging pendulum" and "my heart appeared to sink within me, independently of the doubts raised by Father's dislike to the scheme. I could scarcely make up my mind to leave England even for the time which I then thought the voyage would last." The sensation of his heart "sinking" within him was a depressed feeling, that he would often experience when first confronting a new situation.[3]

After 1 September, the intensity of the "sinking" lessened, and he began making plans for the *Beagle.* On 6 September, he was in London, purchasing equipment he would need with money advanced by his father. After writing to Susan about his hand disorder, he asked her to ask their father whether he should take "Arsenic for a little time" for the disorder. When their father apparently disapproved, he informed Susan, "I do not think I shall take any Arsenic." For the rest of his stay in England he would make no further mention of hands or arsenic. On 17 September he stated to Susan his resolve to go on the voyage: "I dont care whom you now tell; for all is fixed & certain.—& I feel *well up to it* not but what this has often been a difficult task & my reason has been the only power that was capable of it: for it is most painful whenever I think of leaving for so long a time so many people whom I love."[4]

On 24 October, he moved from London to Plymouth where the *Beagle* was preparing to depart. When the *Beagle* twice attempted to sail but was driven back by heavy gales, there was a delay of two months. During these months, he suffered what he later rated as a "most miserable" illness, consisting of a mixture of fluctuating psychiatric and psychosomatic symptoms: a "wearisome anxiety," "giddiness" and feeling "giddy & uncomfortable" in the head, "palpitations and pain about the heart," along with the conviction that he had heart disease, and feelings of depression that caused him to regard the weather as "inexpressibly gloomy" and to feel disinclined to wash his hands or read a book. Occasionally he "felt some of the same heart-sinking sensations" of fear that he had experienced when he first learned of the voyage, and he became seasick when the *Beagle* attempted its two sailings.[5]

The causes for the illness were mental conflicts between his resolve to go on the voyage, despite "all hazards," and his burgeoning realizations and apprehensions of its hardships and hazards. These included daily experiencing the "evil" of the "absolute want of room" of his ship quarters, the "rough" manners and grumbling and growling of the ship's crew, persistent anticipations of becoming homesick for family and friends, and a dread that future seasickness would incapacitate him from doing work.[6] He also contemplated the various dangers of death from heart disease,[7] tropical diseases,[8] and drowning.[9] He had probably never before confronted death in so many forms nor made a resolution that involved the possibility of being killed.[10]

On 27 December, the *Beagle* sailed out of Plymouth and across the North Atlantic Ocean. Over the following week Darwin recorded in his diary that he was "wretchedly out of spirits & very sea-sick." He first worried whether the flogging of several *Beagle* sailors, for their "crime" of drunkenness on Christmas Day, made the crime "more or less excusable." Then he was "haunted" by "dark & gloomy thoughts" that he should have "repented" of the whole *Beagle* undertaking, and he greeted the new year of 1832 with gloom and "jaundiced senses." Yet when he reread "Humboldt's glowing accounts of tropical scenery," he commented that "nothing could be better adapted for cheering the heart of a sea-sick man."

"The misery I endured from sea-sickness," he wrote in his first *Beagle* letter to his father, "is far beyond what I ever guessed at. I believe you are curious about it. I will give all my dear-bought experience. Nobody who has only been to sea for 24 hours has a right to say, that sea-sickness is even uncomfortable.

The real misery only begins when you are so exhausted—that a little exertion makes a feeling of faintness come on." He added that he was treating himself by taking father's "receipt of raisins, which is the only food that the stomach will bear." Susan would then write him: "Papa was much interested by your miserable account of the sea sickness you had endured & not a little proud of his prescription of the Raisins answering so well. I think he should publish such a discovery for the benefit of all such sufferers."[11]

On 8 January, he experienced a bitter disappointment when the *Beagle* reached Teneriffe but was unable to land because of a quarantine against cholera. However, during the subsequent months his gloomy thoughts waned, he developed warm friendships with his *Beagle* shipmates, and his confined ship quarters forced him to develop "methodical habits of working." His seasickness became less intense but continued to be intermittent, causing him to feel "squeamish & uncomfortable" and painfully indolent.[12] In addition to raisins, he treated the sickness by eating unspecified amounts of a very hot mixture of "Sago, with wine & spice," and later he may have taken, separately or in different combinations, peppermint, hops, carbonate of soda, laudanum, and lavender water.[13] The "only sure" treatment that he used constantly was to lie in the horizontal position, preferably in a hammock. His shipmate, John Lort Stokes, recollected how after he had worked for about an hour at a table in the poop cabin of the *Beagle*, he would say to Stokes, "Old fellow, I must take the horizontal for it," and then stretch out on one side of the table. After a while he would resume his work, until he again had to lie down. Referring to these treatments he wrote: "It must never be forgotten the more you combat the enemy the sooner he will yield," and by following them he was able to accomplish a good deal of work when at sea.[14]

After seeing tropical vegetation on the island of St. Jago, he recorded in his diary that it had been for him "a glorious day, like giving to a blind man eyes.— he is overwhelmed with what he sees & cannot justly comprehend it." Six weeks later, when he visited the Brazilian port of Bahia, he recorded that the reality of seeing a Brazilian tropical forest surpassed the glory of Humboldt's descriptions of tropical scenery. When he first explored the forest, for three days the "acute" and almost continuous "chaos of delight" he experienced appears to have been a "violent fatigue." Undoubtedly because of exhaustion, he became "idle" and unable to work for two days. He was soon able to work in the forest for many hours at collecting objects in natural history and not have any violent fatigues, while continuing to have "unspeakable" feelings of pleasure.[15]

He recorded in his diary that, "exempting when in the midst of tropical scenery," he experienced feelings of homesickness. He described these feelings as "painful" and the "greatest drawback" to going on with the voyage. Although he would have these feelings throughout the voyage, he would hold them in check for several years.[16]

During his sojourn in Brazil, from March through July 1832, he had severe inflammations of a knee and then of his arm, each of which lasted about one week. He observed, "Any small prick is very apt to become in this country a painful boil."[17] On 11 April 1832, while journeying through a Brazilian forest, he began to feel "feverish, shivering and sickness [vomiting]," with exhaustion and loss of appetite. He stayed for the night in a Brazilian country house, feeling sick and fearful of more sickness. "It did not require much imagination," he wrote, "to paint the horrors of illness in a foreign country, without being able to speak one word or obtain any medical aid." In the morning he treated himself by "eating cinnamon & drinking port wine," and reported that this "cured me in a wonderful manner."[18] His choice of medicine may have been influenced by his father, who prescribed port wine for fevers in children and cinnamon teas as a daily drink.[19]

After he returned to Rio de Janeiro, he walked to the Botanic Garden and studied the "trees" of camphor, sago, cinnamon, tea, cloves, and pepper. He was interested in these plants because of their medicinal use—what he called their "notorious . . . utility"—and he smelled and tasted some of their leaves.[20]

On 6 June 1832, he sent his family in Shrewsbury some "calamitous" news. "A large party of our officers & sailors before leaving Rio, went a party in the Cutter for snipe shooting up the bay. Most of them were slightly attacked with fever: but the two men & poor little Musters were seized violently & died in a few days. . . . What numbers snipe shooting has killed & how rapidly they drop off." Before receiving this news, he had "very nearly" joined another snipe-shooting party. "My good star," he commented, "presided over me when I failed."[21]

When Susan read his June letter, she wrote him first of her worry that his "over tiring" himself would bring on a fatal fever and then that his family would all feel happy if he would put aside "false shame" and become "inclined" to return home.[22] In May 1833, he replied to his family while he was exploring the coast of Argentina. After stating the need to "go on" with the work he had done in zoology and geology, he emphasized his evolving sense of the value of this work: "I trust & believe, that the time spent in this voyage, if thrown away for all other respects, will produce its full worth in Nat: History: And it appears to me, the doing what *little* one can to encrease the general stock of knowledge is as respectable an object of life, as one can in any likelihood pursue."[23]

He also asked his father to pay for a member of the *Beagle* crew to become his servant and to aid him in scientific work.[24] One reason for the confident and assertive tone in his letter was that at this time he had been free from illness for over a year. His father, who had previously paid for his scientific expeditions, then agreed to pay for a servant, and for a time his family did not further press him to come home.

Months after writing his letter, he began to have brief episodes of illness. On 2 October 1833, while horseback riding from Buenos Aires to Santa Fe in Argentina, he felt "very weak from great heat," and "unwell and feverish, from having exerted myself too much in the sun."[25] This may have been a heat stroke.[26] The next day, feeling "very weak" and with a "headach," he reached Santa Fe where he got himself into a house and bed. He later recollected how he was cared for by "a good natured old woman," who wanted to treat him with several odd remedies, such as placing a bit of black plaster on each of his temples, or splitting a bean into halves and placing one on each temple.[27] "Many of the remedies used by the people of the country are ludicrously strange," he wrote, "but too disgusting to be mentioned. One of the least nasty is to kill and cut open two puppies and to bind them on each side of a broken limb. Little hairless dogs are in great request to sleep at the feet of invalids."[28] On 5 October, he was well enough to move out of his Santa Fe house and bed. Then, "not being quite well" and "unable to ride a horse," he returned to Buenos Aires in a small boat.[29]

On 16 October 1833, while in Montevideo, Uruguay, he felt "not . . . quite well" and "stomach disordered," and he stayed for a day in a house. The following day he had no complaints and was able to travel.[30]

On 11 January 1834, the *Beagle* anchored at Port Saint Julien, in southern Argentina, and Darwin, FitzRoy, and a group from the *Beagle* went on a walk into the interior country. The day was very hot, the group became "excessively tired"—several collapsed and were unable to walk—and suffered a "most painful degree of thirst." After several hours they were able to obtain some water and returned to the *Beagle*. During this time, Darwin showed more endurance and was able to be more physically active than the others; he was one of the first to reach the *Beagle*'s boat, and he reported that he felt "not much tired." However, for the next two days he was "very feverish in bed," which was in contrast to the other members of the *Beagle* group, who suffered no after effects. By the third day he felt well and "went out walking."[31]

In September 1834, while visiting gold mines in Chile, he drank "some sour new made" Chichi wine. "This half poisoned me," he wrote sister Caroline. "I staid till I thought I was well; but my first days ride, which was a long one, again disordered my stomach & afterwards I could not get well; I quite lost my appetite & became very weak. I had a long distance to travel & I suffered very much." He became so exhausted that he was unable to ride his horse and had to hire a carriage to carry him back to the Chilean port of Valparaiso, where the *Beagle* was and where he bedded in the house of Richard Corfield, an Englishman from Shrewsbury. His illness lasted from 20 September to the end of October. It "disturbed every secretion of his body," and then stopped after one relapse (the longest and most severe illness he had during the *Beagle* voyage). He was treated by Benjamin Bynoe, the *Beagle's* surgeon, with rest and a "good deal of Calomel."[32] The use of calomel (mercurous chloride) suggests that Bynoe thought the illness was a fever. Calomel was prescribed by Darwin's father for some fevers.[33] Although it appears likely that the illness was typhoid fever, other causes have been suggested.[34]

Early in November, Darwin felt "quite well again," and rejoined the *Beagle* while it explored the Chilean coast. On 10 March, however, he wrote Caroline, "My stomach, partly from sea-sickness & partly from my illness in Valparaiso, is not very strong. I expect some good rides will make another man of me." He then went on a strenuous three-week horseback expedition to the Andean Mountains and the interior of Chile. In this expedition, along with making important observations on the geological origins of the mountains, he recorded in his diary that looking at the view caused him to have a feeling that was "like watching a thunderstorm, or hearing in the full orchestra a chorus of the *Messiah*." (This last referred to the violent fatigue he had experienced on hearing the *Messiah* on 8 October 1829 in Birmingham.) He also later recollected that he felt as "if his nerves had become fiddle-strings, and had all taken to rapidly vibrating." After experiencing the tiredness that followed this violent fatigue (a tiredness also caused by moving about the mountain tops, and by the high altitude), he soon went to sleep.[35]

Five days after leaving the Andes summit, on 26 March 1835, Darwin recorded in his diary that when he was in bed for the night, in a house in the village of Luxan (in Argentina), he "experienced an attack and it deserves no less a name of the Benchuca, the great black bug of the Pampas. It is most disgusting to feel the soft wingless insects, about an inch long, crawling over one's body. Before sucking they are quite thin, but afterwards they become round and bloated with blood, and in this state are easily crushed." There can be no doubt Darwin was attacked by several *Triatoma infestans,* which can be a carrier of the protozoa *Trypanosoma cruzi,* the causative agent of Chagas' disease.[36] He may have been exposed to Triatomas previously, and he was definitely exposed to them on two subsequent occasions. (Triatomas were endemic in the parts of Chile, Argentina, and Peru that he explored).[37]

On 9 April, two weeks after the "attack," Darwin wrote in his diary that until he reached Corfield's house in Valparaiso on 17 April, he "was not very well & saw nothing & admired nothing." These eight days of unwellness may have been an acute episode of subclinical Chagas' disease, which then subsided, so that for the next several years Darwin might have had latent Chagas' disease without any outward symptoms.[38]

He continued to travel in Chile from April through July 1835 and was in Peru in August, where he received a disquieting letter from sister Catherine.[39] After expressing sorrow over the suffering he had experienced in his Valparaiso illness Catherine wrote: "Papa charges me to give you a message from him; he wishes to urge you to think of leaving the *Beagle,* and returning home, and to take warning by this one serious illness; Papa says that if once your health begins to fail, you will doubly feel the effect of any unhealthy climate, and he is very uneasy about you, and very much afraid of the fevers you are liable to incur in those Countries. . . . Do think of what Papa says, my dear Charles; his advise is *always* so sensible in the long run, and do be wise in time, & come away before your health is ruined; if you once lose that, you will never recover it again entirely."[40]

Darwin replied to Catherine's letter soon after receiving it by writing to his Shrewsbury family (Caroline and Susan had also urged him to return home) as follows: "Capt Fitz Roy . . . has just stated five minutes ago on ye Quarter Deck that this time year we shall be very near to England.[41] I am both pleased & grieved at all your affectionate messages, wishin[g] me to return home.—If you think I do not long to see you again, you are indeed spurring a willing horse; but you can enter into my feelings of deep mortification, if any cause, ev [en] ill-health should have compelled me to have left the Beagle.—I say, should have, because you will agree with me, that it is hardly worthwhile, now to think of any such step."[42]

At the end of the letter he wrote his father that he was drawing a bill for thirty pounds to cover expenses on the Galapagos Islands, which the *Beagle* was preparing to visit. His father paid for this, and all his subsequent bills for the last year of the voyage, and during that year he remained free from febrile illnesses, and his father and sisters stopped urging him to leave the *Beagle*.[43]

As the voyage drew to a close, his homesickness returned. In December 1835 he wrote to Caroline: "For the last year, I have been wishing to return home & have uttered my wishes in no gentle murmurs. But now I feel inclined to keep up one steady deep growl from morning to night. I count & recount every stage in the journey homewards & an hour lost is reckoned of more consequence, than a week formerly." Two months later he wrote Catherine: "I confess I never see a Merchant vessel start for England, without a most dangerous inclination to bolt. . . . There never was a Ship so full of home-sick heroes, as the *Beagle*. We ought all to be ashamed of ourselves." Along with homesickness, he complained of suffering from seasickness more than he had three years previously.[44] At this time Captain FitzRoy, in a letter to Captain Beaufort at the Admiralty, tersely summed up the health of Darwin and others on the *Beagle*: "My messmate Mr. Darwin is so much the worse for a long voyage that I am most anxious to hasten as much as possible. Others are ailing and much require that rest which can only be obtained at home."[45]

Despite homesickness Darwin explored the new lands the *Beagle* visited, and reexperienced past feelings of pleasure for tropical scenery when there was a revisit to Bahia Brazil. (Before the revisit, he had written Caroline that "one glimpse of my dear home would be better than the united kingdom of all the glorious Tropics.")[46]

From May until October, as the *Beagle* made its return to England, he was able to keep thinking and writing despite seasickness and to prepare for meetings with geologists and zoologists in England, by revising old geological notes and writing up new geological theories, and by composing a catalog of his many zoological specimens.[47]

Of the need to continue his *Beagle* methodical habits of work and of his *Beagle* discovery he also thought "the golden rule for saving time was taking care of the minutes."[48] As the *Beagle* neared England he was influenced by these thoughts to write Susan that he had formed the following resolve about doing scientific work: "I shall act, as I now think.—that a man who dares to waste one hour of time, has not discovered the value of life."[49]

3

Hard Work, Occasional Unwellness, Discovering the Theory of Natural Selection, and Marriage

He returned to England on 2 October 1836, and for the next two months he went "backwards and forwards several times between Shrewsbury, Maer, Cambridge and London." He met with family and relatives, Professor Henslow and other old friends, and some of London's scientific men. The most intellectually exciting was Charles Lyell, England's leading geologist and president of the London Geological Society, who took a warm interest in Darwin's geological work and encouraged him to become an active member of the Geological Society.

From December 1836 through February 1837, Darwin lived in Cambridge, seeing Henslow, organizing his *Beagle* collections, and beginning to revise his *Beagle* diary and notebooks into a book, *Journal of Researches*, which would be a narrative of the *Beagle* voyage. Throughout these first five months, he made no complaints about health.[1]

On 7 March he took lodgings in Great Marlborough Street in London, and in the next twenty months he became "engaged" (a word he used in a letter to Fox) in doing an ever increasing amount and variety of scientific work. This included writing *Journal of Researches*, beginning to edit a zoology of the *Beagle* voyage, preparing accounts of the geology of the islands and countries the *Beagle* had visited, and serving on the Council of the Geological Society. And from July 1837 onwards, his work included secretly writing a succession of notebooks on the "Transmutation of Species," where he passionately struggled to develop a theory that would explain the evolution of new species. While his public work led to being elected to the Royal Society in January 1839, the mental pressures from both public and secret work and his resolve to work as hard as he could disturbed his health.[2]

In March 1837, he was invited by William Whewell to be a secretary to the Geological Society. (Whewell had become president of the society after Lyell.) At first Darwin refused, explaining, "I am not accustomed to write, and still less to use the faculty of digestion in that high degree, which drawing up even small reports, requires." When Whewell asked him again, he reluctantly accepted the position.[3]

On 20 September, when he was engaged in correcting the proof sheets of *Journal of Researches* (work which he found "very difficult"), he wrote Henslow that he had "not been very well of late with an uncomfortable palpitation of the heart." He added, "I feel I must have a little rest, else I shall break down." He further wrote that he had consulted London doctors—probably Henry Holland and James Clark—and agreed with their urging that he stop all writing and leave London to "live in the country for a few weeks."[4] This was the first of what would become many consultations with doctors where he would give an account of his chief complaints and what seemed to cause them, the history of other complaints and their treatments, and a summary of his daily activities, eating habits, and the quality of his sleep and bowel movements. The physician, lacking such medical tools as a thermometer to measure the temperature or tubes and lights with which to examine the stomach and colon, was largely confined to listening to what Darwin told him, taking his pulse, observing his appearance and behavior, palpating parts of his body, and then prescribing a treatment. (In Darwin's later years physicians would test his urine for acidity and alkalinity and for the presence of uric acid and albumen).[5]

Following his medical consultations, Darwin then sojourned with his father and sisters at Shrewsbury for twenty-four days (25 September through 19 October). His father appears to have treated his illness by having him rest from work. On returning to his lodgings in Marlborough Street in London, he did not complain of palpitations, and on 19 November he told Henslow that the *Journal of Researches* was very near completion, and he hoped to turn to other work.[6]

From December 1837 through May 1838, he stayed in London, determined not to interrupt a regimen of preparing works on *Beagle* geology and zoology, and writing in "Transmutation of Species" notebooks. On January 1838, he declined an invitation to visit Henslow's home in Cambridge, telling Henslow: "I should much like it, but as long as I continue well, I cannot bear to leave my work even for half a day." In March and April he went on regular horseback rides, which (he reported to Susan) did him a "wonderful deal of good." This appears to have been his first attempt at treating his illness by riding.[7]

About this time, in a letter to Caroline, he described some of the difficulties in completing geological and zoological writing. "You being my Governess, I am bound to tell you how my books go on. I find rather to my great grief, that they grow steadily in size, and I can see no prospect of their being finished, let me work ever so hard, before three or four years—I hope to bring out one Geological work on 'Volcanic Is^{ds}. and Coral Formations' this autumn or winter.—I have every encouragement to work hard in finding my opinions are thought at least worthy of attention. . . . I hope I may be able to work on right hard during the next three years, otherwise I shall never have finished,—but I find the noddle & stomach are antagonist powers, and that it is a great deal more easy to think too much in a day, than to think too little—What thought has to do with digesting roast beef,—I cannot say, but are brother faculties."[8]

He did not mention to Caroline the pressures he was also experiencing in work on *Species*. Early in his February–July 1838 "Transmutation of Species" notebook, referring to his search for plausible causes of evolution, he wrote: "This multiplication of little means & bringing the mind to grapple with great effect produced, is a most laborious, & painful effort of the mind . . . & will never be conquered by anyone . . . who just takes up & lay down the subject without long meditation—His best chance is to have [thought] profoundly over the enormous difficulty of reproductions of species & certainty of destruction; then he will choose & firmly believe in his new faith of the lesser of the difficulties."[9]

By "painful effort of the mind," he meant headaches. Several pages after this passage, referring to the prevailing opposition to evolutionary ideas, an opposition held by Henslow, Lyell, and the members of the Geological Society, he stated: "Mention persecution of early Astronomers.—then add chief good of individual scientific men is to push their science a few years in advance only of their age. . . . must remember that if they *believe* & do not openly avow their belief, they do as much to retard, as those, whose opinion they believe have endeavoured to advance cause of truth."[10]

On 1 May 1838, he noted he was "unwell," meaning that he occasionally suffered from palpitations, headaches, and a disordered stomach, which occurred as single symptoms or in varying combination with each other. He then rested by leaving London and residing for four days in Henslow's house in Cambridge. There he was treated as "a lion" by Henslow and other old friends, and he had convivial conversations with brilliant Cambridge academics. On returning to

Marlborough Street he wrote Susan that being in Cambridge had improved his health and desire to do more work. He now planned to go to Scotland to try to explain the geological origins of the parallel roads of Glen Roy.[11]

After working hard for several weeks, he again became "unwell" in June. His decision to suddenly leave London by a steamship for Edinburgh earlier than he had planned may have been motivated by a desire to see how the change of climate would affect his illness. The result was another rapid improvement in health and spirits, which he reported in a letter to Lyell: "Here [at Glen Roy] I enjoyed five days of the most beautiful weather, with gorgeous sunsets, & all nature looking as happy as I felt. I wandered over the mountains in all directions & examined that most extraordinary district." He was happy because he believed he had been able to show that the parallel roads were old sea beaches, which had been formed by the subsiding ocean. (This was in accord with his theory that in the past there had been global eras of geological upheaval and subsidence.) In his letter to Lyell he proudly reported how his trip on the steamship from London to Edinburgh "was absolutely pleasant, & I enjoyed the spectacle, wretch that I am, of two ladies & some small children quite sea sick, I being well. Moreover on my return from Glasgow to Liverpool, I triumphed in a similar manner over some full grown men."[12]

He visited Shrewsbury from 16 through 29 July. There, in the course of talks with his father and family, he started a new "M" notebook on the biological origins of behavior, where he noted several observations about his illness. Rephrasing what he had written to Caroline on the "antagonism" between "noddle" and stomach, he now wrote that "hardness of thought" caused "weakness of my stomach" but that "the capability of such . . . thought makes a discoverer." "Fear," he wrote several pages later, "must be simple instinctive feeling: I have awakened in the night being slightly unwell & felt so much afraid though my reason was laughing & told me there was nothing, & tried to seize hold of objects to be frightened at.—(again diseases of the heart are accompanied by much involuntary fear)." The belief that fear without a known cause could be a sign of heart disease (another sign being cardiac palpitations) prompted him to fear that he might soon die from this disease.[13]

At this time he may have discussed future prospects of scientific work and marriage with his father, and then written notes—entitled "This is the Question"—in which he made two prescient observations about his health. First, "it is very bad for ones health to work too much." Then marriage, although it would mean "*terrible loss* of *time,*" would also offer "Children—(if it Please God)—Constant companion, (& friend in old age) who will feel interested in one,—object to be beloved & played with.—better than a dog anyhow. Home, & someone to take care of the house—Charms of music & female chit-chat.—*These things good for one's health*" (my emphasis). In these notes he does not seem to have had any definite prospect for a wife in mind. However, from Shrewsbury he visited the home of his Wedgwood relatives at Maer, and while there, he thought of asking his cousin Emma Wedgwood to marry him. But then he did not speak to her about marriage.[14]

On returning to London in August, while he worked mainly at writing up his Glen Roy theory, on 12 August he interrupted this work to go to the library of London's Athenaeum Club, where he read an essay in the *Edinburgh Review* that discussed the ideas in the French philosopher Auguste Comte's book *Cours de philosophie positive*. In his "M" notebook he first reported how this reading caused him to "remember, & to think deeply," and "to be very much struck with an intense headache." He added that "the immediate manner in which my head got well when reading article by Boz [Charles Dickens's *Sketches by Boz*]—now in this I was interested as was I in the other, & read so intently as to be unconscious of all around, yet there was no strain on the intellectual powers—the difference is of a man wagging his foot & working with his toe to perform some difficult task."

Reading the *Edinburgh Review's* account of Comte's *Cours de philosophie positive* caused Darwin to have a severe headache for several reasons. The account was almost forty pages long, and understanding its closely argued contents required an intense and sustained mental effort. Yet Darwin was drawn to make this effort because in learning about Comte's ideas he was encouraged in his evolutionary thinking and able to advance this thinking by seeing that a theory of evolution should have quantitative elements in it, be able to make definitive predictions, and be supported by the model of artificial selection. Although he was able to effectively check his headache by turning from Comte to reading something that was engrossing but less mentally stressful, he went on fruitfully reflecting about Comte for many weeks after 12 August.[15]

From late September through October, as a result of reading Malthus's *Essay on Population,* he originated the theory of evolution by natural selection in the third "Transmutation" notebook and began to develop it into a "theory by which to work" in the fourth.[16] Although he had begun keeping a journal in which he recorded events in his life and episodes of ill health, he did not make any record of discovering natural selection or having any change in health or mood at the time he made the discovery.[17]

Doubts over whether he should marry Emma Wedgwood may have caused him to become "unwell" on 6, 7, and 8 November. On 9 November, he then traveled to the Wedgwood home of Maer, where, on 11 November, he asked Emma to marry him and was joyfully accepted by her. In an ecstatic 14 November letter to Emma that urged her to agree to an early wedding two months hence, he concluded by expressing concerns about the nearness of death: "You must be absolute arbitress, but do dear Emma, remember life is short, & two months is the sixth part of the year." Nine days later, after first writing his Cambridge friend Whitley that "I have a busy & therefore happy life before me," he added: "that is, if I have the luck to live so long."[18]

In November and December he was sometimes troubled and "unwell," from the pressures of doing *Beagle* zoology, searching for a London house, and working on a theory of evolution. At a 19 December meeting of the Geological Society, he had observed when Robert Grant (who had been a mentor at Edinburgh) suffered a savage public attack for espousing the evolutionary ideas of Lamarck. Darwin doubtless knew that, although the theory of natural selection differed from that of Lamarck, he would have been as savagely attacked as Grant were his theory to become publicly known. He remained silent during the attack on Grant, while secretly continuing to make notes on natural selection in his fourth "Transmutation" notebook.[19]

Emma visited him in London from 6 to 21 December, and on returning to Maer she wrote: "Tell me how you are. I do not like your looking so unwell & being so overtired when I come & look after you I shall scold you into health like Lady Cath. de Burgh used to do to the poor people."[20] A week later, after further reflection on his health, she wrote him less humorously and at greater length: "You have looked so unwell for some time that I am afraid you will be laid up if you fight against it any longer. Do set off to Shrewsbury & get some doctoring & then come here & be idle.... I am sure it must be very disagreeable & painful to you to feel so often cut off from the power of doing your work & I want you to cast out of your mind all anxiety about me on that point & to feel sure that nothing *could* make me so happy as to feel that I could be of any use or comfort to my own dear Charles when he is not well. If you knew how I long to be with you when you are not well! You must not think that I expect a holiday husband to be always making himself agreeable to me & if that is all the 'worse' that I shall have it will not be much for me to bear Whatever it may for you. So don't be ill any more my dear Charley till I can be with you to nurse you & save you from bothers."[21]

At this early stage of their relationship with each other, his unwellness had already become a force that drew her closer to him, bringing out her qualities of being a "nurse" and comforter, qualities she had developed in caring for an invalid mother. And despite her fears that he would become "laid up" and his fears of early death, both had already begun to share an optimistic belief that his episodes of unwellness could be managed by changes in work routine and her caring for him.

From 3 December 1838 through 2 January 1839, he moved his *Beagle* collections from Marlborough Street into a new house on London's Lower Gower Street, which he had rented for himself and Emma. He reported to Emma that "the three days of moving my goods rested me almost as much as a visit in the country" and enabled him to work "very hard" and finish correcting the proofs on his Glen Roy paper by 9 January. He also told her that he was pacing for half an hour in their ninety-foot garden, which he then may have continued to do as a daily exercise. At this time, he appears to have stopped horseback riding.[22]

Following his January visits to family at Shrewsbury and to Emma at Maer, he and she exchanged letters articulating apprehensions about their differences and their anticipations of coping with these differences in their marriage. After writing her of his fear that she would be unhappy because of his need for solitary thinking, he commented: "I think you will humanize me, and soon teach me there is greater happiness than building theories and accumulating facts in silence and solitude." She replied that her only unease was over his lack of religious faith, and she hoped "that though our opinions may not agree upon all points of religion we may sympathize a good deal in our feelings on the subject."[23]

They further differed in the plans they each wanted to make following their wedding, which was to be at Maer on 29 January. Fearing the ceremony as an "awful" event that would upset his health, he desired to go "straight home" to London as soon as it was over.[24] Emma desired to delay departure, so she could say extended farewells to her family. When they learned of these differences, while each then wanted to comply with the desires of the other, it was Emma's compliance to his needs that prevailed. It was a compliance that drew on her empathy and sensitivity for his fears (she told him that he wanted to be "married like a royal Prince without being present" at his wedding) and her great "dislike" of doing what he did not like. Both agreed in not finding "the steam" for a honeymoon at Warwick Castle or anywhere else.[25]

The differences with Emma caused him to have what he described to her as "a bad headache, which continued two days & two nights, so that I doubted, whether it ever meant to go & allow me to be married." He added that taking a train from London to his family in Shrewsbury "quite cured me." He was at Shrewsbury 25–27 January, then traveled to Maer.[26]

On 29 January he and Emma were married quietly at Maer Church. She and her husband then took a train to London and arrived the same day at their Lower Gower Street home.

4

Malaise, Vomiting, and the Beginning of "Extreme Spasmodic Daily & Nightly Flatulence"

In the first weeks of married life at Lower Gower Street, Darwin participated in social events and parties with Emma, continued a regimen of scientific work, and recorded no change in health. Then, on 10 March 1839, when he and Emma were attending a service in Kings' College Church, he complained of feeling "very cold" and became (what she described as) "very unwell" for five days, so that they cancelled a social visit. On 1 April, they gave a dinner party for the Lyells, Henslows, and other scientific friends. The next day she reported he was "dreadfully exhausted" and "rather ashamed of himself for finding his dear friends such a burden."[1]

From April to December, while Emma was sometimes "not very well from her first pregnancy," Darwin often suffered from a malaise that depressed his capacities for socialization and work. From April through May, while he was at Maer and Shrewsbury for about four weeks, he was "unwell almost the whole time," and he did "very little" work. At Shrewsbury he received "doctoring" of an unspecified nature from his father, which at first made him feel better. But in August and September, again at Maer and Shrewsbury, he wrote in his journal: "During my visit to Maer, read a little, was much unwell & scandalously idle.—I have derived this much good, that *nothing* is so intolerable as idleness."[2] In September he was seen briefly, while traveling in a coach, by Thomas Butler, an old acquaintance, who later recollected that he appeared "obviously very ill & looking like a shadow."[3]

In October 1839, he returned to Lower Gower Street. From there, he reported on himself and Emma in a letter to Fox: "I am now getting on steadily, though very slowly with my work . . . on Coral Formations. . . . Emma [in her third trimester] is only moderately well & I fear what you said is true 'she wont be better till she is worse.'—We are living a life of extreme quietness. . . . We have given up all parties for they agree with neither of us." He concluded, "My dear Fox, excuse this letter—I am very old & stupid." He also wrote his naturalist friend Jenyns that "a succession of headaches" had delayed his meeting with another naturalist.[4]

In 1840 his illness worsened in two ways. At first he had two new symptoms: periodic vomiting and flatulence, which began on 24 December, three days before Emma gave birth to a son, and continued for about two months.[5] During this illness, Emma became his closest and most constant companion. After he had been ill for six weeks, she wrote her aunt: "It is a great happiness to me when Charles is most unwell that he continues just as sociable as ever, and is not like the rest of the Darwins, who will not say how they really are; but he always tells me how he feels and never wants to be alone, but continues just as warmly affectionate as ever, so that I feel I am a comfort to him. And to you I may say that he is the most affectionate person possible."[6] Emma would nurse her husband for the rest of his life.

In March 1840, Darwin wrote letters to the Geological Society, stating that illness "compelled" him to resign the position of secretary to the society. He explained that he had not been able to attend the last four secretarial meetings and that in 1839 he had "never once attended [a meeting], without having suffered the next day." What he did not mention in the letters was how his fear of public speaking had caused him to suffer mental symptoms as he was speaking to groups of geologists. Many years later he told his son William: "When I was Secretary to the Geolog. Soc., I had to read aloud to Meeting M.S. papers; but I always read them over carefully first; yet I was so nervous at first, I somehow could see nothing all around me, but the paper, & I felt as if my body was gone, & only my head left." Although the Geological Society accepted his 1840 letter of resignation, it requested that he allow his name to remain as secretary until February 1841.[7]

At this time he had three consultations with Dr. Henry Holland, and at first reported that the latter "thinks he has found out, what is the matter with me, & now hopes he shall be able to set me going again." How Holland explained the illness, and what he prescribed for it, are not known. Emma then commented that his treatments were "without much good effect."[8]

Early in April, Darwin went to Shrewsbury for a week by himself to consult with his father. Soon after arriving, he reported on his health to Emma. He was "surprisingly well" and had "not been sick [vomited] once." Father had weighed him and found him a "good deal thinner." He now weighed 148 pounds, having lost 10 pounds and 6 ounces since September 1839. Father had "recommended nothing in particular," but said he "may often take Calomel." This is the only reference to his using Calomel at this time. As his health continued to improve, he credited this improvement to his consulting with his father, and in June, he wrote to Fox: "My Father, who has certainly in a quite unexpected degree put me on the course in getting well (having put a stop to periodical vomiting to which I was subject) feels pretty sure that I shall before long get quite well."[9]

Then in the summer and fall of 1840, when he was with Emma in Maer during the first trimester of her second pregnancy, he had a second worsening of illness, which he later rated as the longest and most serious of all his London illnesses.[10] His symptoms from the end of July through most of September, as recorded in Emma's diary, comprised "great flatulence," languor, and vomiting in the day and night, which was more frequent than it had been previously. Eleven years later, when he was nursing his dying daughter Annie, he described to Emma how Annie had "vomited a large quantity of bright green fluid," and then commented that "her case seems to me an exaggerated one of my Maer illness."[11]

Emma's diary shows that from July to September, her pregnancy had caused her to have some of her husband's symptoms of flatulence, weakness, and vomiting. While both he and she were visited by Dr. Darwin on 8 and 21 August, there is no record of what he said or prescribed. Emma improved in the later part of her pregnancy and had an uneventful confinement in early March 1841, giving birth to Annie.[12]

In the four months after 28 September, the information known about Darwin's illness is fragmentary. On 13 and 14 November, he and Emma left Maer and returned to their Lower Gower Street house. On 14 November his father directed that he take a prescription containing logwood, cinnamon, and potassium bicarbonate, which was intended to relieve his stomach. It is not known with what effect, or for how long, he took it.[13] On 22 December, he wrote to a correspondent that he had "been prevented by long continued illness from not having many months since sent you my sincere thanks for your most valuable pamphlets," and he added, "As I am yet far from recovered, I beg you will excuse the lateness & briefness of this letter."[14] About this time the novelist Maria Edgeworth, an old friend of the Wedgwoods, visited Emma in Gower Street and then in a letter reported on Darwin's illness: "His stomach rejects food continually; and the least agitation or excitation brings on the sickness directly so that he must be kept as quiet as is possible and cannot see any body."[15]

By January 1841, Darwin's months of acute illness had subsided, and he wrote to Fox in a positive mood: "I was at one time in despair & expected to pass my whole life as a miserable useless valetudinarian but I have now better hopes of myself." He reported that his strength was "gradually, with a good many oscillations, increasing" so that he could "work an hour or two several days in the week."[16] But he continued to suffer daily symptoms of physical and mental fatigue and both daily and nightly flatulence. The persistence of these symptoms marked the beginnings of the chronic illness that would dominate most of his adult life. He would remember these beginnings many years later, when on three occasions he would state that his decades of chronic illness began in the year 1840.[17] Darwin would also later recollect that during these years of acute and chronic illness—"the three years and eight months" after his marriage to Emma—he did "less scientific work . . . than during any other equal length of time in my life."[18]

There were two possible causes for these years of illness. First were mental stresses from Darwin's family life and his scientific work. His sensitivity to pain and bleeding in others made him especially sensitive to his wife's sufferings in her two pregnancies and to the dangers of her confinements. His onset of illness began three days before Emma gave birth, which probably meant that her signs of birth were imminent. Months later, Darwin complained to Fox: "What an awful affair a confinement is: it knocked me up, almost as much as it did Emma herself." His second illness began about the time Emma began her second pregnancy, and during the first trimester of this pregnancy, his and her symptoms were similar. In the third trimester of her pregnancy, he told Fox that he "most devoutly wish[ed]" that her confinement would be over."[19]

He tried to continue working on his *Beagle* zoology and geology and developing his theory of natural selection. As increase in illness interfered with this work, he "work[ed] as hard as [he] possibly could." This increased effort at trying to do more work then became another cause for increasing illness.[20]

A second possible cause for illness was that, along with mental stresses, he suffered from infection with Chagas' disease. As has been seen, he had been bitten on at least one occasion in 1835 by several possible carriers of the *Trypanosome cruzi* protozoa that cause Chagas'. The onset of his 1839–40 illness is compatible with the four- to five-year latent period for some cases of Chagas'. The clinical history of the illness, its period of malaise followed by exacerbations of vomiting, may be explained as being two phases of Chagas'. First, there was the invasion of Darwin's systemic circulation by the *T. cruzi* protozoa and his immune response to this invasion. Then there was the localization of the protozoa in the stomach, with permanent injuries both to the stomach and its parasympathetic nerves. While injury to the stomach produced flatulence, injury to the parasympathetics had effects that were more complex. Since the parasympathetics normally oppose the actions of the sympathetic nerves, their injury made Darwin more sensitive to the stimulation of the sympathetics and thus more sensitive to such mental stresses as attending meetings and conversing with visitors.[21]

Dr. Jared Goldstein has summarized the effects of Chagas' disease as follows: "Darwin's gastrointestinal symptoms . . . may be explained by a diffuse motility disturbance of the stomach, small intestine, and gall bladder that resulted from denervation, impaired peristalsis, and gastrointestinal endocrine dysfunction. It is likely that a chaotic mixture of local hyper and hypomotility and secretion caused his daily suffering. It would worsen at times of anxiety or stress, simply from unopposed sympathetic stimulation of a parasympathetically denervated gut, and improve at times of relative emotional calm." Goldstein believes that Chagas' disease did not further progress and that its damage then became arrested.[22]

Although there are those who have argued that Darwin did not have Chagas' disease, and although arguments for and against Chagas' have become part of an unresolved controversy regarding Darwin's illness, since Chagas' explains some of the main symptoms of his onset of illness, it will be accepted as a possible cause.[23] While Darwin at times may have had an increase in illness because of toxins in London's Athenaeum Club, the evidences for this are problematic.[24]

In July 1841, while visiting his family in Shrewsbury, Darwin informed Lyell: "My Father scarcely seems to expect that I shall become strong for some years—it has been a bitter mortification for me, to digest the conclusion that the 'race is for the strong' & that I shall probably do little more, but must be content to admire the strides others make in Science."[25]

Dr. Darwin had reversed his July 1840 positive prognosis—that his son would "before long get quite well"—into what was possibly a recognition that the latter had a chronic illness. For Darwin, who thought that his father could "predict with remarkable skill the course of any illness," to now hear that he would remain ill and weak was probably the greatest despair he could feel. In September, he told Fox: "But I am grown a dull old spiritless dog to what I used to be.—One gets stupider as one grows older I think."[26]

Despite these negative feelings, in 1842 he was able to make plans to move from London to a house in the country and to do three kinds of scientific work. Near the end of July 1841, he had recommenced writing his book on coral islands, and by continuing to write "daily for a couple of hours," along with taking "a little walk or ride every day," he was able to send a manuscript of the book to the printers in January 1842. On 6 May, he completed correcting proofs of the book, and although he knew that his theory of how coral islands had been formed was well regarded by Lyell and other geologists, the completion of the book prompted him to write Emma (who was visiting her family in Maer) on 9 May with lugubrious retrospective thoughts on lost time and illness: "On Saturday [6 May] I went in City & did a deal of Printing business—I came back gloomy & tired. . . . I will give you statistics of time spent on my coral volume, *not* including all the work on board the Beagle—I commenced it 3 years & 7 months ago, and have done scarcely anything besides—I have actually spent 20 months out of this period on it! & nearly all the remainder sickness & visiting!!!" Near the end of the letter he reported that an "hour's hard talk" about the affairs of the Geological Society with his old geological friend Leonard Horner had "quite knocked me up & this makes my letter rather blue in its early part."[27]

From 18 May through 17 June, when he was in Maer and Shrewsbury, he wrote a thirty-five-page "pencil sketch" of the ideas and evidences for his theory of evolution by natural selection. He was able to do this because, as he noted in his autobiography, he had continued "collecting facts on the origin of species . . . when I could do nothing else from this illness." Thus he first recorded in his journal that in April 1839, when he was ill at Maer, he did "some reading connected with species, but did very little on account of being unwell" and that in his first vomiting, he "read a little for transmut[n] theory" but otherwise was unable to work. During his illness he was collecting evidence for his theory by making notes on the various expressions first shown by his son William. As he explained in his autobiography, "I felt convinced, even at this early period, that the most complex and fine shades of expression must all have had a gradual and natural origin." He noted in his journal that in the six months of his second vomiting, "when well enough did a good deal of species work." After he had recovered in 1841, he reminded Fox on 25 January that he was continuing to collect "all kinds of facts about 'Varieties & Species,'" and he went on collecting, and organizing what he collected, for the following year. Now, in the spring of 1842, he felt the "satisfaction" of first writing out his theory in the form of a "brief abstract."[28]

From 18 June through 29 June, feeling an increase in his physical strength, he made a geological excursion to the glacial sites of North Wales where he identified the signs of past glacial actions. However, despite his increase in strength, he found that his stamina had greatly decreased from what it had been four years earlier when he did geological work at Glen Roy. Following his trip to Wales, he decided that he would not undertake any further geological excursions, although he continued to find pleasure in taking daily walks.[29]

The decline in physical vigor that he observed in himself at the age of thirty-three was the result of his experiencing frequent episodes of mental and physical fatigue, along with the discomforts and pains of daily and nightly episodes of flatulence.

Moving to Down and Developing
a "Profoundly Tranquil" Routine of
Work, Rest, and Walks around the Sandwalk

In his September 1841 letter to Fox, Darwin wrote that he and Emma were planning to move from London and were in the "turmoil" of searching for a country house in which to live. Some of the reasons for this change in living were the need for more space in which to raise a growing family and Darwin's enjoyment of being in the country. "I long to be settled in 'pure air,'" he told Fox, "out of all the dirt, noise, vice & misery of this great Wen [London]."[1]

Several individuals had formed his belief in the goodness of "pure" country air. Doctors Holland and Clark, who had previously urged him to live in the country, both held this belief.[2] Clark had stated that a change from city to country ameliorated many diseases, including "dyspepsia and various nervous disorders," and that London's air was a "destructive malady. . . justly termed Cachexia Londinensis, which preys upon the vitals and stamps its hues upon the countenance of almost every permanent resident in this large city."[3] (This term reflected the prevailing idea that many disorders were caused by miasmas in the air arising from decaying organic matter, especially from decaying human excrement in London's sewers.)[4] Emma, who had an "inclination" for living in the country, thought that London's air had a "bad effect" on the development of her son's speech.[5] Dr. Erasmus Darwin had written that air was "nutritious" and that "constant immersion in pure air is now known to contribute much both to the health of the system, and to the beautiful color of the complexion."[6] Dr. Robert Darwin most likely held similar views.

From the fall of 1841 to the summer of 1842, Darwin and Emma's search for a suitable country house was "fruitless," and they were disappointed when they were unable to acquire a beautiful house at Woking called "The Hermitage."[7] In July 1842, they first visited Down House and its estate of eighteen acres, near the village of Down (Downe today) in Kent. In a letter to his father and sisters, Darwin expressed strong feelings of pleasure for the house and its environs: "On the road to the village, on *fine day* scenery absolutely beautiful. . . . The charm of the place to me is that almost every field is intersected . . . by one or more foot-paths—I never saw so many walks in any other country—The country is extraordinarily rural & quiet with narrow lanes & high hedges & hardly any ruts—It is really surprising to think London is only 16 miles off." Although Emma was first "a good deal disappointed" in Down (her opinion would later change), she took pleasure in doing what gave her husband pleasure. In August he purchased Down House and estate for the sum of £2,200, advanced him against his inheritance by his father.[8]

For him, possessing Down meant several advantages for health and work: having pleasures of varied country walks and varied country scenery and being separated from the demands of society and from London's polluted air, dirt, and noise. Since Down was near London, he could easily visit the city's scientific institutions and scientific men.[9]

From 14 to 17 September 1842, he and his family moved to Down, where he would live for the remaining forty years of his life. During the move, Emma had suffered much from the third trimester of her third pregnancy, and on 23 September, she gave birth to Mary Eleanor, who lived only three weeks and was buried on 19 October in the churchyard of Down's parish church.[10] After the burial, Emma told a relative: "Our sorrow is nothing to what it would have been if she had lived longer and suffered more. Charles is well to-day and the funeral over, which he dreaded very much." She added, "It will be long indeed before either of us forget that poor little face."[11]

Two days before Mary Eleanor died, Darwin had distracted himself by writing about volcanic islands, the second volume of the geology of the *Beagle* voyage. Occupying himself with scientific work would become one of his main defenses against distressing events.[12] Two months after Mary's death, he expressed positive thoughts about Down and his family to Fox: "Our removal has answered very well; our two little souls are better & happier—which likewise applies to me & to my good old wife."[13] He was also pleased that Emma had made a quicker recovery from her third pregnancy than from her two previous pregnancies, which he attributed to "country air."[14]

Within a year after settling in Down, he started making a number of changes in house and grounds that were financed by loans from his father, including building a wall to create privacy in part of the house that was exposed to another man's field (he had told his father and Susan that "the publicity of the place at present is intolerable"); altering old rooms and building new rooms for his servants, children, and wife (Emma was again pregnant); and making what he called the house's "Capital study" into his own study for reading, writing, microscopy, and dissecting.[15]

A study with an armchair in one corner, between fireplace and windows, tables close by, an alcove for books and folios containing notes, with pictures on the wall of Lyell, his father, and two grandfathers. In one curtained off corner was a "personal privy" containing water, bowls and towels, where, when his flatulence increased, he could retire and retch. Between two windows was a small mirror that enabled him to see visitors approaching the front door. In the hall he kept a jar of snuff, which had become an essential stimulant for his work. In 1846, when Emma persuaded him to leave off snuff for a month, he became "most lethargic, stupid & melancholy in consequence," and he had to go back on it.[16]

In December 1843, he began to correspond about his still largely unexamined *Beagle* plant collections with Joseph Hooker, a rising young botanist and son of Sir William Hooker, director of the Royal Botanic Gardens at Kew. In a letter dated 11 January 1844, Darwin revealed that he had recently developed a theory of evolution: "I am almost convinced (quite contrary to opinion I started with) that species are not (it is like confessing a murder) immutable. Heaven forfend me from Lamarck nonsense of a 'tendency to progression' 'adaptations from the slow willing of animals' &c, but the conclusions I am led to are not widely different from his—though the means of change are wholly so—I think I have found out (here's presumption!) the simple way by which species become exquisitely adapted to various ends."[17]

In making this revelation he was motivated by hopes and fears. He hoped that sharing his theory with Hooker would gain him information on his *Beagle* plants and their geographical distribution that would support the theory. He feared that Hooker would judge the theory as if he were "confessing a murder." He enclosed these last words in parentheses, as he would do with other statements expressing truths that were painful but that he had to confront. With the parentheses he was perhaps trying to circumscribe and wall off his pain.[18] For him, "confessing a murder" expressed most immediately and directly his fear that—in the ideological climate of his time—his theory would be viewed with an opprobrium equivalent to that attached to murder.

Hooker replied to Darwin in a letter that remained silent about "confessing a murder," while stating a belief in separate creations of species, along with "a gradual change of species," and then added, "I shall be delighted to hear how you think that this change may have taken place, as no presently conceived opinions satisfy me on the subject." Throughout 1844, Darwin pressed Hooker with questions about a steadily increasing range of botanical subjects. Hooker sent him detailed replies that drew on information from scientific friends and on Kew Garden's plants and books. "Your queries & remarks," Hooker wrote him in April, "have opened a wide field for research & investigation, for which I am truly obliged. These are all subjects, which I ought to have attended to, without requiring to be reminded of them by a more industrious Naturalist."[19]

From February through July 1844, after completing the geological volume on *Volcanic Islands*, Darwin enlarged the 1842 abstract of his evolutionary theory into a longer and more coherent essay that was suitable for reading by others. On 5 July, the day he finished the essay, he wrote Emma a letter stating that if the theory were to be accepted "by one competent judge" it would "be a considerable step in science," and that it was necessary to make plans for preserving transmutation ideas in the event of his "sudden death." He was probably thinking of his fear of dying from heart disease or perhaps from a fever, and of the sudden deaths of friends and relatives.[20]

In his letter he first instructed Emma to devote £400 to posthumously publishing the essay, to promote his notes and annotated books, and to have her brother Hensleigh Wedgwood aid her.[21] After anxiously considering, and reconsidering, who among several scientific colleagues might best do this work, he tentatively wrote in a postscript to the letter, "Lyell, especially with the aid of Hooker (& of any good zoological aid) would be best of all."[22] While it has been held that the letter to Emma was an attempt to avoid responsibility for publishing controversial ideas, a more plausible view is that it was the effort of a man, facing the possibility of premature death, to assert his priority in originating these ideas.[23]

On 14 July, Darwin wrote Hooker a note announcing that he planned to visit the latter at Kew Gardens on Thursday morning at about 10 a.m. on 18 July. At the end of the note he wrote: "As my health is always extremely uncertain, you must not be surprised if I fail: if I am not with you before eleven, you will understand that my health is to blame." In this instance, he was able to have a first meeting with Hooker, whom he described afterwards to Lyell as a "most engaging young man." On the weekend of 7 December, Hooker visited him at Down.[24] Over the following years, Hooker became Darwin's intellectual confidant, although he continued to believe in "immutability" of species and was not impressed by the ideas of the 1844 essay when Darwin gave it to him to read.[25]

Like Darwin, Hooker had trained to be a physician and had experienced psychosomatic symptoms. As a result of giving a public talk, he suffered from "violent palpitation," "physical nausea," and "severe nervous reaction." Doctors had told him that he had a "slight disease" of the heart and that he "need not expect ever to attain a freedom in public delivery."[26] He soon developed a sympathetic interest in the nature and course of Darwin's illness. Darwin responded to this, and in March 1845 wrote Hooker: "You are very kind in your enquiries about my health; I have nothing to say about it, being always much the same, some days better & some worse.—I believe I have not had one whole day or rather night, without my stomach having been greatly disordered, during the last three years, & most days great prostration of strength: thank you for your kindness, many of my friends, I believe, think me a hypocondriac [*sic*]." He was mainly describing the day and night fluctuations of flatulence, which resulted in "prostration of strength" because of their pains and interference with sleep.[27]

In June 1845, Darwin reported to Hooker that he had been working too hard and had "some unwellness." Hooker, impressed by the contrast between Darwin's chronic day and night illness and his own occasional illness, then replied: "I am sorry to hear that you have been still suffering a little. I would willingly take a little bad health (temporarily only) to let you work a bit in comfort, you do so richly deserve a little peaceful working." Hooker would become, along with Fox, Darwin's medical confidant.[28]

From 1844 through 1847, Darwin on several occasions invited Hooker to visit him for several days at Down. During these visits it was Darwin's established rule that on every morning, for about twenty minutes after breakfast, he would "pump" Hooker (as he called it) with long lists of queries that Hooker described as "botanical, geographical &c," which Hooker would then answer.[29] Hooker recollected:

> These morning interviews were followed by his [Darwin's] taking a complete rest, for they always exhausted him, often producing a buzzing noise in the head, and sometimes what he called "stars in the eyes," the latter too often the prelude of an attack of violent eczema in the head during which he was hardly recognizable. These attacks were followed by a period of what with him was the nearest approach to health, and always to

activity. Shortly before lunch I used to hear his mellow voice under my window, summoning me to walk with him. . . . This walk was repeated in the afternoon; on both these occasions his conversation was delightful, animated. It turned naturally on the scenes we had witnessed in faraway regions and anecdotes of our seafaring lives [Hooker had made a voyage to Antarctica], and on discoveries in science.[30]

It seems likely that Darwin's attacks of "violent eczema" were psychosomatic symptoms caused by a controversy with Hooker over "questions botanical geographical." Whereas he was influenced by his theory to believe that species of plants had been able to migrate across oceans from their lands of origin, so as to settle new lands and attain their present geographical distributions, Hooker, the nonbeliever in natural selection, questioned whether migration was a "sufficient agent" to explain these distributions.[31] While the controversy went on without being resolved, Darwin's attacks of eczema stopped when he stopped talking with Hooker about controversial topics. Because Hooker gave him facts—and Darwin's main purpose was to accumulate facts bearing on natural selection—Darwin persisted in his morning talks and braved having the attacks of eczema.

After several years of communicating with Hooker, he felt the shortcomings of his scientific knowledge and wrote his young friend: "How painfully (to me) true is your remark that no one has hardly a right to examine the question of species who has not minutely described many."[32] In October 1846, after finishing *Geological Observations on South America* (the third and last volume of his *Beagle* geology), instead of further developing his 1844 essay, he began to work on classifying barnacles.[33]

At this time, he suffered from criticisms of his Glen Roy theory. In 1847, David Milne published a paper postulating that the roads of Glen Roy had been formed not by the sea or glacial lakes (as had been propounded by Darwin and Agassiz) but by lakes formed by dams of "detrital matter." After reading this paper, Darwin confided to Hooker: "I have been bad enough for these few last days, having had to think & write too much about Glen Roy (an audacious son of dog, Mr. Milne) having attacked my theory which made me horribly sick." There was then a discussion on Glen Roy, and Darwin told Hooker that "the confounded subject has made me sick twice."[34] He recognized the force of the arguments against his Glen Roy theory, yet persisted in believing in it. One reason for his persistence was deep commitment to his theory that the formation of Glen Roy's parallel roads had been part of past eras of global upheaval and subsidence.[35] Over the next fourteen years the subject of Glen Roy would continue to cause him uncertainty, anxiety, and perhaps further episodes of vomiting.[36]

In addition to meeting individually with Hooker and other friends and acquaintances, Darwin participated in meetings of scientific organizations. For several years (fortnightly, or for every three weeks) he regularly attended London meetings of the Council of the Geological Society as well as meetings of the Royal Geographical Society and Royal Society, even though traveling to and from London (by coach and train) greatly fatigued him, and attending scientific meetings was a strain on his health even when he did not speak. Thus when an acquaintance asked him to take the chair of a natural history meeting, he refused, explaining: "Very little fatigue, or excitement or anxiety (of which I s[hd]. have plenty) almost invariably brings on so much swimming of the head, nausea, & other symptoms, that the effort of sitting for 2 or 3 (or even less) [hours] in a public chair would be quite intolerable to me." After attending London meetings, he was able to refresh himself by sojourning in the London home of brother Erasmus.[37]

In June 1847, making plans to attend the Oxford meeting of the British Association, and with no familiar home to reside in, he arranged by correspondence with Hooker to be allowed to stay alone and dine alone in the home of Hooker's uncle, "for as you know, my odious stomach requires that" and "what a ridiculous fuss I do make about my precious self." During his sojourn at Oxford, while he refused to dine outside of his own room because of fear of being knocked up, he enjoyed listening to organ music at Oxford's New Chapel. His health remained well, and on returning home to Down he was "*extra* well."[38]

On two occasions he hosted weekend meetings at Down for the purpose of having scientific talks. In December 1845, he conversed with Hooker and two other colleagues, had no health disturbances, and later told Hooker he enjoyed "all our raging discussions."[39] On 12–15 February 1848, his thirty-ninth birthday, he arranged a meeting with Lyell, Mrs. Lyell, and three other colleagues. The conversation was convivial, and one guest reported how there was a "nice cosy chat. . . before and after dinner." However, three days after the last guest left, Darwin suffered a belated reaction to the meeting, consisting of three days of vomiting, headache, and depression. What caused him to be well and then ill on each of these occasions is not known.[40]

Anticipating a visitor could also be stressful to him. In June 1847, Bernhard Studer, a professor of geology in Switzerland, wrote him about making a geological tour of England early in August and requesting that they meet. In July, apprehensive over the meeting, yet unable to refuse it, Darwin wrote Studer about his infirmities:

> Shortly after my return from my long voyage, I had a tedious & severe illness, & have never since recovered my strength & suppose I never shall. . . . I appear quite well, but from being a strong man, I am become incapable of any continued muscular exertion; or indeed of much exertion of mind, for even conversation, if it excites me, tires me in a very short time, so that I am compelled to live a most retired life. . . . I must apologise for troubling you with so many particulars about myself, but I thought it better to forwarn you that I am incapable of being of much service.

On 12 August, he told Hooker that "the foreigner [Studer] has not appeared, deuce take him" and that his stomach had been "wretchedly bad" for a week. The next day, Studer wrote him from London, and the two met at Down on 16 August, without any apparent serious upset in Darwin's health. Two days later, he wrote Hooker: "My stomach is extra well, & as I have had an extra long bad batch [of stomach illness], I have little fears of failing." On 20 and 21 August, he had an "enjoyable" two-day visit with Hooker at Kew.[41]

While conversation with scientific acquaintances varied greatly in their impacts on his health, he would frequently tell visitors that such conversations were health hazards, and his fear of these conversations became one of his strongest and most lasting fears and one of the main differences between his illness and the illnesses of his friends and acquaintances.

During his first six years of living at Down, when he was not traveling, he developed a routine in which he divided every day into periods when he did scientific work—he worked for one to one and a half hours at a time, in the early morning, late morning, afternoon, and early evening—and periods when he rested from science by doing various mental and physical activities.

One of his most frequent nonscientific activities was listening to Emma read three to four times a day, for about an hour each time. They shared similar tastes in books of history, biography, travels in foreign lands, and in novels. Reading a novel caused Darwin to experience what he described as "a wonderful relief and pleasure." He eagerly entered into the novel's unfolding plot, insisting that the ending not be revealed until the reading of the novel was finished and hoping it would be a happy ending. He would discuss, with Emma and their family, the charms and attributes of the novel's heroine. His daughter recollected that he was "often in love with the heroines of the many novels that were read to him," and he would imagine that some heroines were more beautiful than they were actually portrayed. Sometimes, during his afternoon reading period, a novel that at first stimulated him would relax him so he would briefly fall asleep.[42]

The one nonscientific reading he did by himself was the *Times*. Every day he read through it for its reports on topics that included news events, debates in parliament, law cases he had become interested in following, and movements in the stock market (informing him of the value of his investments). He became so accustomed to the *Times* that he once would jokingly call it "meat drink & air."[43]

In 1846, he had created the sandwalk, a 1.5-acre strip of land that he planted with trees and circled with a sandy path. This became his favorite walking place, although he would also sometimes walk on some of Down's many other footpaths. He walked with members of his family, friends, or by himself. When alone he would sometimes stop and observe plants or animals, or he would become preoccupied with thoughts on a variety of subjects that were unrelated to his surroundings. Walking stimulated him to think, and the sandwalk has been called his "thinking path." He walked in the morning, at noon, and at four in the afternoon. At noon he walked around exactly five times to complete a mile.

These walks also became a daily ritual of exercising and thinking that he forced himself to do even when the weather was bad or when he felt weak. Near the end of his life when he was unable to go to the sandwalk, he became deeply depressed.[44]

In the early evening, he would play two games of backgammon with Emma. If he won, he would jokingly proclaim how much his score had exceeded her score, and he would chaff Emma and tell her that she believed that backgammon was "all luck."[45] If he was losing, he would let himself go in loud complaints to her, exclaiming, "Bang your bones" and "Confound the women."[46] This humorous anger (he always had difficulty in expressing serious anger) may have cleared his mind and mentally refreshed him, for after backgammon he did some German scientific reading by himself—reading which he found especially onerous.[47]

After this reading he would listen to Emma play the piano. He complained that as he grew older, his appreciation of music had waned and that "music generally sets me thinking too energetically on what I have been at work on, instead of giving me pleasure."[48] Yet as he listened to Emma play—as she played both he and she were silent[49]—he was affected by what he heard, and he once made a list of the compositions that he especially liked and the impression each made upon him. (The list, which probably included compositions from Handel and Beethoven, has since been lost.)[50]

During most of his indoor leisure—when reading the *Times* or listening to Emma read or play the piano—he would recline on a sofa or bed, always lying flat on his back, and sometimes putting his hands under his head.[51] Lying in this horizontal position eased his flatulence and was perhaps a carryover from the days when he treated his *Beagle* seasickness by "taking the horizontal for it." However, in the evening when conversing with family or friends, he would sit "very erect" in a high chair made still higher by being placed on a footstool.[52] He told visitors that this particular way of sitting was to "guard his weakness," "to guard against . . . digestive trouble," and "to keep off giddiness and nausea." Why this way of sitting should so affect him is unknown.[53]

During his first six years at Down, he described himself as being in "a profoundly tranquil state," and living "like clock work. . . in what most people would consider the dullest possible manner." By this he meant that every day (including holidays and weekends), he followed the same routine of alternating periods of work and rest from work. This routine enabled him to do three hours of morning work on most days. He frequently experienced pain and fatigue, which he tried to assuage by taking various treatments.[54]

In these six years, his work was only seriously interrupted on one occasion because of a severe episode of boils. "I am suffering," he told Hooker on 7 April 1847, "from four boils & swellings, one of which hardly allows me the use of my right arm & has stopped all my work & damped all my spirits." After "several weeks," the boils subsided and he was able to resume work.[55] In 1847, he also suffered from boils that were less severe in February, July, and October. The causes of these boils are not known, and there is no record of how they were treated.[56] He would continue to have boils for many years.

Treatments from Father, Father's Death, Prolonged Vomiting, and Treatments from Dr. Gully with Hydropathy at Malvern

Darwin's 1842–45 letters to his Shrewsbury family reveal how he continued to depend on his father for advice, assistance, and medical treatments. In a September 1842 letter to Catherine, he requested his father's opinion on a letter he had written to Mr. Cockell, a surgeon at Down whom he had decided to employ. He then asked his father to pay for medicines sent to him by the Shrewsbury chemist Thomas Blunt and to write the dosages for children on a list of medicines that he used. (At this time, his son William was three years old, and his daughter Annie, eighteen months.)[1]

In November 1844, he wrote Susan: "Thank, also, my Father for his medical advice—I have been very well since Friday, nearly as well as during the first fortnight & am in heart again about the non-sugar plan.—I am trying the very bitter, weak, but thoroughly fermented Indian Ale, for luncheon & it suits me very well."[2] Indian Ale, also called bitter ale, was bitter because it contained hops, a plant which was "stomachic and tonic" and "slightly narcotic" and which belonged to a class of vegetable medicinal substances known as "bitters."[3] Darwin may have used hops at least once previously in 1836.[4] The "non-sugar plan" may refer to the prevailing medical notion that "in some constitutions there is a peculiar tendency to an abnormal oxidation" of sugar into poisonous oxalic acid, and that because of this, these individuals were sometimes benefited by an injunction to abstain entirely from sugar.[5] Darwin had a strong penchant for eating sweets, and it is not known for how long he was able to follow Dr. Darwin's sugar-free diet.[6]

In a September 1845 letter to Susan, he reported to his father: "I have taken my Bismuth regularly, I think it has not done me quite so much good as before;

but I am recovering from too much exertion with my Journal."[7] Emma's diary records that he had previously taken bismuth on six days in September 1840. Bismuth nitrate was used to treat stomach pains and chronic vomiting. It was held that, since bismuth was apparently not absorbed by the intestines, it exerted its therapeutic effect "by simply cloaking some of the delicate or irritable portions of the mucous surface with an insoluble white covering." At this time bismuth presumably did not benefit Darwin, for he makes no further reference to it.[8] The "Journal" that he mentions was the second edition of his *Beagle, Journal of Researches*, where he presented some of the evidence for transmutation that had especially influenced his thinking, while carefully refraining from mentioning the possibility of transmutation. Emma observed that he had taken "a great deal of pains" in preparing the edition and that writing it had "overtired him a good deal."[9]

In November 1845, Darwin informed Hooker that he was undergoing a new kind of treatment. "I have been unusually well for a week past, owing, I believe, to what sounds a great piece of quackery, viz twice a day passing a galvanic stream through my insides from a small-plate battery for half an hour. I think it certainly has relieved some of my distressing symptoms." He was describing the application to his body of an electric current from a voltaic battery, a treatment known as "galvanisation" that was popular during the first half of the nineteenth century. In January 1846, Emma observed that he continued to be "unusually well" and "in good heart about galvanism." A month later, he stopped galvanism, when it did not prevent him suffering "three days bad sickness."[10]

In the summer of 1846, he alternated treatments. On 24 June, he first reported to Emma (who was away from Down), "I was sick in middle of day, but two pills of opium righted me surprisingly afterwards." He rarely used opium, probably because he feared its dulling effects on thinking.[11] The next day he wrote Emma: "I have been stomachy & sick again, but *not* very uncomfortable: I will take bluepill again." While his use of the blue pill, mercuric chloride, was a change over his past use of calomel, he would continue to use calomel. It is not known when or why he made this change or how frequently he then used each of these mercury medications.[12] In July, having had a "good deal more sickness than usual," he recommended a course of galvanism, evidently hoping that he would again experience its positive effects. This did not occur, however, and he probably stopped galvanism sometime in 1846.[13]

Darwin's custom was to visit his Shrewsbury family for about two weeks, in the spring and fall, and often report on his visits to Emma. When he was at

Shrewsbury in October 1843, he wrote her the following: "By the way I told him [Dr. Darwin] of my dreadful numbness in my finger ends, & all the sympathy I could get, was 'yes, yes exactly—tut-tut, neuralgic, exactly yes yes'—Nor will he sympathise about money 'stuff & nonsense' is all he says to my fears of ruin & extravagance." While Father was trying to reassure him that the paresthesia of his hands and fears of financial ruin should not be taken seriously, he regarded this reassurance as lacking the sympathy he received from Emma. His finger numbness was probably a psychosomatic symptom resulting from the anxieties he was feeling at this time.[14] A year later, after writing to Emma of the admiration Susan and his father had expressed for her, he added his own thoughts about being her invalid husband: "I did not require to be reminded how well, my own dear wife, you have born your dull life with your poor old sickly complaining husband. Your children will be a greater comfort to you than I ever can be, God bless them and you."[15]

During these years, Darwin's father remained in good health and spirits. However in 1846 and 1847, when he was eighty and eighty-one, he had periods of illness. This caused Darwin to have accentuations of illness and to begin to realize that "Father's death [was] drawing slowly nearer & nearer."[16]

In 1848, Darwin visited Shrewsbury in the last two weeks in May, and from there he wrote Emma a succession of letters reporting Dr. Darwin's failing health and his fluctuations of illness. At first he wrote that, although his father had an occasional "dyeing sensation," he "thought with care he might live a good time longer, & that when he dyed, it would probably be suddenly which was best." In later letters, he wrote that his father's health was "rapidly breaking up" and that while he was "very cheerful at cards . . . the day here is almost continual anxiety." In his last May letter to Emma, he reported in detail how he experienced a sudden attack of illness that "came on with fiery spokes & dark clouds before my eyes: then sharpish shivery & rather bad not very bad sickness." He added, "Yesterday . . . I felt rather faint & had a slight shaking fit & little vomitting and & . . . slept too heavily; so today am languid & stomach bad, but I do not think I shall have any more shivering & I care for nothing else." Shivering, perhaps, exhausted him more than his other symptoms. Then he wrote Emma that while sister Susan had been "very kind" in her care of him: "I did yearn for you. Without you, when sick I feel most desolate. . . . Oh Mammy I do long to be with you & under your protection for then I feel safe."[17]

After returning to Down in June, he again visited Shrewsbury from 10 to 26 October, and later recollected that he found his father "comfortable" and appearing "serene & cheerful."[18] Three weeks later, Catherine wrote him that

Dr. Darwin had died on the morning of 13 November and that his funeral would be on 18 November. Because of illness, Darwin did not leave Down until 17 November, and he arrived too late to attend the funeral. After a week at Shrewsbury, he returned to Down on 26 November.[19]

From July 1848 through March 1849, he suffered from attacks of "violent vomiting," once or twice a week, that along with shivering, trembling, and languor were associated with a "swimming" head and black spots before his eyes.[20] The apparent causes for these attacks were feelings of grief and loss over the loss of his father, on whom he depended for so many things in life, and his work of classifying barnacles, which he found arduous, frustrating, time-consuming, and of questionable value. In 1848, he told acquaintances that most of his friends laughed at his barnacle work and that "in truth never will a mountain of labour have brought forth such a mouse as my book on the Cirripedia."[21] However, in letters to Fox and Hooker, while he reported grief over his father's death, he did not state that this grief was a cause for his illness.

Because of the attacks of violent vomiting, he had several changes in his activities and thoughts: he was only able to work on barnacles one out of three days, he came to fear that he was now "rapidly" dying (a change from his previous fears of dying from heart disease), and he became so depressed and "dispirited" that he did not answer letters from Hooker and other friends and withdrew from most social activities.[22] Many years later, he recollected that at this time, in addition to vomiting, dizziness, fears of death, and depression, he had nocturnal obsessional thoughts, so that "whatever I did in the day haunted me at night with most vivid & most wearing repetition."[23] These obsessions may have been stimulated by his daily worries over time lost in work on barnacles and by worries over not replying to information in the letters from Hooker and others.[24]

In December 1848, a month after his father's death, he consulted Dr. Henry Holland, who became his main doctor until February 1849. Dr. Holland told him his illness was not quite dyspepsia "but nearer to suppressed gout" and that he had never seen such a case.[25] He treated him with varying doses of calomel and then bismuth. These treatments did not alleviate the distress of the illness.[26] On 1 January 1849, Darwin began keeping a daily diary of his health, perhaps because he thought that it would be a source of information for Dr. Holland and other physicians he might consult. From January through March, he only reported a few observations on his illness: the times that he vomited, the appearance of boils, and times when he felt "poorly."

The ineffectiveness of Dr. Holland's treatments inclined Darwin to think of trying Dr. James Gully's hydropathy treatment, which he had been urged to try by his *Beagle* friend Bartholomew Sulivan and then by Fox.[27] In 1842, Dr. Gully and Dr. James Wilson had founded hydropathic establishments in Malvern, which in several years had become famous for successfully treating many ordinary and eminent Victorians (including Tennyson, Carlyle, Dickens, Edward Bulwer Lytton, and Wilkie Collins).[28] In 1846, Dr. Gully had published a book, *The Water Cure in Chronic Disease*, that was widely read and that appeared in two editions within nine months after publication.

In this book, he argued that disease was caused by a faulty supply of blood to the internal viscera and that hydropathy—the application of cold water to the body—corrected this fault by shifting blood from the viscera to the less important body parts of the skin. He reported how at Malvern he had successfully treated cases of long-standing dyspepsia with a daily regimen of hydropathy, early rising, walks, a diet of plain food, and drinking spring water. Dr. Gully asserted that this regimen was superior to other treatments for dyspepsia, which he called "violent and irrational," and that "I cannot but repeat the strong conviction I have that *medication never did, never will, never can, cure a case of chronic dyspepsia, and that short of organic change, the hygienic water treatment seldom, if ever, fails to cure it.*"[29]

By the middle of February 1849, Darwin had read *The Water Cure*, communicated with Dr. Gully, and decided to go to Malvern and try hydropathy for about two months, a decision not supported by Dr. Holland. "It will cause a sad delay in my Barnacle work," he told a scientific colleague, "but if once half-well I c^d do more in six months than I now do in two years."[30]

On 10 March, with Emma and their six children, a governess and servants, he moved to Malvern. Here he rented the Lodge, a large villa, and attended Dr. Gully's establishment as an outpatient.[31] Although he had no faith in Gully's homeopathic medicines, he quickly formed a warm respect for him. "I like Dr Gully much," he wrote Susan, "he is certainly an able man: I have been struck with how many remarks he has made similar to those of my Father."[32] (He and Gully had been contemporaries at Edinburgh Medical School and were only one year apart in age.) Gully diagnosed Darwin as suffering from a form of indigestion he called "nervous dyspepsia." In *The Water Cure*, he described this disorder as a "chronic excess and congestion of blood in the nutritive blood vessels . . . of the stomach, or . . . the ganglionic nerves that supply the stomach. The effect of this congestion is to interfere with the quality of the blood, and its organic sympathy with the vessels which contain it . . . forming the acidity so much talked about dyspeptics . . . and the much-dreaded *flatulence*." He believed that "the close application of the mind to any one subject, whether it be abstruse or superficial . . . ranks among the frequent causes of nervous dyspepsia."[33]

In *The Water Cure*, he delineated a course of treatments for nervous dyspepsia, which he began at once to apply to Darwin, who then recounted them in a letter to Susan that was written nine days after he arrived at Malvern:

> As you say you want my hydropathical diary, I will give it you . . . —1/4 before 7. get up, & am scrubbed with rough towel in cold water for 2 or 3 minutes, which after the few first days, made & makes me very like a lobster—I have a washerman, a very nice person, & he scrubs behind, whilst I scrub in front.[34]—drink a tumbler of water & get my clothes on as quick as possible & walk for 20 minutes—I c[d]. walk further, but I find it tires me afterwards—I like all this very much.[35]—At same time I put on my compress, which is a broad wet folded linen covered by a mackintosh & which is "refreshed"—ie dipt in cold water every 2 hours & I wear it all day, except for about 2 hours after midday dinner; I don't perceive much effect from this of any kind.—After my walk, shave & wash & get my breakfast, which was to have been exclusively toast with meat or egg, but he has allowed me a little milk to sop the *stale* toast in. At no time must I take any sugar, butter, spices tea bacon or anything good.[36] At 12 oclock I put my feet for ten minutes in cold water with a little mustard & they are violently rubbed by my man; the coldness makes my feet ache much, but upon the whole my feet are certainly less cold than formerly.[37]—Walk for 20 minutes & dine at one.—He has relaxed a little about my dinner & says I may try plain pudding, if I am sure it lessens sickness.
>
> After dinner lie down & try to go to sleep for one hour.—At 5 oclock feet in cold water—drink cold water & walk as before.[38]—Supper same as breakfast at 6 oclock.—I have had much sickness this week, but certainly I have felt much stronger & the sickness has depressed me much less.[39]

One reason for feeling stronger and less depressed, despite still vomiting, was that Malvern treatments had "at once relieved" him of the nocturnal obsessions that interfered with sleep.[40]

As his health continued to improve, he resumed correspondence with friends, and eighteen days after arriving at Malvern he wrote Hooker (who was in India) the following:

I . . . now have had no vomiting for 10 days. D.ʳ G. feels pretty sure he can do me good, which most certainly the regular Doctors could not. At present, I am heated by Spirit lamp till I *stream* with perspiration, & am then suddenly rubbed violently with towels dripping with cold water.[41] . . . I mention all this to you, as being a medical man, you might possibly like to hear about it. I feel certain that the Water Cure is no quackery. How I shall enjoy getting back to Down with renovated health, if such be my good fortune, & resuming the beloved Barnacles.

To this, Hooker replied:

Your bettered health rejoices me greatly, I pray God Malvern & the cold water will do you good, I do indeed court all the medical details you send, & boring though it be to recapitulate such things, would beg you to continue to me particulars of your case. I read that part of your letter with as much interest as any other, & that is saying a great deal, for all your gossip is dearly welcome to me.[42]

In the following months, as a result of the Malvern treatments, his health and mood improved in a variety of ways. He remained free of vomiting, and his appetite and strength increased, so that he gained weight and went on daily walks of seven miles. In addition, he began to more closely scrutinize how he felt, so that in his health diary he recorded his daily health, whereas previously he had recorded only days when he was ill. He resumed correspondence with friends, talked to Susan when she visited him at Malvern, remembered his father with the "sweetest pleasure," and probably stopped fearing he was dying. In several letters, he reported that he was feeling "indolence & stagnation of mind," which meant that for a time he was freed from many anxieties.[43]

His health improvements resulted from a combination of several causes, in addition to the effects of hydropathy: He was free from the pressures of scientific work. By living in his own house, he avoided being exposed to the stresses of conversing with strangers. There was the daily solace of Emma, whom he described as thinking "as much about me as I do even myself."[44] Of special importance were his feelings for Dr. Gully.

In his sojourn at Malvern, he was impressed by Dr. Gully's attentiveness, kindness, flexibility, and "caution" (a word he used several times about Dr. Gully) in making large and small changes in his treatments.[45] He developed a confidence in Dr. Gully resembling the confidence he had in Dr. Darwin, which enabled him to persevere in carrying out unpleasant treatments.[46] His eight-year-old daughter, Annie, told her governess how he "liked" hydropathy, but that it sometimes made him "so angry" and "cross." While he first complained of the "excessive irritation of skin brought on by rubbings and cold water baths," he believed (with Dr. Gully) that this would pass, and then he came to believe that "the violent excitement of the skin" had rested his stomach and checked vomiting.[47]

He was also impressed that there were "many patients" at Malvern and that Dr. Gully "must be making an immense fortune." At Malvern, he paid Dr. Gully two to three guineas a week, plus a weekly payment of four shillings to his washerman.[48]

At the end of his stay at Malvern, in a letter to Fox after first reporting how Dr. Gully had directed that he continue to take hydropathy treatments at Down for a year, he then summed up his thoughts on the condition of his stomach, the value of hydropathy, and his medical debt to Fox:

> I consider the sickness [vomiting] as absolutely cured. And 3 weeks since I had 12 hours without any flatulence, which showed me that it was possible that even that can be cured, as Dr. G. has always said he could.
>
> The Water Cure is assuredly a grand discovery & how sorry I am I did not hear of it, or rather that I was not somehow compelled to try it some five or six years ago. Much I owe to you for your large share in making me go this Spring.[49]

On 30 June, he and his family returned home.[50] He had stayed at Malvern for sixteen weeks, the longest continuous period he would ever be away from Down.

7

Self-Observation and Doing Dr. Gully's Treatment at Down and Then Self-Observation and Treating Himself

On returning home, Darwin followed Dr. Gully's directions and adapted Malvern treatments to Down living. He went on early morning walks around the sandwalk, rode a horse bought in Malvern, and on 24 July resumed work on barnacles, which was limited by Dr. Gully to two and a half hours per day.[1]

He trained his butler Parslow to be a washerman and had hydropathy in a small church-shaped hut built for him near Down's well by the village carpenter, John Lewis. The hut contained a tub with a platform on it and a huge cistern above that held 640 gallons of water. The carpenter's fifteen-year-old son, also named John Lewis (then a page to the Darwin family), recollected: "I had to pump it [the cistern] fully every day. . . . Mr. Darwin came out and had a little dressing place, and he'd go out on the stage . . . pull the string, and all the water fell on him through a two-inch pipe. A douche, they called it." Young Lewis also remembered how he helped to prepare Darwin's early morning lamp bath: "At seven . . . I had to have the big bath outside the study on the lawn . . . and Mr. Darwin would come down [into his hut] and sit in a chair with a spirit lamp and all rolled round with blankets till the sweat poured off him in showers when he shook his head. . . . I've heard him cry to . . . Parslow, 'I'll be melted away if you don't hurry!' Then he'd get into the ice-cold bath in the open air."[2]

Darwin's daughter Etty remembers how she and other children would stand outside the hydropathy hut listening to the "groans" of their father as he took his cold water treatments.[3] Etty's brother George writes that his father would have hydropathy at noon every day even in the coldest weather. "I remember well one bitter cold day with the snow covering everything waiting outside [the hydropathy hut] until he had finished & that he came out almost blue with cold & we trotted away at a good brisk pace over the snow to the Sandwalk."[4]

In his health diary, Darwin recorded that over a period of twenty-one months, from July 1849 until April 1851, he treated himself with several combinations of hydropathy, usually consisting of lamp baths, douches, shallow baths, foot baths, and being rubbed with dripping sheets and that he varied these combinations every three to six weeks.[5]

Although he never found a combination of hydropathy that freed him from flatulence, he came to accept the limitations and benefits of hydropathy, and in May 1850 he wrote to Fox that even with the persistence of flatulence, he felt "*infinitely* better than before I commenced the W[ater] Cure." Several months later, in reply to arguments made by Fox against the efficacy of hydropathy, he wrote: "Your aphorism that 'any remedy will cure any malady' contains, I do believe, profound truth, whether applicable or not to the wondrous Water Cure, I am not very sure. The Water Cure, however, keeps in high favour, & I go regularly on with douching &c &c."[6]

One reason for continuing to use hydropathy was a continuing confidence in his Malvern physician. All during the above period of twenty-one months, Darwin regularly reported in letters to Dr. Gully, who then wrote back instructions for changes in treatment. In September 1849 and June 1850, according to his health diary, he visited Gully in Malvern. However, in a September 1850 letter to Fox, he criticized Dr. Gully for believing in homeopathy, mesmerism, and clairvoyance, and commented: "It is a sad flaw, I cannot but think in my beloved Dr. Gully that he believes in everything."[7] Many years later, George Darwin recollected:

Dr. Gully . . . bothered my father for some time to have a consultation with a clairvoyante, who was staying at Malvern, and was reputed to be able to see the insides of people & discover the real nature of their ailments. At last he consented to pacify Dr. Gully, but on condition that he be allowed to test the clairvoyante's powers for himself. Accordingly, in going to the interview he put a banknote in a sealed envelope. After being introduced to the lady, he said, "I have heard a great deal of your powers of reading concealed writings & I should like to have evidence myself; now in this envelope there is a banknote—if you will read the number I shall be happy to present it to you." The clairvoyante answered scornfully, "I have a maid-servant at home who can do that." But she had her revenge, for on proceeding to the diagnosis of my father's illness, she gave a most appalling picture of the horrors which she saw in his inside.[8]

In June 1850, the Darwin's nine-year-old daughter Annie began suffering from a malaise that persisted into the first months of 1851. When she was not helped by medications from Dr. Holland, her father placed her under the care of Dr. Gully, who then suggested that Darwin treat Annie with daily hydropathy at Down and report to him on the effects of these treatments. At this time, Darwin also continued to report to Dr. Gully on how hydropathy was affecting his illness. After several months of hydropathy failed to improve Annie's malaise, Darwin brought her to Malvern on 24 March 1851 for further treatment by Dr. Gully, while he returned to Down to be with his pregnant wife. (On 13 May 1851, Emma would give birth to her ninth child and fifth son, Horace.) Weeks later, Annie developed a low-grade fever with bilious vomiting that caused Dr. Gully to fear for her life and to write her father to come immediately.[9]

Darwin arrived at Malvern on Thursday, April 17. Over the next six days, as he experienced one of the most painful events of his life, he found it was a relief to write Emma detailed accounts of Annie's condition, while Emma felt a similar relief after reading what he had written. On Friday, he wrote: "It is now from hour to hour a struggle between life & death. . . . Sometimes Dr. G[ully] exclaims she [Annie] will get through the struggle; then, I see, he doubts. . . . She has vomited a large quantity of bright green fluid. Her case seems to me an exaggerated one of my Maer illness."[10] On that Saturday, he was joined at Malvern by Fanny Wedgwood, Emma's sister-in-law, who came at Emma's request. Emma, who believed her husband's health was "always affected by his mind," now feared that his anxiety over Annie would make him ill, and she hoped Fanny would comfort him and aid in the care of Annie.[11]

On 21 and 22 April, although Annie appeared somewhat better, Darwin wrote Emma, "I must not hope too much. These alternations of no hope & hope sicken one's soul." Although he was so restless that he could not sit still and was "constantly up & down," he took part in Annie's nursing, bathing her in a mixture of vinegar and water, giving her water and brandy to drink, and applying poultices to her abdomen. Fanny Wedgwood stayed by Darwin and Annie's side, and Darwin told his wife they were "under deep obligations to Fanny never to be forgotten."[12]

On Tuesday morning, Darwin wrote an optimistic letter to Emma, but soon doubted his hopes and did not send the letter.[13] Later in the day, Fanny reported that he was "very ill . . . with one of his stomach attacks" and that "it's most affecting to me how he suffers constantly crying—but he says it's a relief."[14] By that evening, Annie was "sinking," and Dr. Gully declared she was "in imminent danger."[15]

Annie died at noon on Wednesday. Dr. Gully recorded the cause of death as "bilious fever with typhoid character."[16] In the afternoon, Darwin wrote to Emma that Annie "went to her final sleep most tranquilly, most sweetly. . . . We must be more & more to each other my dear wife. . . . I am in bed not very well with my stomach."[17] During his stay at Malvern, Darwin's stomach illness appears to have consisted of fits of flatulence that were not associated with vomiting.[18]

On Wednesday evening, Fanny informed Emma that she had been sitting with Darwin, who had been "able to find relief in crying much." At the same time, Emma wrote to Fanny: "I cannot help all sorts of fears for Charles which I know are not reasonable. . . . I know he must be ill. . . . My first feeling of consolation will be to have him safe home again." Darwin and Fanny then arranged for him to return home on Thursday, 24 April, while she would remain at Malvern and be present at Annie's burial in the yard of Malvern's Priory Church on 25 April. Darwin arrived home at 6:30 p.m. Thursday. On Friday, Emma again wrote Fanny: "I cannot tell you the surprise and joy it was to see poor Charles arrive. . . . He is much better bodily than I had any hopes of and not worse in spirits." By "better bodily," Emma meant that despite the stresses of Annie's death and of traveling from Malvern to Down, her husband's stomach complaints and dizziness were not as severe as she had feared. Emma added: "We have done little else but cry together and talk about our darling. He cannot express what a comfort you were."[19]

Five days later, Darwin wrote down those memories of Annie that brought out his deepest feelings so that he would always remember her.[20] His weeping for her, first with Fanny and then with Emma, perhaps was the most heartfelt weeping he had ever experienced. It was probably because of this weeping that his illness did not become more severe and that his physical health remained relatively stable during the period of Annie's death.[21]

Darwin kept up his health diary through January 1855, a period of almost four years, during which he stopped corresponding with Dr. Gully and became his own physician.[22] The diary records that from 26 April to 21 June 1851, he took daily shallow baths, and then for about two months he had no hydropathy. From 28 August to 7 October he had what he would describe as *moderately severe treatment*," consisting of lamp baths, douches, shallow baths, and foot baths. From 8 October 1851 to 14 January 1852, his hydropathy was limited to daily shallow baths. From 15 January to 28 February, he had "*moderately* severe treatments" of lamp baths, douches, foot baths, and shallow baths, and then told Fox that these treatments were "always with good effect."[23]

From 1 March to 10 June, his treatment was limited to either daily shallow baths or daily dripping sheets. From 11 to 20 June he had "moderately severe treatments," followed by daily treatments of either shallow baths or dripping sheets from 21 June to 11 July, and then moderately severe treatments from 12 July to 21 August. After this last treatment he wrote at the end of the August page of his diary: "Six weeks of treatment: not much good effect extremely tired in Evening. I do not think last treatment did me much good."

From 22 August through December, he had daily shallow baths. For almost a year he then had no water treatment. From 13 November to 25 December 1853, he had six weeks of moderately severe treatment. Water treatments then ceased for several years. Darwin had come to recognize that he was well enough to do without hydropathy, while continuing to believe in its beneficial effects should his illness worsen.

The diary records that occasionally, and for very brief periods, he used several nonhydropathy forms of treatment. On 24 December 1850 he began rubbing tartar emetic ointment into his skin, and on 27 February 1851 he began using it in the evening. His reasons for taking the ointment were not known.[24] On 4 March 1851 he treated his flatulence by taking Croton, a medicinal substance found in plants that was used as a tonic and for treating dyspepsia.[25]

On 16 October 1851, he wrote in the diary, "(Electric Chains to Waist)," and on 19 October, "do [ditto] neck." A hydroelectric chain was composed of alternate brass and zinc wires which, when moistened with vinegar, gave out electric shocks.[26] It was applied to different body parts for varying lengths of time and was used to treat "cases of partial paralysis, neuralgic headaches, and many other nervous diseases," and cases where the muscles were too relaxed.[27] This was his second attempt, in five years, to treat himself with currents from electrical appliances.

For several days in December 1853, he noted the nocturnal effects of coffee and tea: coffee usually caused him to be "wakeful," but with tea, the "wakeful" effect was not as pronounced; with both beverages he was usually able to have a "good" night.[28] For several months in 1854, for unknown reasons, he recorded consuming lemons two or three times a day: 23 January, "1/2 lemon thrice"; 24 January, "Whole Lemon Twice a day"; 8 March, "*Left off Lemon*"; and 5 April, "Half Lemon."[29]

On 31 August 1854 his daily diary entry read: "Well . . . as far as stomach. But very p [poor] from S.E. [Seldom Evacuating]." The night entry read, "wretched." He then recorded in the diary, for 6–8 September, the cathartic effects of decreasing doses of Cordial Aloes: 6 September, "30 drops of Aloes no work"; 7 September, "20 drops . . . no work"; 8 September, "10 drops purged 5 work." Alongside these three entries he wrote that "10 drops twice a day w^d. be enough." However, he still had bowel complaints, and on 22 September Emma wrote in her diary that his taking rust of iron chalk and rhubarb had not done "any good." In November he evaluated the cathartic effects of decreasing and increasing the doses of Liquor Infusion Aloes: 17 November, "20 drops Aloes"; 19 November, "1 work"; 20 November, "4 work?"[30] These entries on Aloes are the last medical observations in the health diary.

The diary's most commonly reported symptoms were "fits" of flatulence, occurring with a frequency of one to seven times in a period of twenty-four hours, of varying (largely unknown) durations, and greatly varying intensities that Darwin variously described as "almost," "barely," "very slight," "slightest," "slight," "moderate," "good deal," considerable," "much," "rather bad," "baddish," "not bad," "bad," "very bad," "sharp," "sharpish," and "excessive." It will be seen that when Darwin wrote "excessive" he was really experiencing an excessive amount of pain. Many "fits" would make him feel "fatigued," "oppressed," or "heavy." Along with the fits, he sometimes had nausea, vomiting, "retching," and retching up "acid & slime."

Next to "fits," his most frequently described symptoms were boils, ranging in severity from "little" and "small" to "bad." Less frequent symptoms were skin disorders he called "rash," "erythema," "eruption," that sometimes may have been caused by mechanical irritations of hydropathy treatments; headaches he usually described as "slight"; his "colds" mostly appear to have been afebrile and uncomplicated. On 20 April 1853, however, he wrote in the diary that he had a cold with mild fever and "chest-pain." This lasted only a day.

Other symptoms included being "tired" in the evening, "shivering" that was sometimes "slight" and at other times "fatiguing," but never as severe as the shivering he had in his violent vomiting of 1848–49, and being "weakish," "languid," "weak & languid." On several occasions, he recorded a diminution in his old feeling of "sinking" by writing "sinking slight." On 8 June 1851, he described himself as "squashy," a term he never defined but sometimes used to describe a particular negative feeling.

When Darwin wrote to Fox in March 1852 that "my nights are *always* bad, & that stops my becoming vigorous," he was referring to three nocturnal disturbances that occurred singly or in combinations with one another: having flatulence, and other day symptoms; being "heazish," or "heazyish," which described breathing difficulties and coughing; and having obsessions over events that had occurred during the day: an unresolved scientific problem, failing to answer a troubling letter, a disturbing passage he had read in a book, or a troublesome conversation.[31] These nocturnal thoughts would often cause him to lie awake or sit up in bed for hours.[32] Sometimes when he was troubled by what he had said to a person, he would get up from his bed at night so as to further explain to the person exactly what he had meant to say.[33] He was especially vulnerable to nocturnal obsessional thoughts because, when he was lying in bed, he lacked distractions (reading, music, and backgammon).

In most of the diary entries he adapted a method of summarizing his health by writing "well" or "well very," and further delineating the degree of wellness by underlining the "very" with one or two dashes. At the end of each month, at the bottom of the diary page, he counted the number of "double-dash" days, valuing these days for their feeling of well-being and for the work he had accomplished. However, although on most double-dash days he had a diminution of flatulence, on other double-dash days in 1850 and 1851 he had "occasional" flatulence, and in August 1853 he wrote at the bottom of the diary page: "17 Double-Dashes, but I think I am not as strict as I used to be." On April 1854 he wrote at the bottom of the diary: "Only 3 Double Dashes & two of these not good!" On the two "not good days" he had "occasional flatulence."

Collating Darwin's increases in illness with what is known about events in his life, it can be seen that a frequent cause for these increases were his travels from Down. On 16 August 1849, he dined and visited at the home of Lord Mahon at Chevening, which was about three miles from Down. In a September letter to Lyell he reported how, during the visit, Lord Stanhope (father of Lord Mahon) had "abused geology & zoology heartily," "describing *species* of birds & shells &c [as] all fiddle faddle." While the visit was not mentioned in the health diary, the diary records that the day after the visit Darwin had "3 its of fl night rather wakeful much fl."[34]

On 11 and 12 September 1849, Darwin and Emma went to Birmingham for a meeting of the British Association for the Advancement of Science. When he was there, he thought that the meeting place was "large & nasty" and the meeting "not very brilliant," and he had increasing day and night flatulence. After eight days, he and Emma started for Warwick and Kenilworth, but he "broke down" and returned to Down, where he spent a day in bed feeling "poorly" and with "a good deal of ft." He then told Henslow: "I think I stand any change, even worse than formerly & my stomach has not gotten over the excitement of Birmingham as yet."[35]

On 28 January and 16 November 1850, when he traveled to the preparatory school attended by his son William, located in Mitcham in Surrey, he suffered "continued" flatulence.[36] On 4 September 1850, he reported to Fox that he was considering the "awful experiment" of sending William to the Bruce Castle School, which had many educational innovations in its curriculum. In his diary entry for 6 September, he recorded his visit to the school, which was at Tottenham in the environs of London, as follows: "London. Well not quite. Excessive ft." At night: "excessive ft." Following this, he had increased flatulence for several nights, probably from worrying about the Bruce Castle School and William, and then decided to send William to Rugby.[37]

From 30 July to 10 August 1851, the Darwin family went to London for three weeks and visited the Crystal Palace and Great Exhibition of 1851 in Hyde Park. This was the first great "World Fair," seen daily by enormous crowds and remembered "with wonder and admiration by all."[38] Although Darwin "intensely" enjoyed the Exhibition, he told an acquaintance that he had "many bad headaches" from "heat & fatigue" and that "London . . . always makes me unwell."[39]

From 23 to 27 March 1852, he visited William at Rugby, and the diary shows that he had "well very" health. When he went on to visit his sisters Catherine and Susan at Shrewsbury, he became "not well" and had fits of flatulence. On 17 November 1852 (the fourth anniversary of the death of his father), he visited London for the day with Hooker, and with crowds estimated at hundreds of thousands viewed the body of the Duke of Wellington lying in state in the hall of Chelsea Hospital.[40] He then reported in the diary that he had two fits of flatulence and a "poor" night. In 1853, he twice visited the Crystal Palace, which was being built anew at Sydenham, and each time he had some accentuations of his flatulence.[41]

From 13 to 17 August 1853, he and his family stayed at The Hermitage, home of his brother-in-law Harry Wedgwood. Nearby was Chobham Camp, where since June, a force of about ten to sixteen thousand English soldiers and dragoons had been engaged in mimic warfare (the first protracted large-scale mimic warfare in the history of the peacetime British army).[42] For three days, Darwin watched this "warfare" with "intense enjoyment" and "happy excitement," and was "keener than anyone in his interest."[43] On this occasion, "excitement" did not disturb his health. In the diary, he described himself as "well *very*." His nights, however, were either "goodish" or "indifferent." On 10 June 1854, he,

Emma, and Emma's sixty-one-year-old sister, Elizabeth Wedgwood, traveled to Sydenham to watch—along with tens of thousands of spectators—Queen Victoria open the new Crystal Palace.[44] It was an event which Darwin, in a letter to his son William, described as follows: "I did not much care for it: it was so hot that Aunt Elizabeth fainted dead away & it was very frightening & disagreeable; and we had to lay her flat on the ground."[45] In the diary, he recorded his health as "Poorly & sickness & bad headache"; his night was "good." From 13 to 15 July 1854, he sojourned at Hartfield, which was the home of several Wedgwood relatives.[46] Here there was a wild forest that he greatly enjoyed walking in alone.[47] In the diary, he described his health as "well" and "well very," and his nights as "goodish" and "good."[48] The diary showed that in travels to London (some of which were to attend scientific meetings, or study barnacles at the British Museum), while he frequently had increases in flatulence, he sometimes remained well.

Although traveling did not always make him sick, he came to believe that all travels were hazardous to his health. He excused himself from visiting Fox by writing his old friend: "Very many thanks for your most kind & large invitation to Delamere, but I fear we can hardly compass it. I dread going anywhere, on account of my stomach so easily failing under any excitement." Several months later, he told Fox that because of his "dreadful flatulence," he could "in fact . . . go nowhere."[49]

Visitors had variable effects on his health. On 2 November 1849, when he was visited at Down by Fox, the visit was constrained by his having "excessive" day and night flatulence. Two months later he wrote Fox that his health was "better than when you were here," and that despite illness he and Emma had "both much enjoyed" the visit. In March 1851, in a letter to Fox, he commented on the influence of illness on his friendships: "long continued ill-health has much changed me, & I very often think with pain how cold & different I must appear to my few old friends to what I was formerly; but I internally know that the inner part of my mind remains the same with my old affections."[50] When he was visited by Lyell from 15 to 18 October 1849, and from 28 to 30 April 1850, while there was no record of what they talked about, the diary shows that his health remained good. When Lyell visited him on two occasions in 1851—22 February and 22–25 October—they talked about controversial aspects of his transmutation theory (Lyell did not believe in transmutation) and the diary showed an increase in his flatulence.[51] On 27–30 November 1851, when he was visited by his *Beagle* friend Captain Sulivan, the diary shows an increase in flatulence. On 17–26 April 1852, when Hooker and Hooker's wife stayed at

Down, the diary shows that Darwin was sometimes ill and sometimes well. On 26–28 October 1854, when Hooker and Lyell visited him, he had no illness.

The diary recorded several illnesses and their causes: 17 May 1850, one fit of flatulence "from excitment," without specifying what the excitement was; 22 July 1851, three fits of flatulence from being visited by two acquaintances, Daniel Rowlands and George Armstrong; and 6 January 1854, "several fits" of flatulence from attending a party given by the Fry family, who lived near Down village. On January 1850, a week before and a week after Emma gave birth to a fourth son, Darwin had a good deal of nocturnal flatulence. In May 1851, a week before and a week after Emma gave birth to a fifth son, he had "slight Eruption." On 15 and 23 October 1852, when he was at two "Dinner Parties," the first given by the Normans (who were friends and neighbors) and a second attended by unidentified individuals, he did not have significant ill effects.

On some occasions the diary recorded illnesses from foods: 30 August 1849, "*much fl.* From spice"; 24 June 1850, "2 long fits of fl Evening (Salad)"; 27 April 1853, "Poorly sickness frm indigestion"; and 15 July 1853, "Dreadful vomiting from Crab" [after supper when the Darwin family was staying at Sea Houses, in Eastbourne].

While boils and colds would sometimes not much disturb Darwin, at other times they resulted in the following diary entries: 15 April 1850, "(Boil) night at first very much fl," and on 20 April, "Boil broke night, later much fl."; 18 May 1850, "2 rather bad fits of fl (Got Boil)," and on 22 May, "6 or 7 bad fits of fl (Boil first broke)." On 10 November 1850, "Poorly bed. Much continued fl. (cold)," and at night "some bad fits of fl"; 21 January 1851, "Poorly headache, excessive fl from Boils"; 10 March 1851, "1 baddish fit (new Boil)"; 14 July 1851, "occas. fl (small Boil broke)"; 17 April 1852, "several fits slight headache Cold," and on 21 April, "1 baddish fit (slight cold)"; 4 January 1853, "Poorly a little not much fl. Boil"; 6 February 1854, "i fit (slight cold)"; 30 March 1854, "much vomiting Bad Boil"; 2 July 1854, "Well not quite, 2 Boils"; and on the next day, "Poorly, *sickness.*"

Let us now consider what the health diary reveals, and does not reveal, about some of the overall patterns of Darwin's illness between 1849 and 1854. The diary shows that almost any physical, mental, or medical event that disturbed Darwin's daily routine could cause an increase in his flatulence. He lived under the tyranny of day and night "fits" of flatulence and apprehensions of the flatulence becoming worse and leading to uncontrolled vomiting. However, despite "excessive" episodes of flatulence and occasional vomiting, his vomiting did not become uncontrolled as in 1848–49, so that he was able to return to his pre-1848 routine of work. In an 1850 letter to his ex-servant Covington, he wrote: "I am sorry to say that my health keeps indifferent, and I have given up all hopes of ever being a strong man again . . . but natural history fills up my time."[52] In 1852 he wrote to Fox: "not that I am at all worse, perhaps rather better & lead a very comfortable life with my 3 hours of daily work, but it is the life of a hermit."[53] One reason for his illness not worsening was that he appears to have been careful not to work on barnacles for more than three hours daily (doubtless influenced by Dr. Gully's advice on not working too hard).

What the diary does not reveal is the effects of barnacle work on Darwin's flatulence. Nowhere in the diary is this work mentioned as a possible cause for his episodes of flatulence. And yet the work, although limited, occurred almost daily and was often found by Darwin to be wearying and more difficult than he had expected,[54] and it became one of the main stresses in his life. Perhaps one reason he did not acknowledge this stress is that he wanted to show Dr. Gully that he was not being hurt by his work. He also may not have mentioned his visits with Lord Mahon, Fox, and others because he feared these visits detracted from his doing hydropathy at home. Thus, in his previously quoted September 1849 letter to Lyell, he commented that his visit to Lord Mahon was "against all rules," meaning the rules established by Dr. Gully for how he should do hydropathy at Down.

In a May 1854 letter to Hooker (who had recently complained of stomach illness), Darwin explained some of the reasons for keeping his health diary: "I am really truly sorry to hear about your stomach. I *entreat* you to write down your own case,—symptoms—& habits of life, & then consider your case as that of stranger; & I put it to you, whether common sense w.d not order you to take more regular exercise & work your Brains less.—(N.B. take a cold bath & walk before breakfast) I am certain in the long run you would not lose time. Till you have a thoroughly bad stomach, you will not know the really great evil of it, morally physically & every way. Do reflect & act resolutely. Remember your troubled heart-action formerly plainly told how your constitution was tried. but I will say no more, excepting that a man is mad to risk health, on which everything—including his *children's inherited health* depends.—Do not hate me for this lecture." At the end of the letter, he wrote: "Adios, my dear Hooker; do be wise & good & be careful of your stomach, within which, as I know full well, lie intellect, conscience, temper & the affections."[55]

Following this letter to Hooker, Darwin went on writing a daily health diary for a period of seven months, June 1854 until the middle of January 1855. While the diary entries showed his health remained relatively stable, he noted that from 14 through 29 December, his children were ill.[56] Hoping that they would benefit from a "change of air" (even if the new air was London air),[57] he moved with his family to London from 18 January through 14 February. On returning to Down he reported to Fox that the move "turned out a great failure, for the dreadful frost just set in when we went, & all our children got unwell & Emma & I had coughs, & colds, & rheumatism nearly all the time." His health became better when he returned home.[58]

The move to London coincided with changes in the diary. After writing an entry for 16 January 1855, he wrote no further entries, but recorded the daily dates until 31 January. Following this, six years after he had begun writing the diary, he stopped. His reasons for stopping are not known. In the future, although he would make some occasional medical notes in a "private diary," he would not again attempt to keep a daily health diary.[59]

Working "Too Hard" on *Natural Selection* and Treatments at Moor Park

In September 1854, on completing the work of describing all known living and fossil barnacles, Darwin somewhat unhappily recorded in his journal that it was now eight years since he had begun the work.[1] However, his descriptions of barnacles (along with previous work in geology) won him the Royal Medal of the Royal Society of London, the first public recognition of his scientific achievements. This award caused him to feel great and unusual happiness when he received a letter of approbation from Hooker.[2] He then vomited and felt "poorly" when he had to receive the medal in a public ceremony organized by the Royal Society.[3]

Delineating the anatomies of species of barnacles had shown him that every species varied in "some slight degree," and suggested that over time these variations could evolve into new species. This encouraged him to move forward with his evolutionary theory.[4] In his journal he noted that, after finishing with barnacles, he had immediately begun "sorting notes for Species Theory."[5] And from the fall of 1854 to the spring of 1856, he searched for evidence for the theory in ways that included trying (at first without success) to elucidate how species could be transported to new lands, visiting pigeon shows and keeping pigeons at Down so as to study the variations between breeds, studying variations in plants by conducting hybridizing experiments with more than thirty varieties of peas, and corresponding with scientists.[6]

In a letter to Hooker, he expressed mixed feelings about his work: "I sh^d. have less scruple in troubling you, if I had any confidence what my work would turn out; sometimes I think it will be good; at other times I really feel so much ashamed of myself as the Author of The Vestiges ought to be of himself."[7] *Ves-*

tiges of the Natural History of Creation, a much discussed book by an anonymous author, had propounded a theory of evolution that had been vilified by theologians and criticized by leading scientific men (including Hooker, Lyell, and other friends of Darwin) as not being up to their professional standards. Darwin feared that when he published his work, it would receive a similar reception. He also hoped that, by learning from the shortcomings of *Vestiges*, he could shape his theory of evolution so that it would meet scientific standards.[8] Throughout this period he described his health as "better," while noting that he had "a few bad days almost every fortnight." In March 1856, he told Fox that he was "able decidedly to work harder." But he also wrote: "Sometimes I fear I shall break down for my subject gets bigger & bigger with each month's work."[9]

On 16 April 1856, in a talk with Lyell at Down, he disclosed the main tenets of natural selection. Lyell did not become a convert to the theory, yet he urged that it be made public. "Out with the theory," Lyell wrote Darwin on 1 May 1856, "& let it take date—& be cited—& understood."[10] Darwin then began to write what he hoped would become a comprehensive and very big book entitled *Natural Selection*, and from May 1856 through June 1858, he wrote up about two-thirds of the topics he intended to discuss.[11]

As his writing progressed—"sometimes in triumph & sometimes in despair"[12]—he expressed, to old friends and new acquaintances, some of his different fears. In June 1856, referring to the evidences he would muster for his theory, he told Fox that "my work will be horridly imperfect & with many mistakes, so that I groan & tremble when I think of it."[13] In July of that year, he wrote Hooker: "What a book a Devil's Chaplain might write on the clumsy, wasteful, blundering low and horridly cruel works of nature!" In calling himself a "Devil's Chaplain" who writes a book about the cruel works of nature, he was expressing two of his most troubling feelings: horror over the suffering and death of ill-adapted species in the war of nature, and apprehensions that in Victorian society his scientific ideas would be considered immoral and irreligious so that he would be judged as having an identity that was socially reprehensible.[14]

His fear returned that his belief in evolution would estrange him from those scientific men he most respected and whose help he most needed. In October 1856, after first revealing his evolutionary views to the American geologist James Dana, he commented: "I groan when I make such a confession, for I shall have little sympathy from those, whose sympathy I alone value." Months later, after making a similar "confession" to the American botanist Asa Gray, he told Gray: "I know that this will make you despise me."[15]

For a time he continued to be painfully perplexed over understanding how species could be transported to new lands. On 3 October 1856, he told Fox, "No subject gives me so much trouble & doubt & difficulty, as means of dispersal of the same species of terrestrial productions on to oceanic islands.—Land Mollusca drive me mad, & I cannot anyhow get their eggs to experimentise on their power of floating & resistance to injurious action of salt-water." He told Hooker that the transport of land mollusks "tormented & haunted" him. In a letter to Hooker, in which he discussed species transport, he called himself "Your insane & perverse friend."[16]

Some of his experiments were then successful, and early in 1857 he told Hooker that mollusks could be transported over distances by adhering to the feet of ducks. He had earlier shown how millet seeds could be transported by being carried in the stomachs of birds and fish. Discovering these and other means of transport caused him to "feel as if a thousand pound weight was taken off my back."[17]

Along with work, he worried about the health of his eight living children. In the early 1850s he had written that his "dread" and "bug-bear" was that they would inherit his ill health and that "even death [was] better" for his children than to have his kind of illness.[18] Now he began to feel that his "dread" was becoming a reality. In letters to Hooker and Fox, he reported how several of his children were having episodes of "irregular & feeble pulse" and that this was "strange & heart-breaking."[19]

Despite anxieties over work and children, he did not have a serious increase in illness, and his main complaints about his health were of working "too hard" on *Natural Selection* and of sometimes being "overdone" because of his work. By "overdone" he meant mental fatigue and increases in flatulence. Occasionally he considered stopping work and consulting Dr. Gully, but he feared that being at Malvern would "revive" disturbing thoughts of Annie. He also considered trying hydropathy at Moor Park, in Surrey, but then held back from going there.[20]

In February 1857, he told Fox: "I do not think I shall have courage for Water Cure again: I am now trying mineral Acids, with, I think, good effect."[21] "Mineral Acids" probably meant a mixture of muriatic (hydrochloridic) acid and nitric acid.[22] It was believed that in some cases of "dyspepsia" the stomach did not secrete acids and that treatment should consist of replacing these missing secretions. Acids were also thought to act as "tonics."[23] It is not known for how long Darwin took "mineral acids." Apparently, their "good effect" had ceased by April.

On 13 April, he informed Lyell: "My health has been very poor of late, & I am going in a week's time for a fortnight of hydropathy & rest.—My everlasting species-Book quite overwhelms me with work—It is beyond my powers, but I hope to live to finish it."[24] Nine days later, he went by himself for two weeks to the hydropathic establishment at Moor Park, Farnham, Surrey, a place once famous as the home of Sir William Temple and his secretary, Jonathan Swift.[25] At Moor Park—after a week of daily shallow baths, douches, and sitz baths—he reported to Hooker that he had "already received an amount of good, which is quite incredible to myself & quite unaccountable. I can walk & eat like a hearty Christian; and even my nights are good." He commented to Hooker that the hydropathy of Moor Park (like hydropathy during his first visit to Malvern) "dulls one's brain splendidly, so that I have not thought about a single species of any kind, since leaving home." He returned to Moor Park in June and November 1857 for periods of one or two weeks of treatments.[26]

He found in Moor Park additional benefits and attractions that, Emma would recollect many years later, caused him to feel "rested and improved and full of enjoyment."[27] He was separated from the pressures and concerns of his Down family (except for June 1857 when he was with his sick daughter Etty, who was a hydropathy patient at Moor Park from 29 May to 7 August).[28] He was also relieved from the pressures of writing *Natural Selection*, while he could continue to think about aspects of his theory in more relaxed ways. "Moor Park," he wrote Fox, "I like *much* better *as a place* than Malvern."[29] He found that Moor Park's woods were "very pleasant for walking."[30] He would describe these woods as "very wild & lonely, so just suits me. . . . There is an exquisite mixture of ancient Scotch Firs & very old magnificent Birches."[31]

The physician to Moor Park, Dr. Edward Wickstead Lane, was only thirty-five years old (thirteen years younger than Darwin, probably the youngest physician he had yet consulted), and he lacked the national prominence of Dr. Gully. In 1850, he had studied law at Edinburgh University, and in 1853, he obtained his medical degree from Edinburgh University. He had come to Moor Park in 1854. He was charming, and he had read widely in medical and general literature and thought deeply about the philosophy and efficacy of different medical treatments.[32] After first meeting Dr. Lane, Darwin reported to Fox: "I like D^r. Lane & his wife & her mother, who are the proprietors of this establishment very much. D^r. L. is too young,—that is his only fault—but he is a gentleman & very well read man. And in one respect I like him better than D^r. Gully, viz that he does not believe in all the rubbish which Dr. G. does; nor does he pretend to explain much which neither he nor any doctor can explain."[33]

The patients in Moor Park were accommodated in the same building as Dr. Lane and Lane's family, and during his second Moor Park visit, Darwin told Hooker: "D^r. Lane & Wife, & mother-in-law Lady Drysdale are some of the nicest people, I have ever met."[34] He read Dr. Lane's 1857 book on hydropathy and commented that it was "very good & worth reading."[35]

In the book, Dr. Lane summarized what he called "the philosophy of hydropathy" as follows:

Hydropathy . . . is based on one . . . distinctly characteristic idea . . . that nature possesses . . . in the original construction of the living organism, her own means of restoration, when that organism is overtaken by disease; that she is constantly endeavoring to work out her own cure; that she frequently succeeds in her efforts . . . when her powers are not sufficient the aid of art is to be invoked, the aid must be founded on a consideration of the primary laws of health as unfolded by physiology . . . hydropathy is grounded . . . on the belief that the mass of chronic diseases are most effectually and most safely cured . . . by the identical means . . . modified . . . according to circumstances, that are requisite for maintaining the animal economy in health. . . . Its cardinal medicines are the apparently simple medicaments of air, exercise, water, and diet . . . along with healthy moral influences.[36]

Dr. Lane later published an account of Darwin at Moor Park, the only recollection of Darwin by a physician who treated him. In it he emphasized the severity of the episodes of acute flatulence that his patient would sometimes experience:

Mr. Darwin was . . . a great sufferer of dyspepsia of aggravated character. . . . In the course of a long professional experience, I have seen many cases of violent indigestion, in its many forms, and with the multiform tortures it entails, but I cannot recall any where the pain was so truly poignant as in his. When the worst attacks were on, he seemed almost crushed with agony, the nervous system being severely shaken, and the temporary depression resulting distressingly great. I mention this circumstance because it was then that I first perceived the wonderful sweetness and gentleness of his nature, his patience, and the gratitude with which he received the most ordinary services and tokens of sympathy. . . . Of course such attacks as I have spoken of were only occasional—for no constitution could have borne up long under them in their acute phase—but he was never to the last wholly well.[37]

Lane recalled that Darwin—"apart from his feeble health, and constantly in spite of it"—would eagerly socialize with the many people who were at Moor Park. Conversing and joking, "he dearly loved a joke, seeming to enjoy it to his heart's core," laughing "with a mock-mischievous expression that took you captive."[38] Darwin told his family how he made friends with Mary Butler, an Irish lady and the sister of Richard Butler, vicar of Trim, Ireland. Darwin and Miss Butler had the same habit of putting salt on the tablecloth to eat with their bread. She amused him with "bright anecdoty," telling ghost stories (she claimed to have seen the ghost of her father "when he didn't die") and nonsense stories of "honey suckles turning into oaks . . . & new species springing up on every Railway embankment." In the absence of family and friends, she became a solace and comfort.[39]

Dr. Lane had vivid recollections of the walks that he and his patient took in Moor Park's woods:

Darwin was then literally "all eyes." Nothing escaped him. No object in nature, whether Flower, or Bird, or Insect of any kind, could avoid his loving recognition. He knew about them all . . . could give you endless information in his own graphic way about them . . . a question of comparative Botany or Zoology would crop up and carry him aback to his great voyage in the "Beagle," with countless anecdotes of all he saw of nature and of men in the course of it—the whole delivered . . . in a manner so full of point and pith and living interest, and so full of charm, that you could not . . . fail to feel . . . you were enjoying a vast intellectual treat to be never forgotten, and that these were indeed red letter days in your calendar.[40]

After a sojourn at Moor Park, Darwin returned to Down and, feeling better, resumed work on his species book, only to feel ill yet again. Attributing his illness to "nothing but mental work," he went on working.[41] In June 1857, he had written Hooker: "It is most provoking that a cold on leaving Moor Park suddenly turned into my old vomiting, & I have been *almost* as bad since my return home as before, notwithstanding the really surprising state of health I was in there. I fear that my head will stand *no* thought, but I would sooner be the wretched contemptible invalid, which I am, than live the life of an idle squire."[42] In these self-punitive, rough, and eloquent words, Darwin was stating what had become one of his main credos. He was also grimly anticipating a future of work and suffering.

On January 1858, in a letter to Hooker in which he mentioned illness in himself and his family, he let himself go in a sudden burst of feeling: "Oh health, health, you are my daily & nightly bug-bear & stop all enjoyment in life." Then he quickly apologized: "But I really beg pardon, it is very foolish & weak to howl this way. Everyone has got his heavy burthen in this world."[43] By mid-April, his health had become "very bad from overwork," and so for two weeks—20 April through 4 May—he sojourned at Moor Park, where he had hydropathy three times a day each day.[44]

When Emma wrote him that she was "headachy," he wrote back suggesting that when he returned home she and Etty should come to Moor Park for hydropathy while he stayed with their children. He added: "Ah Mammy, I wish you knew how I value you; & what an inexpressible blessing it is to have one whom one can always trust—one always the same, always ready to give comfort, sympathy & the best advice.—God bless you my dear, you are too good for me." He reported to Emma how he had on one day journeyed from Moor Park to the military camp at Aldershot, a distance of about four miles, so as to see Queen Victoria review troops. But watching the review had upset his health, and he felt "poorly" for the day (he did not specify the reasons for this upset).[45]

During his sojourn in Moor Park, while he relaxed from writing *Natural Selection,* he was able to advance his work. By "loitering about the Park" woods and observing its trees and plants, he reflected "with astonishment" on how the war of nature had determined "the presence & relative number of . . . the plants." When not looking at plants, he would spend "hours" looking at "many thousands" of ants, intent on observing the different kinds of work done by each, and believing that he had found "the rare slave making species."[46] At first, he believed that the division of labor among ants was a "grave difficulty" to the theory of natural selection, and then he came to realize that it was really an example of the "efficiency" of how the theory worked.[47] Writing up notes on his observations on the plants and ants of the Moor Park woods, which were intended to be added to *Natural Selection,* did not disturb his health.

There were also times when being in the woods enabled him to stop thinking about natural selection and experience a state of happiness and tranquility. On 28 April, he wrote Emma how, after enjoying an "excessively pretty view" of different colored trees, he "fell fast asleep on the grass & woke up with a chorus of birds singing around me, & squirrels running up the trees & some

Woodpeckers laughing, & it was as pleasant a rural scene as I ever saw, & I did not care one penny how any of the beasts or birds had been formed."[48]

On several occasions, he had verbal "battles" about natural selection with the novelist Georgiana Craik—who was a patient at Moor Park—without having an upset of health.[49] He went on corresponding with scientific friends, and enjoyed a visit from Fox, who brought him information on traits in different species of birds and whom he introduced to Dr. Lane.[50]

Two activities that gave him much pleasure and much relaxation from the fatigue of work were playing billiards, in which he was instructed by Dr. Lane, and reading novels. In separate letters to Emma and his eighteen-year-old son William, he urged each of them to read the just published novel, *Three Chances,* praising it as "a strange powerful novel written by one with plenty of 'gumption,'" and as "very clever, & part very amusing." He sometimes discussed the merits and demerits of a novel with Mrs. Lane.[51]

At first, when he was halfway through his sojourn at Moor Park, he wrote William that "it has not done me so much good hitherto as before, but yet has much rested me." In the last two days of the sojourn he began feeling "splendidly well," was able to make "some splendid strokes" at billiards, and one day walked four miles. "As usual," he told Hooker, "hydropathy has made a man of me for a short time."[52]

It was only for a short time. On 14 May, ten days after returning to Down and resuming work on *Natural Selection,* he informed William: "I have been working as usual too hard, & have almost quite lost the good which Moor Park did me." Four days later, as he went on writing his big book, he commented that he had "to discuss every branch of natural history, and the work is beyond my strength and tries me sorely."[53]

"Dreadfully Up-hill Work" on the *Origin of Species* and Treatments at Moor Park and Ilkley

On 18 June 1858, Darwin stopped writing his big book because Alfred Wallace sent him what he described as "an essay containing my exact theory [natural selection]."[1] He felt "forestalled"[2] and as if he had lost his priority of many years,[3] and he turned to Lyell and Hooker for advice. His two friends arranged that his and Wallace's evolutionary writings—Wallace's essay and excerpts from Darwin's 1844 essay and an 1857 letter to Asa Gray—be publicly read at a 1 July 1858 meeting of the London Linnean Society. This public reading, however, made practically no impact on those who heard it.[4]

At this time, Darwin was troubled not only about the priority of his ideas but about several other events, the most distressing of which were illnesses in his family. At the end of June, his daughter Etty became seriously ill with an attack of diphtheria, and one of her nurses contracted this illness.[5] As Etty and her nurse were recovering, his eighteen-month-old son, Charles Waring, fell ill with scarlet fever and died on 28 June.[6] Four days later, Darwin expressed the grief he felt for his son by writing a brief yet heartfelt memorial. Recollecting that, although Charles Waring was "backward in walking & talking," he was "intelligent & observant . . . of a remarkably sweet, placid & joyful disposition . . . [and] very affectionate."[7] However, one of Charles Waring's nurses had contracted scarlet fever, and it was now feared that a scarlet fever epidemic might break out in Down House and village. "Fear," wrote Darwin to Fox, "has almost driven away grief."[8]

On 2 July, at the urging of Fox and others, Darwin moved most of his family out of Down to the home of his sister-in-law Sarah Elizabeth Wedgwood in Hartfield, Sussex. He wrote Fox that he and Emma would stay at Down "till Etty can move & I of course stay till nurse is out of all danger."[9] On 5 July, with the nurse recovering and Etty becoming stronger, he felt relieved and "more happy." On 9 July, he, Etty, and Emma joined their family at Hartfield. Since the feared epidemic of scarlet fever had become a reality in Down village, the Darwins then spent the early summer at several country houses.[10]

On 21 July, Darwin wrote to Fox, "we are all very fairly well," while at the end of July, he told Hooker that "my stomach [has not yet] recovered all our troubles."[11] This probably refers to an increase in flatulence and was the only observation he recorded about his stomach during the troubles of June and July. Despite the personal and professional stresses of these months, with their feelings of grief, fear, and rivalry with Wallace, he had not suffered from a serious increase in physical illness. One reason for his relative stability of health was, as he expressed it, "the extraordinary . . . kindness" and support he had received from Lyell and Hooker.[12] Early in August, when the fever epidemic had subsided, he and his family returned to Down.

He was also interested and troubled by a much discussed June/July trial in London's Court for Divorce, in which a husband, Henry Robinson, petitioned for a divorce from his wife, on the grounds of her having had an erotic relationship with Dr. Lane when she had been a patient at Moor Park in 1854. She had described this relationship in a diary that her husband discovered and read several years later and that he now brought to the London Court.[13] Darwin followed the events of the trial as they were reported in the *Times,* which cited the sexual passages in Mrs. Robinson's diary and gave evidence for and against their credibility.

In a letter to Fox he wrote that the diary passages were probably an "invent[ed] story prompted by extreme sensuality or hallucination," that the evidences suggested Dr. Lane to be innocent, and that it was a "most cruel case" which he feared would "ruin" Dr. Lane.[14] Fox replied that he also believed Dr. Lane to be innocent (he had recently met Dr. Lane). Darwin wrote back, "I am profoundly sorry for Dʳ. L. & all his family to whom I am much attached."[15] On 3 July, the chief justice at the trial declared "no case had been established" against Dr. Lane.[16] Three weeks later, Darwin happily reported to Fox: "Dʳ. Lane has his house full, I am glad to say."[17] Along with the feelings of friendship and sympathy for Dr. Lane, he went on worrying about the latter's ability to maintain a medical practice.

At some time in the summer of 1858, he began to write what he called "an abstract" of his big book.[18] His usual slow rate of writing now quickened. Although still beset by doubts and fears, he was determined to publish his theory.[19] After a year of "hard" writing, he finished his "abstract," which, when published, would be *The Origin of Species.*

During this year, the mental pressures of writing up his theory often affected his stomach. In November 1858, he wrote Fox: "I am working slowly & steadily at my Abstract & making progress & hope to print in the Spring. My stomach has been bad enough, & I have lately spent a very pleasant week at Moor Park, & Hydropathy & idleness did me wonderful good & I walked one day 4½ miles,—a quite Herculean feat for me!"[20]

As his "abstract" neared completion, his stomach and head symptoms became more severe, and he spent most of February in Moor Park. From there, he reported to Fox:

> I have been extra bad of late, with the old severe vomiting rather often & much distressing swimming of the head; I have been here a week & shall stay another & it has already done me good. I am taking Pepsine, i.e. the chief element of the gastric juice & I think it does me good & at first was charmed with it. My abstract is the cause, I believe of the main part of the ills to which my flesh is heir to; but I have only two more chapters & to correct all, & then I shall be a comparatively free man.

He added: "We are a very pleasant party here and very comfortable & I am glad to say that not one of D^r. Lane's patients had given him up & he gets a few fresh ones pretty regularly."[21]

He probably took pepsine because it was held that his vomiting was caused by a failure of his stomach to secrete pepsine, the same reason for trying "mineral acids" two years earlier.[22] He recorded in his journal that the two weeks at Moor Park "did not do me so much good as usual."[23]

At Moor Park he continued to enjoy playing billiards, and early in 1859 he bought a billiard table for himself—selling a gold watch that belonged to his father and some beautiful and valuable Wedgwood ceramics in order to get the necessary money, and he installed the table in a room in Down House.[24] In March, he reported to Fox that playing billiards at home "does me a deal of good, & drives the horrid species out of my head."[25] For several years, billiard playing would be a welcome diversion from the pressures of his work; then he would largely lose interest in billiards.[26]

In the last stages of the writing of his "abstract," he described his health and the relation between health and work in letters to Hooker:

> 7 April 1859: My God how I long for my stomach's sake to wash my hands of it,—for at least one long spell.[27] ["It" was his abstract, which he had completed and was then correcting.]

12 April 1859: Do not, pray, think of giving up coming here; I sh^d. extremely regret it. With you I can go away the *moment* my stomach feels bad, & that is the important point for me.[28]

Five weeks later, when he had finished correcting his "abstract," he wrote Hooker: My health has quite failed." He described his symptoms as "bad vomiting . . . & great prostration of mind & body." On 21 May, he went to Moor Park, telling Hooker that his "object" in going was "to drive the subject [of the origin of species] out of my head." After six days at Moor park, he reported that "entire rest & the douche & Adam Bede [George Eliot's recently published novel *Adam Bede*] have together done me a world of good."[29]

His health did not remain "good" for long. At the end of May, he began correcting proofs of his book, sent to him by his publisher, John Murray, and he found that the corrections—entailing considerable revision and rewriting—were "terrifically heavy, & . . . most difficult *to me*."[30] On 2 July, he wrote Hooker: "I have been bad, having had two days of bad vomiting owing to the accursed Proofs—I shall have to go to Moor Park before long."[31] Along with nursing him when he vomited, Emma aided him in reading and correcting proof sheets.[32] As his vomiting continued to be "bad," he went to Moor Park from 19 July to 25 July.[33] On 28 July, he wrote to Hooker: "Take warning by me & do not work too hard. For God's sake, think of this.—It is dreadfully up-hill work with me getting my confounded volume finished."[34] On 1 September, he again wrote Hooker: "I had a terrible long fit of vomiting yesterday, which makes the world rather extra gloomy today. And I have an insanely strong wish to finish my accursed Book." He wondered whether, after finishing his book, he would 'ever be good for anything again."[35] He would later tell a friend that, during the year when he was working on the book, he "had seldom been able to write, without interruption from pain [the pain of flatulence], for more than twenty minutes at a time!"[36]

On 10 September, he finished correcting his last proofs—the book was now entitled *The Origin of Species*—and the next day he wrote to Hooker: "Oh good Heavens, the relief to my mind & body to banish the whole subject from my mind."[37]

In the month that followed completion of the book, he took various medicines.[38] He resolved to be "idle" during the winter while telling Fox that he feared "ennui will be as bad as a bad stomach."[39] He also made plans to take several weeks of hydropathy at Ilkley House, near Ilkley, in Yorkshire.[40] Fearing that he would not be able to rent a house in Ilkley for his family, and that he would be alone in a new place, he wrote to his Moor Park friend, Mary Butler:

> My object in troubling you . . . a trouble, which I hope & believe you will forgive—is to know whether there is any chance of your being at Ilkley in beginning of October. It would be rather terrible to go into the great place & not know a soul. But if you were there I should feel safe & home-like. You see that all your former kindness makes me confident of receiving more kindess.[41]

Miss Butler responded to this letter by joining him. On 5 October, two days after arriving at Ilkley, he wrote Fox: "I always hate everything new & perhaps it is only this that makes me at present detest the whole place [Ilkley House] & everything except one kind lady here, whom I knew at Moor Park."[42] Following this, he at first "much" benefited from hydropathy. Occupying himself by "loitering," reading the newspaper and a novel, and playing "the American Game of Billiards." On 17 October, after he had been able to rent a family house in Ilkley, he was joined by Emma & their younger children.[43] For a time, Miss Butler continued to stay at Ilkley, meeting with him & Emma, and then left. At the end of October, Emma told William Darwin, "Miss Butler your father's friend of Moor Park is gone which is a great loss to us as she is very pleasant & lively & kind."[44]

Throughout October, Darwin's long-held forebodings about becoming an object of reprobation increased as he waited for *Origin* to be published. Early in November, after receiving a first prepublication of the book, he instructed his publisher to send additional copies to friends and acquaintances, to all of whom he wrote personal letters.[45] In these letters he sometimes attempted to forestall criticism by expressing contrite fears of the heterodoxical nature of *Origin*'s ideas (without directly mentioning these ideas). To his old friend Hugh Falconer, he wrote: "Lord, how savage you will be, if you read it, and how you will long to crucify me alive!"[46] To the anatomist Richard Owen, he wrote: "I fear that it will be abominable in your eyes"; to Henslow: "I fear . . . you will not approve of your pupil"; to the Oxford geologist John Phillips: "I fear that you will be inclined to fulminate awful anathemas against it"; and to Jenyns: "I may of course be egregiously wrong."[47]

His main defense against the criticism of what he called "the mob of naturalists" was that he hoped he would be supported by Hooker, Lyell, and his new friend Thomas Huxley.[48] In the first three weeks of November, Hooker sent praise,[49] and Lyell raised objections.[50] Huxley remained silent. Waiting for Huxley's opinion made him "excessively anxious," and on 13 November, he told a correspondent: "If I can convert Huxley I shall be content."[51]

He had "a series of calamities."[52] Five days after arriving at Ilkley, on 9 October, he fell and sprained an ankle. This made him temporarily unable to walk and interfered with the hydropathy treatments.[53] After he recovered from the sprain, hydropathy was resumed, with his legs being rubbed with wet sheets so as to draw blood from stomach to skin. On 23 October, he reported to Hooker that because of an "eruption & inflammation" on the legs, he could not move, but that this had done his "stomach truly wonderful good."[54]

Five or ten days later, he told Hooker: "I have been very bad lately; having had an awful 'crisis' one leg swelled like elephantiasis—eyes almost closed up—covered with a rash & fiery Boils." He added that while Ilkley's doctors believed that this "crisis" was part of hydropathy treatments and would do him good, "it was like living in Hell."[55] On 16 November, he wrote Fox that Dr. Edmund Smith, the proprietor of Ilkley's hydropathic establishment, "constantly gives me impression, as if he cared very much for the Fee & very little for the patient." He told Fox that he felt "worse" than when he first arrived at Ilkley.[56]

The different symptoms of the "crisis" resulted from several different causes: The rubbing with wet sheets caused boils to erupt and become infected. The sprain may have caused infection of the veins. Infection caused swelling. (It is not known which leg was sprained and which became swollen.) The swollen eyes were caused by eczema, perhaps produced by Darwin's "excessive anxieties" over waiting for Huxley's reaction to his book. He may also have suffered from losing the consolations of Miss Butler.

By 25 November, Darwin had heard from his publisher that the first edition of *Origin* had sold out on publication day and that a second edition was needed.[57] He had read criticisms of *Origin* in the *Athenaeum* and in a letter from his old geology teacher, Adam Sedgwick.[58] He had continued to receive support from Hooker and (with reservations) from Lyell.[59] He had at last received a letter from Huxley, promising to fight for *Origin*'s ideas with "claws & beak."[60] Soon he humorously referred to Huxley as "my good & admirable agent for the promulgation of damnable heresies."[61] He was happy to anticipate that Huxley would help to shoulder the opprobrium of his being viewed as a "Devil's Chaplain."

The pro-*Origin* opinions of Lyell, Hooker, and Huxley, his "three judges," became for him a "success" that infinitely exceeded his previous wildest hopes for *Origin*.[62] He gratefully wrote Lyell: "I fully believe that I owe the comfort of the next few years of my life to your generous support & that of a very few others: I do not think I am brave enough to have stood being odious without support. Now I feel as bold as a Lion." He added, "But there is one thing I can see I must learn, viz. to think less of myself & My book."[63] A week later he told Huxley: "It will be God's blessing if I do not become the most conceited man in England."[64]

About this time the physical symptoms of the hydropathy "crisis" abated, he described himself as feeling "splendidly well," and he was able to return to hydropathy treatments, which he continued until 7 December when he returned home. From Down he wrote a friend: "Ilkley did me extraordinary good during the latter part of my stay & during my first week at home."[65]

10

Illness and "Anxious Looking Forward"

Weeks after returning to Down, as Darwin worked on a new edition of *Origin* and felt obligated to answer a "Multitude of Letters"[1] from old and new correspondents about the book, his flatulence accentuated. He complained to friends of being "not worth an old button," of "having gone back . . . to my bad way," and of having "incessant discomfort, I may say misery." The increase of illness caused him to change his positive opinions about Ilkley and tell Hooker that "Ilkley seems to have done me no essential good." Four days later he reverted to his previous opinion and wrote Fox that at Ilkley: "I was hardly able from lameness, Boils &c to give Water-cure a fair trial this time, but I think we shall go there again next early summer."[2]

In January 1860, he began consulting about his stomach with a new London physician, Frederick William Headland.[3] Dr. Headland probably diagnosed him as suffering from oxaluria, in which there was an abnormal formation of oxalic acid in the blood and excess of urea in the urine, and treated him with nitro-hydrochloric acid and a diet restricting sweets and wine.[4] In March, he first reported to Fox that this regimen "has done nothing for me as yet & I shall go to my grave, I suppose, grumbling & groaning with daily, almost hourly, discomfort." However, in May he wrote his old friend that his health had been "better of late," and he was "inclined to attribute" this improvement to Dr. Headland's regimen. He then makes no further mention of following a sugar-free diet.[5] This was a second recorded attempt at treating his illness by limiting sweets.

He also suffered briefly from a new symptom. On 2 March, he told the American botanist Asa Gray: "I have had a very short but sharpish touch of illness,—a slight touch of pleurisy, & am weak." The next day, he told Hooker: "I had an attack of fever (with a touch of pleurisy) which came on like a Lion, but went off as a lamb, but has shattered me a good bit."[6]

Early in April, he read an anonymously authored review of *Origin* in the *Edinburgh Review* that he recognized as being written by Richard Owen, and he described it to Lyell as "extremely malignant, clever & I fear ... very damaging." He confided to Lyell that it was "painful to be hated in the intense degree with which Owen hates me," but that after feeling "uncomfortable for one night" he "got quite over it."[7] When Hooker and Huxley (whom Owen had also attacked) told him it was his "duty" to publicly reply to Owen, he refused.[8] Fearing that the effort of making such a reply would upset his stomach, he told Hooker that "to answer and think more on the subject is too unpleasant."[9] He continued to share with his friends the pain Owen was causing him, while Hooker and Huxley shared with him the antipathies they felt for Owen.

He was pleasantly distracted from thoughts of Owen when from 25 April to 1 May he was visited at Down by Mary Butler.[10]

Early in June, he equivocated about whether he would attend the annual summer meetings of the British Association for the Advancement of Science at Oxford,[11] where there were to be confrontations between supporters and critics of *Origin,* including Hooker, Huxley, Owen, and the Anglican bishop of Oxford, Samuel Wilberforce. On 26 June, the day the Association meetings began, Darwin wrote to Hooker: "My stomach has utterly failed; & I cannot think of Oxford."[12] The utter failure of this stomach resulted not only from aversion to attending a public controversy over his book but also from anxiety over eight weeks of persistent fever in his daughter Etty.[13] From 28 June to 7 July, he went for hydropathy to Dr. Lane's new establishment, which had moved from Moor Park to Sudbrook Park, Richmond Surrey.[14]

From there, upon receiving a letter from Hooker reporting how he and Huxley had successfully defended *Origin* against attacks by Bishop Wilberforce, before a crowd of almost a thousand,[15] he wrote Hooker:

I have been very poorly with almost continuous bad headache for 48 hours, & I was low enough & thinking what a useless burthen I was to myself & all others, when your letter came & it has so cheered me. Your kindness & affection brought tears into my eyes. Talk of fame, honour, pleasure, wealth, all are dirt compared with affection; & this is a doctrine with which, I know from your letter, that you will agree from the bottom of your heart ... now that I hear that you & Huxley will fight publicly (which I am sure I never could do) I fully believe our cause will ... prevail. I am glad I was not in Oxford, for I sh^d. have been overwhelmed, with my stomach in its present state.[16]

The next day he worried about the animosities that would arise, and wrote Asa Gray: "My book has stirred up the mud with a vengeance; & it will be a blessing to me if all my friends do not get to hate me."[17]

After leaving Sudbrook Park, he ceased being a patient of Dr. Lane, although he had pleasant recollections of his sojourns at Moor Park and of Lane and his family. The reasons for the cessation are not known.[18] For a time he and Emma would maintain contacts with Miss Butler, who continued to be a patient at Sudbrook Park. (It is not known, however, if she was at Sudbrook Park when Darwin was there.)

Etty continued to be ill with fluctuating fever, vomiting, and weakness for many months. Her illness, along with the demands of scientific work, caused her father to have several kinds of distress. In the summer and early fall of 1860, as he accompanied her to different country houses of convalescence, he had "incessant anxiety."[19] In October, when Etty "suffered pitably," he "almost got to wish to see her die," and "had 9 days of as much misery as man can endure."[20] In December, after telling Hooker, "poor Etty . . . keeps in the same state . . . the Doctors do not despair, I almost do," he added: "I cannot sleep & my heart is almost always palpitating."[21] In January and February 1861, when Etty had "three terrible days of sickness" and then became "rather better," he told Hooker his health was "very bad," and he feared that he would have to go to Malvern for hydropathy.[22] In March, Etty "certainly" improved and then went on improving, and his complaints to Hooker about his health stopped.[23]

All during the period of Etty's illness and improvement, Darwin had been able to carry on (sometimes with delays and interruptions) different kinds of work: intermittently writing parts of the big sequel to *Origin*, *The Variation of Animals and Plants under Domestication*, preparing a third edition of *Origin*, keeping up a "gigantic" scientific correspondence, and doing botanical work on *Drosera* and other plants.[24] His work on *Drosera* was a fresh new interest that was called by Emma "a great blessing to him," because she observed how it distracted him from some of his anxieties.[25]

In March and April 1861, Hooker informed him that Professor Henslow, his old mentor and steadfast friend, was slowly dying from diseases of the heart and lungs. (Hooker was Henslow's son-in-law and was nursing Henslow.) In two letters to Hooker, Darwin delineated the conflict that he felt between feeling that he ought to visit Henslow, and fear that such a visit would egregiously upset his stomach. In March, he wrote that he "would not have missed coming for anything if Henslow had wished to see me," but that he was "not equal to such an exertion." He then reminded Hooker how when he had seen his son

George chloroformed for teeth extraction, it had "immediately . . . brought on my eternal sickness for 24 hours."[26]

In a 23 April letter to Hooker, he tensely stated several more reasons for his reluctance to visit Henslow:

> The journey with the agitation would cause me probably to arrive utterly prostrated. I sh^d. be certain to have severe vomiting afterwards, but that would not much signify, but I doubt whether I could stand the agitation at the time. I never felt my weakness a greater evil. I have just had specimen for I spoke a few minutes at Linn. Soc., on Thursday & though extra well, it brought on 24 hours vomiting. I suppose there is some Inn at which I could stay, for I sh^d. not like to be in the House (even if you could hold me) as my retching is apt to be extremely loud.
>
> I shd. never forgive myself, if I did not instantly come, if Henslow's wish to see me was more than a passing thought.[27]

Darwin did not come to Henslow's home in Hitcham, Suffolk, and he thus spared himself the discomfort and embarrassment of retching and being agitated when he was in the company of his best friend and dying mentor.[28] Several weeks later, when Henslow had died, Darwin wrote to Hooker: "I fully believe a better man never walked this earth."[29]

At some time in June, Emma, torn by her desire to comfort her husband as he confronted stresses and illnesses, and pained by his religious disbelief, wrote him a letter: "I mind your sufferings nearly as much as I should my own and I find the only relief to my own mind is to take it as from God's hand, & to try to believe that all suffering & illness is meant to help us exalt our minds & to look forward with hope to a future state." She begged him to pray to Heaven "for the sake of your daily happiness . . . I feel in my inmost heart your admirable qualities & feelings & all I would hope is that you might direct them upwards, as well as to one who values them above every thing in the world. . . . I shall keep this by me till I feel cheerful & comfortable again about you. . . . I thought I would write it partly to relieve my own mind." She, after writing such a letter, did feel some relief. He, after reading her letter, did not alter his disbelief. Yet, deeply touched by her concern for him, he preserved the letter and wrote on it: "God bless you. C.D. June 1861."[30] Emma's biographer has commented that there would always be a "painful void" of religious differences between Darwin and his wife, "but because it was bridged by a strong and growing love, it never divided them."[31]

In July and August, Darwin and his family visited the seaside town of Torquay, so that Etty could further recuperate from her illness.[32] Soon after returning to Down, he told a correspondent that his visit to Torquay "did my health at the time good; but I am one of those miserable creatures who are never comfortable for twenty-four hours; and it is clear to me that I ought to be exterminated."[33] It was while he was at Torquay that he became "profoundly" engrossed in investigating the various contrivances in orchids for ensuring their cross-pollination by insects.[34] He believed that delineating these contrivances provided evidence for the action of natural selection, and he told Hooker it was "far better" work than writing the *Variation of Animals and Plants* and that it gave him feelings of "delight" and "intense enjoyment," which then effected an improvement in his health.[35] As he went on to examine orchids, he continued to have feelings of pleasure, and his health remained improved. In 1862, he published a book, *On the Various Contrivances by Which British and Foreign Orchids Are Fertilised by Insects, and the Good Effects of Intercrossing*, which was praised by Hooker, Asa Gray, and other botanists.[36]

Early in the spring of 1862, he became "rather extra headachy" several days before going to London to give a paper on *Catasetum* forms of orchids to a meeting of the Linnean Society.[37] Following the meeting he reported to Hooker: "I vomited all night & could not get out of bed till late next evening, so that I just crawled home.—I fear I must give up trying to read any paper or speak. It is a horrid bore I can do nothing like other people."[38] At this time, he also suffered from having an "almost constant fear" about his son Horace, who since the winter had developed "strange" symptoms of "hysterical sobbing" and "semi-convulsive movements."[39] Late in the spring he had new fears about his son Leonard, who came down with scarlet fever.[40] (While Horace had become better, he remained "far from strong.")[41] Fears for his children may then have been a cause for his developing an acute attack of (what his doctors called) "eczema," which lasted about three weeks and which he described to Hooker as "extra bad . . . violent skin inflammation"; and for his "hands . . . burning as if dipped in hell-fire."[42] About this time he also had less severe and more persisting eczema of the face, so that following the suggestion of Emma, he resolved to grow a beard.[43]

In the summer, Leonard's fever developed dangerous complications. In a July letter to Asa Gray, Darwin first reported that because of being in "fearful distress" over Leonard's illness, he had temporarily been unable to do any scientific work, but that Leonard was now recovering and had been happy to look at a three-cent American stamp that Gray had sent him. Darwin then discussed his thoughts about having children and doing scientific work (Gray was married but had no children): "Children are one's gretest happiness, but often & often a still greter misery. A man of science ought to have none,—perhaps not a wife; for then there would be nothing in this wide world worth caring for & a man might (whether he would is another question) work away like a Trojan."[44]

In mid-August Darwin and his family started out for the seaside town of Bournemouth, where Leonard was to convalesce. But after Emma contracted scarlet fever "pretty sharply," they stayed for several weeks in the Southampton home of William Darwin. From there, after beginning a letter to Gray by writing, "We are a wretched family & ought to be exterminated," Darwin went on to write that although Emma was recovering he feared that Leonard "would be an invalid for months, if not years." He added that there was "no end of trouble in this weary world."[45]

Several days after moving into a Bournemouth house, Darwin felt "squashier than ever" and began taking "two shower baths a day" in the hope of gaining "a little strength."[46] This was the only reference to using hydropathy while at Bournemouth, and it may have been the first occasion he used it since being at Sudbrook Park in the summer of 1860. During several weeks at Bournemouth, he described himself to Hooker as having "headach half everyday," and an "intolerably bad stomach," and he wrote to Fox "all Darwins ought to be exterminated." In his letter to Fox, after writing of his hope to see his old friend at a meeting of the British Association that was planned to be held in Cambridge from 1 to 8 October 1862, he recollected their 1828 Cambridge breakfasts, teas, and "beetle-hunting expeditions." And he commented: "There were no fears & anxious looking forward in those days."[47] His feelings of "anxious looking forward" probably largely centered on fears of future illness in himself and his family.

Early in October, soon after returning to Down from Bournemouth, he had another "bad" attack of eczema (location unspecified) that kept him at home "for a week or two" and prevented his attending the Cambridge meeting of the British Association.[48] The causes for this may have been both allergenic and psychological: a change from allergens in the environment of Bournemouth to those at Down, and his being "shaken a good deal" by the "misery" he felt over the illnesses of his family.[49] Although the "bad" attack subsided, Emma reported that he continued to be "constantly plagued with slight attacks of exema," which made him feel "very uncomfortable."[50]

In the months of October through December, he then had three episodes of vomiting that followed conversations with visitors. The first occurred on 21

October when he was visited at Down for an evening dinner by three former officers of the *Beagle*. It was a reunion that was at first pleasant, but after he and his guests had gone to their rooms for the night Darwin became "very ill with violent shaking & vomiting till the early morning; & could not even wish them [the three officers] goodbye next morning." Two days later, Darwin wrote a letter to John Lubbock, his young scientific friend and supporter, recounting the vomiting and specifying the conditions he and Lubbock should follow so they could have a conversation that would not upset his stomach: "If you could any day come & dine & sleep here & let me go away for an hour after dinner & retire to my room at 9 o clock I do not think it would hurt me."[51] Lubbock agreed to these conditions. But a day before he was to come to Down, Darwin worried about their meeting and wrote to his son William: "Heaven knows how I shall stand it."[52] Following the meeting, Emma recorded in her diary on 31 October: "Ch. Attack of sickness in night but not so bad."

Darwin's confidence in his ability to avoid becoming ill from a conversation was now severely shaken. On 14 November, replying to a request from his friend Hugh Falconer that they meet when he was next in London, he wrote:

> I will beat up your quarters if I possibly can; but I do not know what has come over me: I am worse than ever in bearing any excitement. Even talking of an evening for less than two hours has twice recently brought on such violent vomiting and trembling, that I dread coming up to London.[53]

He again resolved (as he had often resolved in the past) that he would converse less with all visitors, including Hooker.[54] When a correspondent whose work on plants he admired suggested a meeting with him, he refused: "I suffer severely from ill-health of a very peculiar kind, which prevents me from all mental excitement, which is always followed by spasmodic sickness, & I do not think I could stand conversation with you, which to me would be so full of enjoyment."[55]

On 29 December, he conversed at Down with his nephew Henry Parker and was pleased to learn that Parker had published an article defending his theory against a critic.[56] Although the talk with Parker lasted only an hour and a half and was broken by his taking tea by himself, it was followed by his "shaking & vomiting half the night." He then humorously and grimly commented to Hooker: "What I shall soon have to do, will be to erect a tablet in Down church 'sacred to the memory &c' & officially die, & then publish books 'by the late Charles Darwin'; for I cannot think what has come over me of late; I always suffered from the excitement of talking, but now it has become ludicrous... it is fearful evil for self & family."[57]

Hooker (who had experienced his old friend's vomiting and retching after conversation as much as anyone) replied: "[I am] extremely concerned to hear [of your] failing powers of enduring [conve]rsation—that will however [soon] come right again as far as [ev]er you can be right: I do not doubt."[58] Hooker was prescient in his reply, for in the following months Darwin did not record any further episodes of violent vomiting after conversation and was able to have brief conversations with friends that did not result in vomiting.

Along with trying to limit vomiting by limiting conversation, Darwin attempted to diminish his ever present flatulence by taking Condy's Water, a solution of alkaline permanganates, "used for the purification of air and water, and sanitary objects in general," but not prescribed as a medicine by physicians. Darwin had read about Condy's in letters he received in June and September 1862 from George Chichester Oxendon, a poet and orchid fancier who had urged him to take Condy's as a "pleasant daily diet drink" that would produce many beneficial effects.[59]

In November 1862, Darwin then wrote to Hooker: "Did you ever hear of Condy's Ozonised Water? I have been trying it with, I think extraordinary advantage to comfort at least, a tea-spoon in water 3 to 4 times a day. If you meet any poor dyspeptic devil like me, suggest it."[60] This "extraordinary advantage" does not appear to have lasted, for there are no further references to Condy's Water in Darwin's correspondence.

About this time, Emma wrote Miss Butler informing her that Darwin was growing a beard because of his eczema and inviting her to again visit Down. Miss Butler replied, "I wish... I could go to you now and have the very great pleasure of being once more amongst you all," but that she was at present too engaged in holiday activities at Sudbrook Park. She closed by writing, "My best love to M^rs. Darwin. I don't like the idea of your long beard. ... Always Sincerely & affectionately yours, Mary Butler." This is the last known communication between Darwin and Miss Butler.[61]

At the end of 1862, in a letter to a scientific friend who lived in India, Hooker depicted Darwin as follows:

Darwin still works away at his experiments and his theory, and startles us by the surprising discoveries he now makes in Botany; his work on the fertilisation of orchids is quite unique—there is nothing in the whole range of Botanical Literature to compare with it, and this, with his other works, "Journal," "Coral Reefs," "Volcanic Islands," "Geology of Beagle," "Anatomy, etc., of Cirripedes," and "Origin," raise him without doubt to the position of the first Naturalist in Europe, indeed I question if he will not be regarded as great as any that ever lived; his powers of observation, memory and judgement seem prodigious, his industry indefatigable and his sagacity in planning experiments, fertility of resources and care in conducting them are unrivalled, and all this with health so detestable that his life is a curse to him and more than half his days and weeks are spent in inaction—in forced idleness of mind and body.[62]

Prolonged Vomiting and Treatments from Doctors Ayerst, Gully, Brinton, and Jenner

On 2 January 1863, after reading how his enemy Richard Owen had menda-
ciously criticized the work of his friend Hugh Falconer, Darwin had feelings of
"burning . . . indignation" that interfered with sleep, and produced an episode
of eczema which took "off the epidermis a dozen times clean off."[1] The eczema
subsided, and he had no further complaints of illness in January.

Emma's diary records that on 2 February he was "very languid" in the morning and on the next day languid and "sick after great faintness." A cause for
these symptoms was that he was scheduled to present a paper on dimorphic
flowers in *Linum* to a 5 February meeting of the London Linnean Society,
and he realistically feared (as he told Hooker) that following the presentation
"bad sickness may come on."[2] From 4 to 14 February, Emma recorded in her
diary, the Darwins stayed at the London home of Charles's brother Erasmus.
Early in the stay he continued to be ill and was unable to give the *Linum* paper,
so that the paper was read for him.[3] After this reading he became better, felt
"wonderfully improved" on returning to Down from London, and was able to
enjoyably converse and dine with Huxley, Fox, and John Lubbock, and to have
no stomach upsets.[4] On 21 February Emma wrote in her diary, "Ch. well all this
fortnight."

His wellness was then sharply broken by the onset of an illness that would
become prolonged and that first resulted from his disturbed feelings on reading Charles Lyell's book, *The Antiquity of Man*. For several years he had hoped
that Lyell, his old friend and scientific mentor, would overcome reservations
and fully support the theory of natural selection. On 4 February, on receiving
a prepublication copy of the *Antiquity,* he had written Lyell that he expected

the book would "give the whole subject of change of species an enormous advance."[5] On 24 February, having finished reading the *Antiquity,* he knew his expectation had been futile, and in a letter to Hooker he wrote: "I am deeply disappointed . . . to find that his [Lyell's] timidity prevents him giving any judgment. The whole discussion I look on as of no more value than a very good Review." He informed Hooker that Lyell and wife would soon be visiting Down: "I dread it, but I must say how much disappointed I am that he has not spoken out on Species, still less on Man."[6]

On 24 February, when Darwin had written Hooker about being "deeply disappointed" in Lyell, Emma wrote in her diary: "Ch. faint in night." Over the next eight days she recorded that he had persisting episodes of "faintness," was "languid & heavy" every morning, and "sick several times."

In a 5 March letter to Hooker, after reporting how he continued to be ill with vomiting and weakness, Darwin mentioned some of his pressing worries: Emma had suggested he might have to go to Malvern for hydropathy treatment, his son Horace was "ailing much," he had not done enough work on the *Variation of Animals and Plants* and doubted whether he would "ever finish" the book, and he feared that he had been "unreasonable" in his criticisms of Lyell to Hooker. He did not suggest (in this or any of his letters to Hooker) that anger at Lyell could have been a cause for his increased illness. "But," he told Hooker, "it is no use complaining. One must grin & bear; but a grumble to you, my dear old friend, does one good. A good severe fit of Eczema would do me good, & I have a touch this morning & consequently feel a little alive."[7] Eczema probably made him feel more energetic because of his strongly held belief that disease of the skin meant a relief of disease in his stomach and internal organs. Hooker replied: "I am atrociously idle & prefer writing to you to anyone else. . . . [P]ray God the Eczema has come out & relieved you."[8]

In a 6 March letter to Lyell, written after he had cancelled the Lyells' visit to Down because of his illness, Darwin wrote: "I have been greatly disappointed that you have not . . . spoken fairly out what you think about the derivation of Species." He added: "I had always thought that your judgment would have been an epoch in the subject. All that is over with me."[9] To this Lyell replied: "I have spoken out to the utmost extent of my tether, so far as my reason goes, and farther than my imagination and sentiment can follow."[10]

On 23 March Darwin told Fox it was now unlikely he would go to Malvern for hydropathy: "I am having an attack of Eczema on my face, which does me as much good as Gout does others; & which renders cold water to my face intolerable; so that I could not stand water-cure of any kind, as I found at Ilkley, when I had first attack of this horrid & blessed eczema."[11] Several days later he consulted James Startin, a London skin specialist who gave him a prescription that, when he applied it locally to his face, he found "*certainly* to me very soothing."[12] His attack of eczema appears to have abated by 5 April.[13] However, on 25 April, Emma wrote in her diary, "Ch skin very bad," and on 26 April she wrote "Ch very poorly."

From 27 April to 13 May, hoping that a fortnight of changes in locales would benefit him and Horace, Darwin and family stayed first for a week at Hartfield (home of the Reverend Charles Langton, married to his cousin Charlotte Wedgwood) and then for a week at Leith Hill Place (home of his sister Caroline Wedgwood). Emma wrote in her diary that at Hartfield, "Ch. poorly & languid all week,"[14] while at Leith Hill he was "better." At the end of the fortnight Darwin told an acquaintance: "Our trip has not done my youngest boy or myself much good in health, I am sorry to say."[15]

Two days after returning to Down from Leith Hill, he suffered greatly from six days of illness, which largely stopped work and confined him to bed and which he described to Hooker as "everlasting sickness & devilish headachs," and to Fox as "my old enemy sickness."[16] Since his eczema had abated, he began to think of seeing Dr. Gully at Malvern, when Fox wrote to him: "I hear D^r. Gully's brain has quite broken down and disabled him from work. He told me when I last saw him that it must do so soon."[17] He replied to Fox: "Gully will be a great loss & I hardly know whom to consult there. I must be under some experienced man, for I could not stand much hard treatment."[18] Following this he made no mention of going to Malvern for several months.

In June he declined to meet with his old Cambridge friend Whitley: "My health has been so bad . . . that . . . for the last two years I have led the life of a hermit, seeing no one & going nowhere; & doing nothing but two or three hours work daily on my good days at natural History. I am become that most wretched & despicable object, a confirmed valetudinarian. I have much, very much, to be thankful for in life; but everyone has his heavy drawbacks & my own health & even more that of my children is our sole drawback. For years we have had one or other of our children invalids."[19]

At this time Hooker wrote, mentioning that he hoped to "steal a Sunday for Down ere long, & see you with my own eyes."[20] In a belated letter of reply, Darwin first expressed feelings of depression: "My eczema is well & consequently till it comes on again, I am languid & bedeviled & [hate] writing & hate everybody. No, that is not true for in my worst state I do not hate you; but I have not had spirit to thank you for two pleasant notes." At the end of the letter he was feeling less depressed: "I shall enjoy extremely seeing you . . . but this gets rarer & rarer with me."[21]

In August Darwin began vomiting every morning, for which he was treated with carbonate of potash. It is not known who prescribed this treatment or how long he took it. When he observed that his vomit contained "vegetable cells," he wrote for information about these to John Goodsir, professor of anatomy at Edinburgh University.[22] On 21 August, Goodsir replied that he would examine his vomit for *Sarcina,* a microorganism that was found in healthy stomachs but that could aggravate existing stomach illness.[23] Darwin then sent Goodsir a vial and slide containing his vomit that Goodsir examined and found to be free of *Sarcina* and pathogenic organisms. Goodsir commented that the carbonate of potash "has no doubt acted beneficially."[24]

On the urging of Hooker he turned for medical advice to George Busk.[25] On 27 August Busk wrote him a letter stating that his stomach complaint was what doctors termed "Waterbrash," about which nothing "very certain is known," and recommended treatments consisting of "light bitters with subnitrate of bismuth & hydrocyanic acid," along with a cup of milk or water, with ten or fifteen grains of calcined Magnesia, and a biscuit taken early in the morning.[26] Such treatments were frequently used and easy to take, but Darwin may not have taken them because when he received Busk's letter he had overcome his past fears about not seeing Dr. Gully and made up his mind to move with Emma and his family to Malvern for hydropathy treatments.

On 4 September, the day after settling into a house in Malvern, Darwin informed Fox that he was placing himself under the care of Dr. Gully's associate Dr. James Ayerst, "though very sorry not to be under D^r. Gully;" and he queried Fox for information about the location of Annie's gravestone. Although Fox had written him years earlier about seeing the gravestone during a visit to Malvern, Darwin and Emma had never seen the stone. Fox promptly provided directions.[27]

On 29 September, Emma wrote Fox that the stone had been found, and this had been a "great relief." She went on to write that Darwin had first been "quite ill," but then had "decidedly improved" in the last five days, that under the supervision of Dr. Ayerst he was taking "2 or 3 wet rubbings in the day & small walks in the garden" of their house, and that he had been visited twice by Dr. Gully, who "quite approve[d] of his treatment."[28]

Darwin's recovery was then painfully jolted on reading a note from Hooker describing the death of his friend's six-year-old daughter, Maria Elizabeth: "My darling little . . . girl died here an hour ago, & I think of you more in my grief, than of any other friend. Some obstruction of the bowels carried her off after a few hours *alarming* illness."[29] In reply, Darwin first tersely compared the deaths of each of their daughters: "I am so deeply glad that she [Maria Elizabeth] did not suffer so much as I feared was inevitable. This was to us with poor Annie, the one great comfort. Trust to me that time will do wonders, & without causing forgetfulness of your darling." He then abruptly stopped his letter, explaining that although he was no longer vomiting, "I am very weak & can write little.—My nervous system has failed & I am kept going only by repeated doses of brandy. . . . My head swims badly so no more."[30]

Over the following ten days, as he went on thinking old and new disturbing thoughts about the deaths of Maria Elizabeth and Annie, he suffered from giddiness and increasing weakness in walking so that (in the words of Emma) "he could not walk a step but from one room to another."[31] He was then seen by Dr. Gully, who concluded that he was "not strong enough to bear" hydropathy, and on 14 October he and his family returned to Down.[32] Although for a time he continued to keep in contact with Dr. Gully and to treat himself with wet compresses (believing he was benefited by the rash the compresses produced), he came to believe that douches and the stronger forms of hydropathy were injurious to his health, and he did not return to Malvern or other hydropathy establishments.[33] However, the sojourn at Malvern had improved his sick son, Horace.[34]

Back at Down, his correspondence with Hooker stimulated him to continue to suffer from thoughts about Maria and Annie, along with the physical illness that had increased when he first had these thoughts. On 23 October Hooker wrote him: "I am very well, but it will be long before I get over this craving for my child, or the bitterness of that last night. To nurse grief I hold is a deadly sin, but I shall never cease to wish my child back in my arms as long as I live."[35] Darwin replied in a very short letter, which mainly read:

> My dear old friend.
> I must just have pleasure of saying this.
> Yours affecty. C. Darwin[36]

Because of weakness, he could only write a few words. Yet the words he did write, "My dear old friend," gave him pleasure because in writing them he was sharing with Hooker (in a way that he could share with no other person) feelings of love and grief. After an interval of several weeks he wrote Hooker that on rereading his friend's letter on the death of Maria he had "shed a few tears" over the memories of Annie, "but believe me . . . these tears have lost that unutterable bitterness of former days."[37] Several days later, at the end of a letter to Hooker, he summed up his thoughts on the relation between love and grief for children. "Farewell my good fellow: I shall be glad to hear sometime about your Boy, whom you love so.—Much love much trial, but what an utter desert is life without love."[38]

From October through December 1863, Darwin's weakness and vomiting, which prevented him from meeting with Hooker and other friends, were described in two letters from Emma to Hooker. Emma first wrote: "I cannot give a very good account of Charles. He has frequent attacks of sickness but recovers from them in a wonderful manner & they are often with very little distress. The stomach retains the food in a surprizing manner which accounts for his not getting thin."[39] This was the first recorded instance where Darwin appears to have digested his food before vomiting. About three weeks later, she wrote in more detail: "One day is a little better & one a little worse but I cannot say that he makes progress at present. He stays in his bed room & gets frequently in & out of bed & occasionally goes down stairs for a very short time. . . . When not very uncomfortable his spirits are wonderfully good, but I am afraid he may remain just as he is very long before there is a struggle in his constitution & that the sickness is conquered."[40]

During the above months, along with correspondence about his medical treatments with Dr. Gully in Malvern, Darwin discussed his illness with Dr. Stephen Engleheart, who since 1861 had been surgeon for Down village and with whom he formed a close medical and personal relationship.[41] At the end of October, he and Engleheart decided that he should consult with Dr. William Brinton in London.[42] Brinton had been recommended to him by George Busk as a specialist in diseases of the stomach and "a sensible & prudent man at any rate not likely to do you any harm."[43] Engleheart then went to London, discussed Darwin's illness with Brinton, and returned to Down with a prescription for treatment with mineral acid and instructions that Darwin would be seen by Brinton after he had taken the treatment for a time.[44]

On 3 November, Brinton visited Down and told Darwin his brain and heart were not "primarily affected," that doing a little scientific work was "not bad, and that he should continue taking mineral acids." This last being in contrast to Dr. Gully, who would write him that he should do no work for six months.[45] On 2 December, Brinton made a second visit to Down, and although Darwin's vomiting was unchecked, Brinton reassured him that he would recover his health. This was a reassurance that Darwin only partly believed, for he told Hooker: "I sh^d. like to live to do a little more work & often I feel sure I shall

& then again I feel that my tether is run out."[46] After 2 December he stopped consulting with Brinton.

For the next several months, although he continued to "be sick," he did not try to consult with a new doctor,[47] but he probably met on a number of occasions with Engleheart. He was daily cared for by Emma and his servant Parslow, only had "very short visits" with his sons,[48] and did not meet with any of his friends. On 24 January, Hooker wrote him: "I want very much to run down on forenoon & see you, but I dread putting you out, as any visitor must: it seems so very long since I have seen you."[49] "Nothing would please me more than to see you here," Darwin replied, "but as it would be very rash in me, as it surely w^d. bring on my vomiting, & I sh^d. suppose few human beings had vomited so often during the last 5 months."[50] In February, after Hooker had asked whether Darwin was actually vomiting or only retching, Darwin explained how vomiting occurred after a meal had been digested: "It rarely comes on till 2–3 hours after eating, so that I seldom throw up food, only acid & morbid secretion, otherwise I sh^d. have been dead, for during more than a month I vomited after every meal & sometimes most nights."[51]

Emma's diary shows that he treated the vomiting by using a compress and taking a succession of medicines, most of which he had taken in the past. Treatments did not check the vomiting for long, but sometimes they gave him short periods of relief.[52]

His longest and greatest relief from illness was in being with plants. He felt "amusement" and "delight" in acquiring new plants from Hooker, in looking at many of these in his bedroom or in a new hothouse that had been built in January, and then in carrying out experiments on plants that resulted in botanical discoveries.[53] "The only approach to work I can do," he wrote to Hooker, "is to look at tendrils & climbers, this does not distress my weakened Brain. My work on climbing plants is getting pretty perfect, & really some of the facts are very curious."[54] After mentioning some of his recent botanical discoveries to a botanist acquaintance, he commented, "Excuse all my boasting. It is the best medicine for my stomach."[55]

On the many occasions when illness prevented work on plants, he obtained relief by reclining on a sofa and listening to Emma and Etty read aloud to him. In February, he told Asa Gray that these readings consisted of a "lot of trashy novels," which he "found more amusing & less tiring" than hearing the newspapers read aloud.[56]

Some of the causes for his continuing illness were continued feelings of disappointment over Lyell's reservations on natural selection,[57] delays in writing the *Variation of Animals and Plants* (he had temporarily stopped this writing to do botanical experiments), and fears that his son Horace had inherited his illness from him and was "becoming a regular dyspeptic invalid."[58]

His recent grief over Annie and Hooker's daughter Maria now took the form of worries over the health of Hooker's young children. "I often get fidgety," he wrote Hooker in January, "& now I fancy that Charlie [Hooker's eight-year-old son] or some of your family [will become] ill. When you have time let me have a short note to say how you all are." He added: "I find it hard to be patient: now for five months I have done nothing but be sick."[59] On 9 March, Hooker wrote him: "I cannot tell which I crave for most, another little girl or for you to get well."[60] About this time Darwin decided to consult with Dr. William Jenner, who had been recommended for him by Dr. Gully, and Engleheart went to London to first meet with Jenner on his behalf. Emma then told her son William that it was "satisfactory to leave no stone unturned," and she wrote Jenner a note on how and when to come to Down.[61]

Jenner visited Down on 20 March and assured Darwin there was "no organic mischief" in his illness, and he would "some day" get over vomiting.[62] In the following five months, Jenner again visited Down on 10 April and 22 May. He placed Darwin on a regimen of treatments that, in contrast to the previous acid treatments of Dr. Brinton, were aimed at making his stomach contents more alkaline.[63] This regimen curtailed intake of fluids, prescribed combinations of several strongly alkaline antacids—chalk, lime water, carbonate of magnesia, and carbonate of ammonia.[64] He also prescribed medicines with different therapeutic uses that included colchicum, podophyllin, taraxacum, and bismuth.[65]

On 13 April, after being on Dr. Jenner's regimen for three weeks, Darwin wrote to Hooker: "Dr. Jenner has done me much good & is, I am sure, a most able doctor." He went on to report how the regimen had "wonderfully" checked his vomiting and increased his vigor and capacity to do botanical work: "I can now read a very little & am beginning a sort of work, (*not exciting!*) viz counting the seeds in capsules of Lythrum. I believe in a fortnight, if I do not go back, I shall dictate my paper on Lythrum!!!!"[66] Hooker replied: "I am so glad that Jenner has done you good. I shall certainly vote him for FRS this year."[67] On 25 April, Darwin wrote Hooker: "I keep going on very well, though weak; I amuse myself with little observations on odds & ends. Some cowslip have just flowered which give a pretty proof of difference of power of so-called homomorphic & heteromorphic pollen."[68] This was the first of Darwin's 1864 letters to Hooker that was not written in pencil or by an amanuensis, and one or two days after receiving it, Hooker began his letter of reply as follows: "It is indeed 'dew in the desert' to see a letter written by you in ink—& in a much improved hand, I am glad to observe, & pat you on the back accordingly!"[69] However, Emma then wrote that her husband had thought that Hooker had been "ironical about his hand writing but I am sure it was a bon fide comp^t." "I was not ironical about your hand-writing," Hooker replied. "I am awfully glad to hear you are so much better."[70]

On 15 May Darwin wrote to Hooker: "I have now been more than a month without sickness, but I do not at all rapidly grow strong, & have to go to bed 2 or 3 times per day.—But it makes a wonderful difference in my life, that I can now occupy myself a little with old pursuits & read a little."[71] On 25 May he finished a draft of his Lythrum paper and began a paper on climbing plants.[72] On 25 June he wrote Hooker: "I do hope you may spare time for a Sunday here. . . . I keep on improving & am now much as usual, except that anything which is hard to understand or which hurries me, knocks me up.—As soon as I have done about climbing plants I shall resume my routine work."[73]

At this time he may have been also "knocked up" by thoughts about Annie's death. On 24 June Emma recorded in her diary the death after a long illness of James Mackintosh Wedgwood, thirty-year-old son of Fanny and Hensleigh Wedgwood. On 28 June, in a brief note to Fanny, Darwin wrote: "The present time has called vividly to my mind, though it is never long forgotten, all that you did for us at Malvern with poor Annie, and the inexpressible stay and comfort you were then to me. I know how bitter your feelings must be; & I can only hope that you will pretty soon recover your bodily strength."[74] On 30 June, Emma wrote in her diary, "C. not very well," and on 4 July she wrote, "C. very unwell and faint &c." Following this she did not record, for over a month, any further illness in her diary. It seems likely that, since her diary had no record of Darwin being ill from 4 to 29 June, his illness of June 30 and July 4 resulted from his equating his feelings about Annie's death with the bitterness that Fanny was feeling over the death of her son.

On Sunday 24 July, Darwin met with Hooker at Down. In the meeting he queried his friend from written lists of questions he had prepared in advance, which were largely about the climbing plants he was working on. Hooker answered some of these at the time and took others home to answer in writing.[75] He reported to Asa Gray that he found Darwin "much better but very thin. He saw me for 10' each time almost a dozen times during the day."[76] After the meeting Darwin wrote Hooker: "Your visit did me no harm; on the contrary it did me good & I enjoyed it beyond measure.—It has done me good mentally &

has interested me in my work.—In fact you have cockered me up to that degree that I want to observe all I can."[77] In September he finished his essay on climbing plants and returned to work on the *Variation of Animals and Plants*.[78] He told Hooker that he was "very weak" and that, while the work was progressing, it was "a good deal harder than writing about my dear climbing plants."[79]

On 16 September, Hooker wrote him that 18 September would mark a year since the death of his daughter Maria: "On principle I think we should not keep anniversarys of great sorrows, but as the day draws nearer I feel all the misery of last year crawling over me & my lost child's face & voice accompany me everywhere by day & by night: So that I now dread an attack of what were more the horrors of delirium tremens than the chastened sorrows of a sensible man. I am sure however that there is no fear of that now; time, as you told me it would, has done its inevitable work." Hooker added: "It is too bad of me to write on such selfish subjects to you . . . but your affection for your children has been a great example to me, & there is no other living soul with whom I can talk of the subject—it would make my wife ill if I went on so to her." At this time Hooker was preparing to attend the annual meeting of the British Association at Bath, and in his letter to Darwin he commented that he had read Lyell's presidential address to the Association and that "on the whole it appears to me a feeble affair, & I seem to see in it (with great sorrow) that Lyell is getting old."[80]

On 19 September, he reported that after Lyell had given this address to the Association he and Mrs. Lyell had become "fairly intoxicated with their popularity & success & can talk of nothing else."[81]

Darwin reacted to Hooker's letters in two stages. First, as recorded in Emma's diary, on 17 September (when he may have received Hooker's 16 September letter) he was "rather bad," and on 18 September he felt "rather poorly," after which there was an interval when Emma did not comment on his health. Darwin's second reaction was to write a 23 September letter to Hooker in which he succinctly expressed support and concern for his friend's grief over Maria, while at the same time holding back from emotionally involving himself with this grief: "I thank you sincerely for your previous letter, your openness towards me gratifies me deeply, & you must know that you have my entire sympathy. I never remember dates for good or evil, & I do believe I have thus escaped many a bitter day. . . . How many anxieties & sorrows there are, great & small as life advances, & nothing to be done but bear them as well as one can, & that I cannot do at all well." He then agreed with Hooker's criticisms of Lyell's British Association presidential address and wrote that he "regretted" some of the geological view Lyell had stated in it.[82] He (doubtless) did not express all of his negative feelings toward Lyell. Several weeks later, Emma wrote in her diary for 12 October: "C. attack of sickness at night," an "attack" that was probably caused by Darwin's troubled anticipations of meeting with Lyell and Lady Lyell at Down on 15 October for a three-day visit.

During the visit the Lyells were "extremely pleasant," but Darwin only saw them "occasionally" for periods of ten minutes. The day after they had left Down, he experienced what he reported to Hooker as "an awful day of vomiting" and what Emma described in her diary as "hysterical crying"—a period of crying that was unusually long. Although Darwin told Hooker he expected to "soon be confined to a living grave & a fearful evil it is," he soon regained the level of improved health he had attained under Dr. Jenner's treatments.[83] Ten days after his "awful day," he wrote Asa Gray that he was having a "uniform life," "plodding on" with writing the *Variation,* doing only a little reading, and living on "endless foolish novels which are read aloud to me by my dear womenkind."[84]

At this time he and Jenner corresponded about the effects of the medicines he was taking.[85] He may have asked Jenner's opinion on continuing to take phosphate of iron pills and on again taking chalk, which Jenner had first prescribed but later curtailed.[86] In a reply written on 15 October, Jenner evaluated phosphate of iron as "a very useful medicine—one I often prescribe—but I am inclined to the opinion that it is the iron which does the good & that the phosphate of iron is a form in which it can some be better or more easily taken into the system. . . . The iron if it agrees will certainly improve the vigour & give you strength." Jenner explained that the objection to taking chalk was its tendency to produce urinary stones by making the urine alkaline. He concluded his letter by advising Darwin to continue the phosphate of iron, take the carbonate of magnesia and carbonate of ammonia, "occasionally add the chalk," and take spirit of horseradish.[87]

Following this letter, Darwin wrote Jenner for information on the composition of a medicine called "Syrup of Phosphates" (the beneficial effects of which had been mentioned by Lady Lyell during her October visit to Down), reported that his urine appeared "turbid," and asked about drinking more water. In a reply written on 9 November, Jenner identified the medicine as "Syrup of Phosphate of Iron" and then gave Darwin the following instructions: "*Not* . . . to drink more water," to continue phosphate of iron pills, treat the turbid urine by taking ten drops of dilute phosphoric acid in water after taking each phosphate of iron pill, and if the urine appeared alkaline to omit the medicines containing potash. Jenner also asked Darwin to send a bottle of his urine for analysis.[88]

Twelve days later, Jenner wrote that the urine had been analyzed, that Darwin should omit all alkaline medicines (presumably because the urine was alkaline), continue on phosphate of iron and phosphoric acid, and in a fortnight send Jenner a report on his condition and another urine sample.[89] On 23 November, Emma wrote in her diary: "C. left off alkali."

In a letter dated 24 November, Jenner again changed opinions on medicines and wrote: "You may take carbonate of ammonia with Horseradish. But had better not take any other alkali till I have again had the urine analyzed." After advising Darwin to stop phosphate of iron and phosphoric acid, he added: "Remain without medicine till we see how you are able to digest—sleep—&c unaided by drugs. . . . Do not resume the evil habit of drinking great quantity of fluid. Keep all rules but leave off medicine."[90] Soon Jenner wrote again, reporting that the urine analysis showed the urine to be "quite natural," its turbidity being "due merely to urates" rather than alkalinity. He therefore advised Darwin to take a "small dose of chalk-potash & ammonia" when "troubled with acidity of stomach," but with this exception to continue to abstain from "all medicines for a short time . . . till you see how you are progressing."[91] Darwin may have remained off all medicine from 23 November to the end of 1864, because Emma's diary records no medicines for this period.

For much of November, Darwin's health was disturbed by events in his scientific life. On 4 November he learned that he had been awarded the Royal Society's Copley Medal, the highest medal the Society could bestow. At first he was excited over the "very great honor" in having the Copley and deeply appreciative of the support he had received in obtaining it from a small group of Royal Society friends, which included Falconer, Busk, Lubbock, and Huxley.[92] However, when on 7 November Falconer wrote him that it would be a "great service" as well as a "comfort and solace" to his friends if he could attend the anniversary meeting of the Royal Society on 30 November and receive the Copley Medal in person, he refused.[93] He explained to Falconer that attending the public meeting "would possibly make me seriously ill" and that one of his friends would receive the Copley for him.[94] "All right," Falconer replied on 10 November, "no one would think for a moment of emperilling your precious health. Any of your friends will be proud to receive the medal for you."[95]

The mental stresses of getting the Copley, and afterwards rejecting the requests of the friends who helped him get it, caused Darwin to experience what he called "extra bad times" from 10 to 15 November.[96] In her 1864 diary, Emma described his health as "poorly," 10 and 11 November; "unwell in bed most of the day," 12 November; "unwell/better in evg-," 13 November; "better at work a little," 14 November; and "at work/very rocking in afternoon," on 15 November. "Rocking" was a symptom that Darwin would then sometimes complain about.

At the 30 November Royal Society meeting, the Copley was accepted for him by George Busk, who wrote him that those at the meeting "deeply" regretted "that you were unable to attend yourself . . . and more especially for the cause that prevented you," and that he "would have been much gratified by the unusually warm & cordial manner in which the announcement of the award . . . was received by the Society."[97] However, Busk did not mention that the eulogium given his work by the Society president, Edward Sabine, omitted any reference to *Origin*. In a letter of reply to Busk, after thanking him for his support, Darwin wrote: "You will remember that you were so kind as to advise me a year & a half ago about my incessant sickness. I have gotten over this, but still keep very weak & fear I shall ever remain so." He added in a postscript: "I do not know whether it is improper, but I have written to Sabine . . . that I sh^d. of course have liked a little more said about the 'Origin.' . . . I then added a few sentences sticking up for the truth of the general principles of the 'Origin.'"[98]

A day before the Royal Society meeting he received a letter from Fox: "I wish I could hear that you were in better health, but I suppose your destiny is to let your Brain destroy your Body."[99] To this he replied: "I fear I have reached my sticking point—I am very weak & continually knocked up, but able most days, to do from 2 to 3 hours of work, & all my Doctors tell me this is good for me; & whether or no, it is the only thing which makes life endurable to me.—I am slowly crawling on in my vol. on 'Variation under Domestication' occasionally recreating myself with a little Botanical work."[100]

For the rest of 1864, along with times when he was "knocked up," he remained at this "sticking point."[101]

Prolonged Vomiting and Treatments from Doctors Jenner, Chapman, and Bence Jones

"You ask how I am," Darwin wrote Hooker on 7 January 1865. "I have now had five pretty good days, but before that I spent fully a third of my time in bed, but had no actual vomiting." He went on to express frustrations over Jenner's frequent changes of medications and with treatments by other doctors. "D^r. Jenner is exhausted as to doing me any good. All Doctors seem to think that I am a case of suppressed gout: do you know of any good men hereafter to consult? I did think of trying Bence Jones; but I know it is folly & nonsense to try anyone."[1] While Henry Holland and perhaps Brinton and Jenner had diagnosed Darwin as having "suppressed gout," this was a diagnosis that was sometimes questioned by those with medical knowledge, as is shown by Hooker's letter of reply: "What the devil is this 'suppressed Gout'? upon which Doctors fasten every ill they cannot name. If it is *suppressed* how do they know it is gout? if it is apparent, why the Devil do they call it suppressed? I hate the use of cant terms to cloak ignorance."[2]

Two weeks later, in a 22 January letter to Lyell, Darwin wrote that, although reading "makes my head whiz more than any thing else," he was able on most days to work two to three hours on the *Variation,* and "this makes all the difference in my happiness."[3]

On 2 February he reported to Hooker that he had heard of the death of their mutual friend Hugh Falconer and had experienced an "extra bad time" of illness.[4] A day later he received a letter from Hooker describing in detail how Falconer had been "fixed with pain, could not move a muscle," and "suffered terribly" before dying.[5] After reading this account he had an episode of illness that he described in a 9 February letter to Hooker as "5 or 6 wretched days, miserable from morning to night & unable to do anything." In the same letter he told Hooker that he was "quite haunted" by thoughts of Falconer's "horrid" sufferings. Transferring these thoughts onto a future of death becoming dominant over life he went on to write: "but everyone has his own pet horror, & ... even personal annihilation sinks in my mind into insignificance compared with the idea, or rather I presume certainty, of the sun some day cooling & we all freezing. ... Sic transit gloria mundi [*Thus passes away the story of the world*], with a vengeance."[6]

In the next two months he did not vomit and was able to work at writing the *Variation*. But this writing appears to have been slow and frustrating. He may also have been frustrated because he still had not been able to decide whether he should write about human evolution and the role of sexual selection as being "the most powerful means of changing the races of man."[7] He summarized his depressed feelings about himself and his work in a 6 April letter to Hooker: "I work a little every day with groans & sighs & am as dull as a pig.—It is hopeless & useless but, *when you meet* Busk, ask him whether any man is better than Jenner for giving life to a worn-out poor devil."[8] Although Hooker contacted Busk, and Busk wrote Darwin recommending Dr. A. B. Garrod, Darwin did not consult Garrod.[9]

He then vomited almost every day from 21 April through 1 May.[10] On 3 May he was visited at Down by Jenner, and the next day he wrote Hooker of the remission of vomiting and a change in attitude toward Jenner: "You will be glad to hear, I know my dear old friend, that my ten or 12 days of sickness has suddenly ceased, & has left me not much the worse: I feared it was the beginning of another six or nine months miserable attack & feared it much: Jenner has been here, & is evidently perplexed at my case; he struck me as a more able & sensible man, than he did before, for then I could not talk with him: I shall consult no one else."[11] After this letter he apparently had no further consultations with Jenner. (The reasons for the cessation of contacts are not known.)

In the same letter of 4 May, he reported his ambivalent feelings, after hearing from Hooker that his ex-*Beagle* captain, Robert FitzRoy, had committed suicide. "I never knew in my life so mixed a character. Always much to love & I once loved him sincerely; but so bad a temper & so given to take offence, that I quite gradually lost my love & wished only to keep out of contact with him."[12] One result of his keeping out of contact with FitzRoy was that the news of the latter's death did not immediately interrupt the cessation of vomiting. However, on 9 May he read a letter from his *Beagle* friend Sulivan that graphically recounted the "trying scene" of FitzRoy's funeral and how FitzRoy's widow and two daughters appeared to be "dreadfully ill" and distraught from grief.[13] This reading may have disturbed his health, so that from 10 to 14 May, Emma recorded in her diary: "C. very unwell all day," "C. poorly," "C. tol," and "C. tol in mg. sick at 5. took blue pill." From this time on, Darwin's daily episodes of vomiting returned and showed no signs of abating.

He then recalled that, several months earlier, Dr. John Chapman—a physician who was unknown to him—had sent him a book that he described as being "on the cure of Sea Sickness," which at first he had not acknowledged receiving or read.[14]

Dr. Chapman was a man of variform parts: editor and publisher of the prestigious literary periodical *Westminster Review,* friend of George Eliot and other literary notables, author of insightful articles on medical education and medical reform, and a practicing physician who had developed a new treatment for several diseases (including epilepsy, neuralgia, paralysis, cholera, menstrual disorders, and dyspepsia and seasickness) which consisted in the application of ice, placed in a specially designed bag, on the spine.[15] This treatment was based on the idea that since most diseases were of nervous origin they could be influenced by application of heat and cold to the spine. In his book, Dr. Chapman had written: "Ice is a direct sedative to the spinal cord, if applied immediately over it: by lessening the amount of blood on it, ice lessens its functional and especially its automatic or excitomotor power. The therapeutic applications of this fact are numerous and immensely important."[16] The book contained the case histories of those who described how their seasickness had been greatly alleviated by the ice treatment.

Darwin now read Dr. Chapman's book, decided to try the ice treatment, and on 16 May asked Dr. Chapman to come to Down, explaining: "My sickness is not from mere irritability of stomach but is always caused by acid & morbid secretions. I am anxious not to try any new treatment unless you have had experience in some similar cases leading you to think it advisable."[17] It was then arranged that Dr. Chapman would visit Down on 20 May. On the day of the visit, Darwin and Emma wrote out on the front and back of a sheet of paper the following account of the symptoms of his illness, which was evidently intended for use in consultation with Dr. Chapman.

Age 56–57.—For 25 years extreme spasmodic daily & nightly flatulence: occasional vomiting; on two occasions prolonged during months. Extreme secretion of saliva with flatulence. Vomiting preceded by shivering, hysterical crying, dying sensations or half-faint. & copious very palid urine. Now vomiting & every paroxys[m] of flatulence preceding by singing of ears, rocking, treading on air & vision. focus & black dots— All fatigues, specially reading, brings on these Head symptoms ?? nervousness when E. [Emma] leaves me.[18]

(What I vomit intensely acid, slimy (sometimes bitter) corrodes teeth.)[19]

Doctors puzzled, say suppressed gout. Family gouty.—No organic mischief, Jenner & Brinton.[20]

Tongue crimson in morning ulcerated—stomach constricted dragging. Feet coldish.—Pulse 58 to 62—or slower & like thread. Appetite good—not thin. Evacuation regular & good. Urine scanty (because do not drink) often much pinkish sediment when cold—seldom headach or nausea.—

Cannot walk above 1/2 mile—always tired—conversation or excitement tires me most.—

Heavy sleep—bad day.

Eczema—(now constant)[21] lumbago—fundament—rash.—

Always been temperate—now wine comforts me much—could not take any formerly. Physic no good—Chalk & Magnesia.—Water-cure & Douche—Last time at Malvern could not stand it.[22]

I fancy that when much sickness my stomach is cold—at least water is very little warmed.

I feel nearly sure that the air is generated somewhere lower down than the stomach & as soon as it regurgitates into the stomach the discomfort comes on—

Does not throw up the food.[23]

At the end of these notes on illness, Darwin queried Dr. Chapman about the ice treatment: "Instruction—How soon any effect? How long continue treatment?"[24]

Dr. Chapman came to Down on 20 May, and after learning about his new patient's symptoms, he started Darwin on a daily regimen of a bag of ice applied to the spine three times a day, for ninety minutes each time. At first, for two days, Darwin was free of flatulence and vomiting, but in the following days these symptoms recurred. Although Dr. Chapman again visited Down on 28 May, there is no record in Emma's diary of what he prescribed during this visit. Four days later, Darwin wrote Hooker that he was trying the ice "at first with strong hope, now with weak hope."[25] On 7 June he reported as follows to Dr.

Chapman: "It is certain that the ice does not stop either flatulence or sickness." He thought the ice caused his pulse to accelerate; "liked" the ice for an hour, then he became "weary of it."[26] By July he had stopped the ice treatment, commenting that "the ice to spine did nothing,"[27] and he stopped contact with Dr. Chapman as well.

Emma wrote: "We liked Dr. Chapman so very much we were quite sorry the ice failed for his sake as well as ours."[28] Dr. Chapman may have been especially disappointed that his ice treatment failed to alleviate distress in a man whose work he esteemed.[29]

In May, although Darwin told Hooker that he had "done nothing" because of sickness, he had written a forty-one-page essay enunciating a theory of heredity that he called "Hypothesis of Pangenesis."[30] On 27 May he wrote Huxley a letter about the essay explaining that, while it was "a very rash and crude hypothesis," he hoped to publish it in his forthcoming *Variation* book, and he asked if Huxley would read it and "give your opinion on whether I may venture to publish it." At the end of the letter, he commented: "I must say for myself that I am a hero to expose my hypothesis to the fiery ordeal of your criticism."[31] Emma's diary shows that on the day he wrote the letter, he had "bad sickness in night." After reading the essay, Huxley wrote Darwin that Pangenesis resembled the ideas of the naturalists Buffon and Bonnet and was too speculative, and he inferred it should not be published.[32]

Darwin replied to Huxley on 12 July, writing that he would read Buffon, and possibly Bonnet, and be cautious and "try to persuade myself not to publish."[33] Emma's diary shows that following his writing (he usually wrote letters in the afternoon) he became "sick" in the evening. After reading Buffon he wrote Huxley that his theory differed from Buffon's views and that he would include Pangenesis in his *Variation* book, "if I ever have strength to publish" it. Huxley then cautioned him that if he published Pangenesis, he should emphasize that it was a hypothesis.[34] Darwin does not appear to have mentioned Pangenesis or his correspondence with Huxley to Hooker or any other friends.

Following the failure of the ice treatments, Darwin's illness ran a fluctuating course marked by daily remissions and exacerbations of rocking, vomiting, and other symptoms, which Emma chronicled in her diary. Some of her entries were 9 July, "v.g. day. bad sickness 12:30 p.m."; 12 July, "v.g. day, sick 10:30"; 20 July, "much better out many times"; 21 July, "uncomf-rocking." On 4 August, Darwin was very good and walking "twice round sandwalk." The next day he went around the sandwalk, but then had attacks of vomiting at 1:15 and 2:30 p.m., and then "3 more times." On 7 August he had a "tolerable morning," followed by "bad shocks & rocking 4 times sick." On 31 August he had "several struggles/much rocking."[35]

In a letter to Hooker, Emma expressed an optimism about the fluctuations of her husband's vomiting: "I do hope Charles is making a little progress in spite of frequent returns of the sickness but there is a degree of vigour about him on the well days which makes me hope that his constitution is making a struggle. If he conquers this sickness I do hope you will be able to come & see him before long & I am sure there is nobody in the world he cares so much to see."[36]

Although Darwin never suggested a cause for his months of illness, two apparent causes were the persistence of frustrations in writing about human evolution and in completing the *Variation* (work on the *Variation* was now complicated by Huxley's reservations over Pangenesis). There were also several other possible causes. In June, Darwin was disturbed by a plagiarism dispute between his friends Lyell and John Lubbock. After telling Hooker that the dispute was "horrid," he went on to express lugubrious forebodings about the future of their friendship: "It will be our turn some day—perhaps we too shall tear each other's eyes out some day."[37] While his forebodings were unfounded, they may have added to his depressed view of life, causing him to tell Hooker in July that he "was disgusted with everything in the world."[38]

His depressed feelings may also have been accentuated by several deaths. On 20 June, Sir John William Lubbock died. While Darwin has left no record of his reaction to this death, he may have felt the loss of an acquaintance who had helped him create his sandwalk in 1846 and with whom he had worked in the 1850s to improve the schools in the village of Down.[39] Darwin's feelings of loss may have been enhanced by the closeness of his friendship for Lubbock's son John, who (according to the latter's biographer) "deeply felt" the death of his father.[40] On 6 July, William Hooker, father of Joseph Hooker, died. Darwin wrote Hooker a letter recalling the "insufferable grief" he had experienced when his daughter died.[41] In another letter to Hooker he reported that he had written to the FitzRoy testimonial fund, which was raising money for FitzRoy's family, and he sadly commented on the "melancholy career" FitzRoy had run "with all his splendid qualities."[42] His account book shows that he made a contribution of £100 to the testimonial fund.[43]

At some unknown time in 1865, Mary Butler died. Although there is no record of Darwin's feelings about her death, he may have suffered feelings of loss over remembering a woman who had been a solace and emotional support for him when he had been ill and separated from Emma and who had then become a welcome visitor to his home.

In her diary for July 1865, Emma noted a succession of medicines (without information on dosage or duration of use), which were probably intended for her husband:

8 July	began bismuth
12 July	began quinine
13 July	took blue pill
14 July	began chalk

On 24 July Emma noted "began diet," which was then "left off" after five days. The failure of these changes in medicines and foods to alleviate Darwin's prolonged vomiting may have been an immediate stimulus for him to consult with Dr. Henry Bence Jones, whom he had once thought it "folly & nonsense" to consult.

Like Jenner and Chapman, Bence Jones was a prominent London physician with a large and ruminative practice. He was also a chemist and physiologist who had made discoveries in physiology and pathology (he had first described the protein in the urine since known as the Bence Jones protein), and he was a friend of several noted scientific men (he would write a two-volume biography of Michael Faraday).[44]

Darwin's account books show that he consulted Bence Jones in July and August. On 15 August he summarized Bence Jones's treatments as "A starving system of cure; eating very little of anything, & that almost exclusively bread & meat."[45] Over the next six weeks, as he continued to follow this treatment and restrict his daily intake of food, the number of entries in Emma's diary on his illness slowly decreased. During this period, according to his account book, he made reports to Bence Jones on 30 August and 12 and 26 September. On 28 September he wrote Hooker: "Did I ever tell you that I have put myself under Bence Jones, & I am sure he has done me good by rigorous diet. I have been half starved to death & am 15 lb lighter, but I have gained in walking power & my vomiting is immensely reduced. I have my hopes of again some day resuming scientific work, which is my sole enjoyment in life."[46] In October he told Huxley he was continuing to "slowly" get better.[47] On 1 November Bence Jones visited him at Down.[48] Later in November, he went to London where he first felt "wonderfully well" and had long talks with Lyell and Huxley, but then caught cold, which, as he told Hooker, "threw me back a whole month." However, on 25 December, he returned to work on the manuscript of *Variation*.[49]

On 3 January 1866 he wrote Dr. Bence Jones a letter,[50] in which he first summarized the positive and negative aspects of his health. "I have a good report to make. I am now able to walk daily on an average of 3 ½ miles & often one mile at a stretch. I feel altogether more vigorous & active. I read more, & what is delightful, I am able to write easy work for about 1 ½ hours every day. The only drawback is that on most days 3 hours after luncheon or dinner, I have a sharpish headache on one side, & with bad flatulence lasting to the next meal."[51] In the rest of the letter he discussed various changes in his treatments and diets.

> One day when my head & stomach were extra bad, in despair I took a cup of coffee without sugar, & it acted really like a charm & has continued to do so; for I now take a cup of coffee each day with luncheon or dinner, & I believe I have never once had headache and flatulence after the meal with coffee. I have transposed luncheon & dinner & made other changes, but so far as I can discover it is the coffee which is effectual. Under these circumstances, may I try coffee with both luncheon & dinner?[52] I have not yet much taste for common meat, but eat a little game or fowl twice a day & eggs, omelet or macaroni or cheese at the other meals & these I think suit me best. I have not taken to [two words illegible] much starch for I have such horror about acid.[53]
>
> There is an odd change in my stomach, for the last 20 years coffee & cheese have disagreed with me, now they suit me eminently well. I took 10g oxyde of Iron for a fortnight but did not miss it when I left it off 10 days ago: I will do as you like about retaking it.[54] I have taken 10 drops of Muriatic acid twice a day (with Cayenne & ginger) for above 3 weeks & it suits me *excellently*. May I continue it longer?[55] I hope you will be pleased with my report. I shall be grateful for any further advice.

The reply to the above has been lost. On 10 February Bence Jones sent Darwin a letter, directing that he continue to take Muriatic acid, along with "a dose of the Potass-ammonia when the flatulence is worst," and enclosing a "model diet."[56] Bence Jones also suggested that his patient "get a rough pony & be shaken once daily to make the chemistry go on better." Darwin would then find that daily horseback rides suited him "admirably."[57] As his health improved, he was able to resume social contacts with friends and acquaintances. In April 1866 he attended a London soirée of the Royal Society where he was presented to the Prince of Wales and saw the leading scientific men in London. Because of his years of withdrawal and his beard, almost none of his old friends recognized him. "His Dr. Bence Jones was there," Emma reported, "and received him with triumph, as well he might, it being his own doing."[58]

When his sisters Catherine and Susan died—in January and October 1866, he expressed feelings of grief to Hooker.[59] But he did not become severely ill or depressed, and he was able to continue regular work activities.

Between 1866 and 1872, he wrote three sequels to *Origin: The Variation of Animals and Plants under Domestication, The Descent of Man and Selection in Relation to Sex,* and *The Expression of the Emotions in Man and Animals,* along with fourth, fifth, and sixth editions of *Origin.* During these years he had brief episodes of illness that did not long interrupt his writing and that he treated either by himself or by consultations with Dr. Bence Jones.

Although Dr. Bence Jones became severely ill in the winter of 1866–67, he partly recovered and was able to offer advice on several of Darwin's symptoms up to 1870.[60] In October 1867, in reply to Emma's queries about her husband's "temporary failure of memory" and his "coming in and out of eczema," Bence Jones wrote that the first symptom was probably "only caused by some irregularities of circulation arising from indigestion" and was not of any concern and that the eczema resulted from the increased mental work of finishing the *Variation* and should be treated by rest from work, outdoor walks, and riding.[61] In August 1870, when Darwin complained of a sensation of "pins and needles" that prevented work on the *Descent of Man,* Bence Jones replied that it was "somehow related" to Darwin's "indigestion" but that he need not stop work on the *Descent,* and that if Darwin could spend ten days with Bence Jones, he would be well and fit.[62]

Three episodes of illness that Darwin treated by himself, aided as always by Emma, were quite different in their causations and nature. First, from 23 June to 16 July 1868, for reasons that are unknown, he had an illness whose symptoms he only described as "so bad that I could do nothing" and "I broke down."[63] As he so often did, he treated himself by changing locales. He moved with Emma and Etty to Dumbola Lodge, Freshwater, on the Isle of Wight. Soon after arriving at the Lodge, he commented that "even two days from home" had made him feel better.[64] He soon recovered his capacity for daily work. During his stay at the Lodge, he was seen by William Allingham, an Irish poet,[65] who in his diary perceptively described Darwin's invalidism and its advantages:

August 11.—To Freshwater; engage bedroom over little shop, and to the Darwins. Dr. Hooker in lower room writing at his Address, going to put "Peter Bell's" primrose into it and wants the exact words.[66] Upstairs Mrs. Darwin, Miss D. and Mr. Charles Darwin himself, yellow, sickly, very quiet. He has his meals at his own times, sees people or not as he chooses, has invalid privileges in full, great help to a studious man.[67]

Darwin's second illness began in April 1869 when the horse he was riding stumbled and fell, rolling on him and bruising him. "He was ill after this," Etty recollected, "and it shook his somewhat re-established health." He continued ill into the summer, when Emma wrote a relative that he was "still very poorly and languid, and not able to walk, so is very disappointed." By the fall he had recovered, so as to become "unusually well."[68]

The third illness occurred in July and August 1871 and was first caused by attacks on the *Origin* and *Descent of Man* by the biologist St. George Mivart, who had "mortified" Darwin more than any previous critic.[69] The main symptom of the illness was giddiness, which prevented Darwin from working and seeing visitors and required him to be supported by Emma when he walked.[70] He does not appear to have had any vomiting.[71] Etty, who was with him during much of the illness, commented, "I don't think he was ever but once nearly so unwell."[72] He treated the illness by going with Emma, Etty, and his brother Erasmus to stay for a month at a house on Albury Health near Guilford in Surrey.

When he returned to Down on 25 August, he confronted the new stress of the marriage of Etty to Richard Litchfield, a scholar and philanthropist, which took place on 31 August. Many years later Etty recollected: "My father was in very bad health at the time of our marriage, and it was with much exertion that he came to [Down] church for the wedding. Any sort of festivity was quite out of the question, and no friends or relations were invited."[73] Francis Darwin remembered that his father "could hardly bear the fatigue of being present through the short service" of the wedding.[74]

By September and October, Darwin had recovered without consulting a doctor or taking medicines, and he completed the sixth edition of the *Origin*, where he answered Mivart's criticisms. At this time he became better able to emotionally bear his antipathies to another of his enemies. Referring to Richard Owen, he remarked to Hooker: "I used to be ashamed of hating him so much, but now I will carefully cherish my hatred & contempt to the last day of my life."[75]

13

Improved Health and Living in a "Perpetually Half Knocked-Up Condition"

In the nine years from 1872 to 1881, the main events in Darwin's health were several acute illnesses, persistent chronic illness, emotional upsets from work and certain social stresses, and an improvement in health.

The first acute illness was in October 1872, when after working on the sundew plant *Drosera* for about five weeks Darwin reported that his "head . . . failed," and he "broke down."[1] Emma told a relative: "I have persuaded Charles to leave home for a few weeks. The microscopic work he has been doing with sundew has proved fatiguing and unwholesome, and he owns that he must have rest."[2] After three weeks of sojourning at Sevenoaks Common and enforced idleness, Darwin recovered. From 12 to 23 December, however, he was often in bed with a cough and a cold.[3]

On 26 August 1873, he experienced what he described as "much loss of memory & severe shocks continually passing through my brain,"[4] perhaps a transient case of cerebral anoxia. Four days later he consulted at Down with Dr. Andrew Clark, a London doctor who at this time, like Jenner, Chapman, and Bence Jones before him, held a leading medical position with a large and prestigious practice.[5] Patients valued Dr. Clark for sympathy, attentiveness, and common sense, and they criticized him for his rigid insistence that a treatment—especially a diet—be carried out in a "minute" manner.

On first examining Darwin, Dr. Clark told him he would be able to do him "some good, and that there was a good deal of work in him yet."[6] After testing his urine and finding that it was loaded with uric acid but free of albumin and that the kidneys were normal, Clark wrote him a letter summarizing the chemical causes for his illness: "There is first of all the acid indigestion, then there is the retention in the blood and in the tissues of acid waste stuffs [i.e., the "gouty" state], and lastly as this retention now & then rises into a big wave it worries the nervous system and then breaks into a shower of uric acid, that fills through the kidney & escapes by the urine." Clark then wrote that the illness would be treated by a special diet that decreased the manufacture and increased the excretion of the acid. He wrote that he would be sending details of this treatment and that "I hope you will practice it [the diet] daily for a few weeks & that you will suspend your judgement of its merits for at least a fortnight to come. It will not suit you at once & even after it may need modification: there will be no getting to paradise without the passage of purgatory."[7]

Several days after starting Dr. Clark's diet, Darwin wrote Hooker: "Dr. Clark is convinced that the brain was affected secondarily for which thank God, as I would far sooner die than lose my mind. Clark is doing me good by an abominable diet."[8] However, a month later he wrote Huxley that he was beginning "to fear that diet will only do a little for me. The great benefit at first was, I believe, merely due to a change & changes of all kinds are at first highly beneficial to me."[9]

Early in January 1874, Darwin was in contact with Dr. Clark.[10] From January through March, he recorded what Clark had prescribed for him in the pages of a private diary.[11] On 20 January 1874: "Began Dr. Clark's Physic. Strychnine & Iodine."[12] On 24 January: "Like all Dr. Clark's Physic did me harm." On 22 February: "Began Dr. Clark's Diet"; 17 March: "Began strict diet again after 1 week of lax diet"; 29 March: "Lax diet." There are no further diary notes. Presumably, after stopping, and again starting Dr. Clark's diet, Darwin finally stopped it, for on 4 March, he had written Hooker, "All the good from Dr. Clark's diet vanished: I fear that it was only the good of my change; but it is a great advantage to have a beneficial change to turn to."[13] From this time on he became a regular patient of Dr. Clark, who also treated Emma and their sons George and William.

In April and May 1875 he wrote up his work on insectivorous plants, and in June and July he went for a holiday to Abinger Hall. He described this period of work and holiday as follows: "I was quite knocked up & worried with the subject. So that I had to take a month's complete rest away from home."[14] At this time he was probably sick not only from work on insectivorous plants but also from stresses over taking a political position on vivisection and from attacks on him and his son George by the biologist St. George Mivart.[15]

Three years later, he was ill with what he described to Hooker as "constant attacks of swimming of the head which makes life an intolerable bother & stops all work." This illness was caused by the mental pressures of the "nonstop" day and night work that he and his son Francis were doing in order to study the movements of plants. He then came to London for a week, writing in his journal that it was "on account of Giddiness" and hoping that a change in locales would help. When the illness persisted, he consulted Dr. Clark, and after several days he reported to Hooker: "Dr. Clark has put me on a dry diet & I would have given a guinea yesterday for a wine-glass of water." Following this he made no further references to head symptoms or to a diet, and for the next three years he had no further episodes of acute illness.[16]

Along with complaining about Clark's diets and physics, he appears to have maintained confidence in Clark as his physician. After his death Emma commented that Bence Jones and Clark were the two doctors who did him "good" and that Clark did him "great good."[17]

While Darwin's two main chronic illnesses were day and night flatulence and daily "extreme fatigue," he was often able to counter the effects of these by doing scientific work.[18] In his 1876 autobiography, he wrote that the "excitment" of work "quite drives away" the discomfort of flatulence.[19] Francis recollected that his father had the habit of "working up to the very limit of his strength" and then stopping by saying, "I believe I mustn't do any more."[20] In following this habit Darwin was influenced by the examples of his father and paternal grandfather, who had also complained of a "sense of fatigue" and yet worked hard.[21]

Although Darwin's youthful sensitivity to stirring music and tropical scenery had declined as he aged,[22] several events that were unusually pleasant, or unusually unpleasant, caused him to have feelings that were just as intense and disturbing. In January 1868, after hearing that his son George had become second Wrangler (or highest-scoring student) at Cambridge University, he hurriedly wrote George a note in which, after expressing feelings of pleasure "with all my heart and soul," he added: "But you have made my hand tremble, so I can hardly write."[23] In November 1877, when he was at Cambridge University receiving an honorary degree, he became so distressed on seeing students publicly mocking his evolutionary ideas that his hand shook when he signed his name to register, causing his signature to become barely legible.[24]

His youthful feelings against acts of cruelty to animals remained unchanged and, in his old age, were expressed in angry attempts to stop these cruelties when he saw them. Francis reports how "he returned one day from his walk pale and faint from having seen a horse ill-used, and from the agitation of violently remonstrating with the man." On another occasion, when he saw a man roughly treating a horse, he jumped out of his carriage and "reproved the man in no measured terms." Horse owners who lived in his neighborhood feared his outbursts.[25] In 1875, in the course of giving testimony to the Royal Commission on Vivisection, he summed up the anger that he felt at cruelty to animals by stating: "It deserves detestation and abhorrence."[26]

He continued to fear that his health would suffer because of talking with individuals who were outside of his family. George Darwin recollected that, while his father much enjoyed conversing with guests who came to Down, such conversation "was always fatiguing him," and that after he had waved farewell to the guests, "he would sigh a sigh of relief" that his health had not worsened.[27] Francis Darwin observed that for his father "half an hour more or less conversation would make . . . the difference of a sleepless night, and of the loss perhaps of half the next day's work."[28]

When Darwin conversed with friends there were occasions when he would enjoy himself by joking and laughing. His laugh has been described "as a free and sounding peal, like that of a man who gives himself sympathetically and with enjoyment to the person and the thing which have amused him."[29] Sometimes, however, these happy occasions would cause him to become alarmed about his health. Laura Forster has recollected how, during an evening at Down:

> When he & I had been in unusually high spirits, & setting no bounds to them had been laughing & telling each other stories to our hearts content, his suddenly getting up & going to his study saying "now I must go & be quiet. If I stop another minute with you I shant work for a week, you will make me so ill." I was leaving after luncheon & he came as usual for his last goodbye at the carriage door & said laughingly "it is a good thing you are going after all, for if you'd stayed much longer you'd have killed me." & seeing I really felt some compunction & feared I had overdone him, he added so sweetly "never mind I shall get over it, & I don't know when I have enjoyed myself so much, or talked such nonsense."[30]

Darwin also continued to fear that participating in public events would upset his health. In January 1875, when he was asked to be one of the pallbearers at Lyell's Westminster Abbey funeral, he refused, saying that he "dared not, as I should so likely fail in the midst of the ceremony, and have my head whirling off my shoulders."[31] He would sometimes suffer when he did participate in these events. Francis Darwin has recollected: "When, after an interval of many years he again attended a meeting of the Linnean Society, it was felt to be, and was in fact, a serious undertaking; one not to be determined on without much sinking of heart [Darwin's sinking feeling] and hardly to be carried into effect without paying a penalty of subsequent suffering."[32] Following his fatigue from attending Etty's wedding, he became fatigued in a similar manner from attending the weddings of his three sons: Francis (1874), William (1877), and Horace (1880).[33]

Despite illness and vulnerability to illness, Darwin told an acquaintance in June 1878 that "my health is better than it was a few years ago"[34] (this was three months after his episode of acute "Giddiness"), and in December 1880 he wrote his old friend Herbert: "My health is better than it used to be, but I live in a perpetually half knocked-up condition."[35] ("Half knocked-up condition" refers to his sense of fatigue.) In the 1870s, his butler Parslow, who had often nursed him when he was sick, told a visitor to Down that Darwin's illnesses "nowadays are nothing to what they used to be."[36] An unusual observation on Darwin's change in health was made by the Swiss botanist Alphonse de Candolle, who had visited him in 1839 and 1880 and who noted that "Darwin at seventy was more animated and appeared happier than when I had seen him forty-one years before."[37]

Emma commented on her husband's improved health several weeks after his death when she wrote her son William, "It is a consolation to me to think that the last 10 or 12 years were the happiest . . . owing to the former suffering state of his health."[38] Several years later she told Etty that Darwin's health had become "much better in the last ten years of his life."[39]

The causes for this small, yet definite, improvement in a long-standing illness were changes in Darwin's involvements with his scientific work.

He became able to avoid or to minimize controversy over his ideas. After 1872 he stopped bringing out new editions of the *Origin* and was under less pressure to defend his transmutation theory because it had become more acceptable and was being effectively defended by others, including his new young colleague and friend George Romanes, who would become known as his "Chief Disciple."[40] Although he published controversial ideas in the second (1874) edition of the *Descent of Man* and upheld his "well-abused hypothesis of Pangenesis" in a second (1875) edition of the *Variation of Animals and Plants,* neither of these publications involved him in serious controversies.[41] When he participated in the controversies over spiritualism and vivisection, he was usually able to limit his participation so his health did not suffer.[42] (An exception was his illness in 1875.) When he followed the advice of Huxley and others and refused to engage in a public controversy with Samuel Butler, he told Huxley he felt "like a man condemned to be hung who has just got a reprieve," and he probably avoided having an accentuation of illness."[43]

As he distanced himself from controversy, his improved health enabled him to be less distracted by illness and to keep (in the words of Emma) "steadier to his work."[44] His main work was on plants, which gave him pleasure both as objects for scientific investigation and as objects he enjoyed looking at and touching. Francis Darwin, who assisted him in botanical work, recollected: "He had great delight in the beauty of flowers. . . . I think he sometimes fused together his admiration of the structure of a flower and its intrinsic beauty. . . . He had an affection, half artistic, half botanical, for the little blue Lobelia. . . . I used to like to hear him admire the beauty of a flower; it was kind of gratitude to the flower itself, and a personal love for its delicate form and color."[45] While botanical investigations sometimes resulted in illness and/or in anguish, Darwin was always able to recover and bring each investigation to a successful fruition, so that in the years 1875–80 he published four botanical books.[46]

In 1881 he published his last book, *The Formation of Vegetable Mould, Through the Action of Worms, With Observations on Their Habits.*

He expressed his feelings about doing work by often quoting the saying, "It's dogged as does it."[47] Francis Darwin has commented on some of the deeper meanings that this saying had for his father: "I think doggedness expresses his frame of mind almost better than perseverance. Perseverance seems hardly to express his almost fierce desire to force the truth to reveal itself. He often said that it was important that a man should know the right point at which to give up an inquiry. And I think it was his tendency to pass this point that inclined him to apologise for his perseverance, and gave the air of doggedness to his work."[48]

Being dogged in work was a habit that gave him a sense of mental well-being, so that in his 1880 letter to Herbert he observed: "I . . . am never happy except when at work."[49] When one of his sons urged him to take a holiday away from home, he replied "that the truth was that he was *never* quite comfortable except when utterly absorbed in his writing."[50] Sometimes when he took a holiday after a period of overwork, "it seemed as though the absence of the customary strain allowed him to fall into a peculiar condition of miserable health."[51]

In his personal life he benefited from several events and from experiencing happiness in his family relationships. His financial income from properties, investments, and the sale of his books steadily increased so that he became "rich."[52] The many painful attacks of boils that had afflicted him in the 1840s and 1850s subsided in the early 1860s. The medical reason (or reasons) for this subsidence are not known. There is no record of any sanitary or plumbing changes in Down that might account for it.[53]

Darwin's family relationships largely centered on his dog Polly, his children, and Emma. Polly was a rough white fox terrier who had belonged to Etty and then become her father's dog after Etty's 1871 wedding. Over the next ten years Polly was Darwin's devoted companion, trotting after him when he went on walks and lying on his sofa or her own rug during his working hours.[54] With Polly he again felt a love he had first felt for dogs as a boy.[55] Francis Darwin has described how he "was delightfully tender to Polly, and never showed any impatience at the attentions she required." When he returned home after a holiday, Polly "would get wild with excitement, panting, squeaking, rushing around the room, and jumping on and off the chairs." He would then "stoop down pressing her face to his, letting her lick him, and speaking to her with a peculiarly tender caressing voice."[56]

Although Darwin told a correspondent that the "inherited" ill health of children was the "greatest drawback in his life,"[57] he enjoyed maintaining close contacts with his adult children. He addressed them in a sentence in the autobiography: "When all or most of you are at home (as, Thank Heavens, happens pretty frequently) no party can be, according to my taste, more agreeable, and I wish for no other society."[58] He was happy when Francis aided him in his work and then came to live in his house. In 1876, noting that his five sons were having successful careers, he exclaimed in a letter: "Oh Lord, what a set of sons I have, all doing wonders."[59] And four years later, when his sons and two daughters had given him a fur coat, he was moved to tears and wrote in a note to his children: "The coat will . . . never warm my body so much as your dear affection has warmed my heart."[60]

During the last decade, without the distraction of caring for children, Emma was able to be more attentive to the needs of her husband. She never left him for a night, and "her whole day was planned out to suit him, to be ready for reading aloud to him, to go on his walks with him, and to be constantly at hand to alleviate his daily discomforts." Francis Darwin has commented that only Emma knew the "full amount of suffering" her husband experienced and that she "omitted nothing that might . . . prevent him becoming overtired."[61] When he would meet at Down with a visitor who came to have a talk with him, Emma would note the time the talk began, and after about forty-five minutes she would enter the room—"smilingly" and without saying a word—and Darwin would then cease his conversation.[62] When Emma observed that he was overworking, she had learned to insist that it was necessary for him to take a holiday with her. He had learned to "submit" to her, and these holidays may have been a major cause for the diminution of his episodes of illness.[63]

Emma also knew that he needed work for his happiness and well-being, and after his death she told Etty "she did not wish him to live without working," that "if it was a condition of his living, that he sh^d. do no work, she was willing for him to die."[64]

In his autobiography, he expressed his gratitude to his wife for her intimate knowledge of his various needs and her care of him: "She has been my greatest blessing. . . . She has never failed in the kindest sympathy towards me, and has borne with the utmost patience my frequent complaints from ill-health and discomfort. . . . She has been my wise adviser and cheerful comforter throughout life, which without her would have been during a very long period a miserable one from ill-health."[65]

14

The Final Illness

From 2 June to 4 July 1881, Darwin and his family took a holiday at Lake Ullswater and lived at Glenrhydding House, Patterdale. One Sunday at Patterdale, Emma wrote that her husband, after climbing some rocks by the side of the Lake Ullswater, had a "fit of his dazzling . . . and came down."[1] In mid-June, Darwin wrote Hooker that being without work made him "despondent," aware of the discomfort of flatulence for every hour, and that "I have not the heart or strength at my age to begin any investigation, lasting years, which is the only thing which I enjoy, & I have no little jobs which I can do—So I must look forward to Down grave-yard as the sweetest place on this Earth."[2] He told Wallace, "I cannot walk and everything tires me, even seeing scenery."[3]

While at Patterdale he consulted Dr. F. C. MacNalty, who thought that he had angina pectoris. "My father," Dr. MacNalty's son wrote, "later told me that he found symptoms of myocardial degeneration in Darwin and considered that his health was precarious."[4]

In the fall of 1881, Darwin did not complain of any symptoms and was able to work on the action of carbonate ammonia on roots and leaves. In December 1881, when he and Emma were staying at the London home of Etty and her husband, he experienced giddiness and an irregular pulse.[5] At first he did not see Dr. Clark, and Emma visited the doctor and reported her husband's symptoms. "Dr. Clark," Emma wrote, "said . . . that there was some derangement of the heart, but he did not take a serious view of it."[6] Dr. Clark then saw Darwin and reassured him about his cardiac condition.

Over the following four days, in talks with the geologist John Judd, Hooker, and Huxley, Darwin intimated "he knew his heart was seriously affected," and he stated his desire to leave money to fund advances in geology, botany, and biology. "I was much impressed," Judd recollected, "by the earnestness and . . . deep emotion, with which he spoke of his indebtedness to Science, and his desire to promote its interests."[7] In his talk with Hooker he "promised" to contribute to the financing of an index on plants.[8] (After his death this would become the *Index Kewensis,* a complete index of the names and authors of the genera and species of plants known to botanists.)[9]

He returned to Down from London late in December, and for about two months he was free of heart symptoms. Early in February 1882, he suffered from a cough, and Emma insisted that he take some quinine. "Though I have very little faith in medicine," he wrote a friend, "this I think has done me much good."[10] On 13 February, replying to an acquaintance who had sent him greetings on his seventy-third birthday, he wrote: "I feel a very old man, & my course is nearly run."[11]

On 3 March, upon coming to Down for a family visit, Etty was told by her mother that her father had been having some pain in the heart nearly every afternoon after walking. Several days later she recorded how he "had a sharp fit of pain in the Sandwalk & got home with difficulty" and that "this was the last time he ever walked in the Sandwalk."[12]

Emma then wrote Dr. Clark a letter asking him to come to Down and telling him he would be paid a fee. Clark came on 10 March. He arrived very late, and his visit was described by Etty as follows: "Dr. Clark arrived in a very excited & hurried state & after saying he wd. never come again if they offered him his fee & that he only had half an hour went into my Father. He there let him quite see that he had angina pectoris." At this time the diagnosis of "angina pectoris" meant coronary thrombosis and organic disease of the heart.[13]

Following this visit Darwin became, in the words of Etty, "excessively depressed." He withdrew to his bed and room and had his meals in his room. He experienced a fit of pericardial pain at least once a day, exhaustion, insomnia, "half fainting feelings"—which he had termed "dying sensations" and which may have been similar to those of his father. He was experiencing the actual effects of heart disease and heart insufficiency. Dr. Clark's diagnosis of "angina pectoris" had convinced him that he would not be able to work again. And he was angry at Dr. Clark—because of the latter's hurried visit, frank diagnosis, and insistence on not being paid. Yet he was unable to openly express his anger, and he may have turned this anger against himself (as is the case with some depressed people) and thus increased his depression. He was also depressed because his daily routine of taking walks on the sandwalk had been interrupted.[14]

His anger at Clark and depression may have further increased when Clark waited some days before sending him instructions for a diet and medicines.[15]

The medicines included amyl nitrate, which had recently come into use as an "antispasmodic" for treating the spasm of the coronary vessels which were held to be a cause of angina pectoris.[16]

Several days after Dr. Clark's visit, Darwin was seen by Dr. Norman Moore, a young and rising London physician, who had told him that he did not have angina "but only weakness."[17] Dr. Moore, however, altered nothing in Dr. Clark's treatments. Darwin was encouraged by Dr. Moore's opinions and seemed to Etty to have a "rallying power." In the next two weeks he resumed family meals, played backgammon with Emma, and walked a little in Down's orchard.[18] Once when he and Emma were sitting at the entrance to the orchard with Laura Forster, who had been invited by them to convalesce at Down from a long illness, he put his arm around Emma's shoulders and said, "Oh Laura, what a miserable man I should be without this dear woman."[19]

He was cheered by seeing Laura recovering from illness, and often sat with her when she had lunch, saying, "My dear Laura . . . in this house you are to be treated like the Queen of England, everything in it is at your command, and anything out of it shall be sent for the moment you ask for it." On some days his depression returned, and he would come into the drawing room where Laura was, saying, "The clocks go so dreadfully slowly, I have come in here to see if this one gets over the hours any quicker than the study one does." After lying down on the sofa, he added, "Ah my dear Laura how terribly slowly the time must have been going for you all these months."[20]

During these weeks he went on with scientific writing, which included "Dispersal of Freshwater Bivalves" and "On the Modification of a Race of Syrian Street-Dogs by Means of Sexual Selection."[21]

On 4 April he noted in his private diary that he was having "much pain." Emma persuaded him not to see Dr. Clark but to consult with Dr. Moore and Charles Allfrey, a surgeon.[22] Since he was determined not to affront Dr. Clark, it was arranged that these consultations be in "nominal conjunction with Dr. Clark." On 5 April, Dr. Moore and Mr. Allfrey examined him, then continued Dr. Clark's treatment (which greatly reassured him) and also tried a little nux vomica, which he found did him no good.[23]

He then went on making medical entries in his private diary: 6 April: "Very tired Pain in evening—2 doses" (this last may have meant two amyl nitrate pills); 8 April: "No dose only trace of pain." He had "no bad pain" on 9 April and "very slight attack Pain" on 10 April, and on neither day did he take any antispasmodics. On 11 April: "Some pain at [illegible word] night & discomfort 2 doses of tr antispasmodics." On 12 April he noted that his son George had returned to England from a trip to the West Indies, and then wrote: "Bad pain at night—2 doses." On 13 April: "Stomach excessively bad—went to bed at 2 but no pain & no dose." On 14 April: "1 attack slight pain 1 dose"; 15 April: "no pain & no dose at Dinner—dropped down." On this occasion he was seized with giddiness while sitting at dinner in the evening, and fainted in an attempt to reach the sofa. Within minutes he recovered consciousness, drank some brandy, was helped to his study by his son George, and seemed relatively well. Etty wanted to send for Mr. Allfrey, but Emma thought that this last medical examination had made him ill, and so no doctor was sent for.

He made two more diary entries: 16 April: "Very slight pain several times before [illegible writing] no dose"; 17 April: "Only traces of pain no dose." These were his final medical notations about himself. The persistence of pain indicated that his coronary arteries were becoming progressively more impaired.

On the night of 18 April, he experienced more pain. He woke Emma and sent her to his study for a capsule of amyl nitrate. When she returned, he was unconscious. She gave him brandy, and he slowly recovered. He thought that he was dying, and after some special words to her he said, "And be sure to tell all my children to remember how good they have always been to me" and "I am not the least afraid to die."[24]

At about 2 a.m. on 19 April Mr. Allfrey arrived (having been sent for by Emma) and was "the greatest possible comfort." He spent the night with Darwin and left Down at 8 a.m. when his patient was asleep.

After Mr. Allfrey left, Darwin began to have nausea and violent vomiting and retching. Emma said she never saw anyone suffer as he did: "He was longing to die."

These symptoms continued through the morning and early afternoon: Mr. Allfrey and Dr. Walter Moxon were sent for, and (as Emma retired to rest) Darwin was attended by Etty and his son Francis.[25] "You two dears," he told them, "are the best of nurses." He went on suffering from "overpowering nausea interrupted by retching." Etty said, "This terrible nausea still goes on." He answered: "It is not terrible. But it is nausea." Several times he said, "If I could but die," and "Oh god, oh god," which was his way of expressing distress. His children gave him sips of beef tea with brandy in it, and then some pure whiskey, which Mr. Allfrey had advised him to try. Francis, who had studied medicine, noted that as the afternoon progressed, he became "more and more pulseless."[26]

At about 3:25 p.m. he said, "I feel as if I should faint." He then became unconscious. Mr. Allfrey and Dr. Moxon arrived at Down House and rushed to his room. "As soon as they came in," Etty recollected, "they saw it was hopeless but the instinct of doctoring prevailed & they ordered a mustard poultice which I rushed off to get—But it was never put on—He was unconscious & there was the heavy stertorous breathing which precedes Death—It was all over before four o'clock."[27]

At the time of his death, Darwin was seventy-three years and two months old. The physicians who treated him diagnosed his final illness as "anginal attacks," with "heart-failure" and signs that his "heart and greater blood vessels were degenerating."[28]

15

Darwin's Use of Snuff and Alcohol

Two substances that Darwin took for most of his life were snuff and alcohol. He first formed the habit of inhaling snuff when he was a teenaged student at Edinburgh and was given snuffboxes—which he valued greatly—by a friend, Squire Owen, and his aunt, Mrs. Wedgwood.[1] During the *Beagle* voyage he made notes to purchase snuff.[2] On several occasions he tried to curb the habit. A month before he married Emma, she wrote him that on their wedding day: "You may be allowed to carry a few pinches of snuff in your pocket for that morning only."[3] In 1846 he was "persuaded" by Emma to stop snuff for a month.[4] In 1849, as part of Dr. Gully's hydropathy treatment, he first limited his snuff to six pinches daily.[5] He then resolved to do without it, and he placed his snuffbox in his cellar and the key to the box in his garret.[6] Soon he began breaking his resolve when he visited the Down home of the Reverend J. Brodie Innes. He would tenderly recollect how his daughter Annie got him snuff: "Her dear face now rises before me, as she used sometimes to come running downstairs with a stolen pinch of snuff for me her whole form radiant with the pleasure of giving pleasure."[7] He may have abstained from snuff for most of 1851–56 because his account books for these years contain no record of purchasing snuff.[8] In May 1857 he abstained from snuff as part of Dr. Lane's hydropathy treatment.[9]

At some unknown time he resumed taking snuff, without serious interruptions, for the rest of his life. He would take a pinch, with "clocklike regularity" at 10:30 every night as he undressed before going to sleep. The amounts of snuff that he took during the rest of the day varied. He tried to limit these amounts by keeping snuff in a jar in the hall, where he would have to walk to get it. In his later years he took two kinds of snuff: a heavy, damp, dark brand, which he greatly liked, and a light, powdery "Irish black guard," which he only took because it was weaker.[10]

He may have thought that taking snuff preventing his having "a cold in his head."[11] He called snuff "my chief comfort" and "that chief solace of life."[12] When he was without it, he felt "most lethargic, stupid and melancholy."[13] Francis Darwin wrote that "snuff stirred him up & kept him going."[14] Regularly inhaling snuff facilitated his daily living and working. His geologist friend Judd, who visited him in his Down study when he was in the last years of his life and working on the earthworms, recollected: "At the side of the little study stood flowerpots containing earth worms, and without interrupting our conversation, Darwin would from time to time lift the glass plate covering a pot to watch what was going on. Occasionally, with a humorous smile, he would murmur something about a book in another room, and slip away; returning shortly, without the book but with unmistakable signs of having visited the snuff-jar outside."[15]

Some brands of snuff—adulterated by red and yellow ocher, red lead, chromate of lead, and bichromate of potash—were thought to cause flatulence, vomiting, and severe gastritis, if taken in large quantities.[16] It is not known whether Darwin ever used any of these adulterated brands. Snuff, because it contained nicotine, may have caused some of his episodes of palpitations.[17] His son Francis thought that snuff may have injured his sense of smell.[18] Since he took snuff for about ten years before he became ill, and then for ten years after his illness had become better, it is unlikely that snuff toxicity was a cause of his illness. (The possibility that he changed brands of snuff, and that a new brand may have caused some of his episodes of illness, cannot be excluded.)

In addition to snuff he sometimes took other preparations of tobacco. During his *Beagle* land explorations, when he was with the Gauchos of Argentina, he smoked what he called cigars and "little cigaritos."[19] He then did not smoke until his later years when he took a little Turkish cigarette at 3 p.m. and again at 6 p.m. as he reclined on the sofa and listened to a novel being read aloud to him.[20] At these times smoking, in contrast to the stimulation of snuff, relaxed him.[21]

His drinking of alcohol, and his attitudes toward drinking, had a long history. In his autobiography, he wrote that, when he was a student at Cambridge, "I got into a sporting set, including some dissipated low-minded young men. We often used to dine together in the evening . . . and we sometimes drank too much, with jolly singing and playing at cards afterwards."[22] He told Francis that "he had once drunk too much at Cambridge."[23] He told Hooker that "he got drunk three times in early life, and thought intoxication the greatest of all pleasures."[24] During his middle age he sometimes curtailed his drinking, and at other times he enjoyed what he drank. In 1854 he wrote Hooker: "My London visits have just lately taken to suit my stomach admirably; I begin to think that dissipation, high living with lots of claret, is what I want, & what I had during the last visit."[25] The next year he wrote Hooker: "N.B. If you want to enjoy perfect health as I do this morning eat turtle soup on two successive days, & drink quantum suffi of wines of all kinds."[26] In December 1858 he told his son William that he had "been rather bad of late" and that the surgeon at Bromley, Mr. Williams, "has ordered me a jolly prescription of two glasses of wine at dinner & he wished me to take three!"[27]

In 1860 Dr. Headland prescribed "drinking some wine" as part of his medical regimen.[28] Over the following years wine comforted Darwin when ill. In 1863, when his "nervous system . . . failed," he was for a time "kept going only by repeated doses of brandy."[29] In 1865, when he was very ill, he wrote about himself: "Always been temperate—now wine comforts me much—could not take any formerly."[30] In his old age he usually drank one glass of light wine and abstained from other liquor.[31] Francis observed that he "enjoyed and was revived by the little he did drink."[32]

He also had a "great horror" that "anyone might be led into drinking too much." He once, "very gravely," told Francis that he was "ashamed" that he had been drunk at Cambridge. After hearing this, Francis wrote: "It made me feel ["solemnly" crossed out] strongly how much ashamed one ought to be of being ["tipsy" crossed out] drunk; and it added to my respect for my father."[33] Darwin's "horror" of drunkenness had several origins: perhaps he feared his tendency to be stimulated by small drinks. A paternal great-grandfather and grandmother had both died from alcoholism, and he may have thought that alcoholism was inherited.[34] And then he was influenced by the anti-alcoholic opinions of his grandfather and father. Dr. Erasmus Darwin had first drunk as a student, later curtailed drinking to prevent his having attacks of gout, and then publicly spoken of the toxic effects of alcohol.[35] Dr. Robert Darwin "was vehement against drinking, and was convinced of both the direct and inherited evil effects of alcohol."[36]

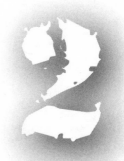

Theories of
the Origins
of the Illness

Theories of Darwin's Doctors, and of Darwin

There is no record of how Dr. Robert Darwin diagnosed his son's illness. Some doctors were "puzzled" by the illness.[1] Others viewed it as a form of dyspepsia: Dr. Gully diagnosed it as "nervous dyspepsia."[2] "Dr. Lane described it as "dyspepsia of an aggravated character."[3] George Busk thought it was "waterbrash,"[4] whereas the *British Medical* Journal reported that Darwin had suffered from "catarrhal dyspepsia."[5] Dr. Holland concluded that Darwin was suffering from a form of gout without joint inflammation, "nearer to suppressed gout."[6] Drs. Brinton and Jenner also suspected "suppressed gout,"[7] and Dr. Clark found manifestations of a "gouty" state.[8]

For several doctors these two diagnoses were related. Dr. Holland believed that gout was "dependent on a *specific material* agent, capable . . . of affecting . . . almost every part or function of the body." He further proposed that there was an "undoubted connection between dyspeptic disorders and the irregular forms of the gouty constitution; a constitution sufficiently close and familiar to observation to justify the belief of relation to some common cause; acting under different modifications from age, sex and other temperament of body; as well as from variations, it may be, in the quality proportion of the morbid matter itself."[9]

Some physicians held that "flatulency . . . generally ushers in an attack of gout."[10] Dr. Alfred Baring Garrod, a leading authority on gout, wrote: "Those varieties of dyspepsia which lead to the excessive formation of uric acids in the system, tend powerfully to the production of gout," "that in gouty cases . . . an excess of uric acid circulating in the blood may itself give rise to a secondary form of dyspepsia, and cause many of the premonitory symptoms referable to the digestive organs, so commonly met with in gouty subjects," and that severe and prolonged study and mental anxiety could cause gout.[11]

Dr. Garrod had shown that in gout the blood uric acid level is elevated, and in 1854 he introduced the following "thread test" for uric acid. Blood was drawn from the patient—since there was a "natural repugnance" to drawing blood, it was sometimes possible to make a blister and draw off its serum—which was then acidified and evaporated; if uric acid was present, crystals formed which adhered to a fine thread. Garrod held that if these crystals did not form, and the results of the "thread test" were negative, the diagnosis of gout was excluded.[12] This "thread test," one of the earliest of bedside diagnostic tests, soon became widely used.[13] It is not known whether any of Darwin's doctors applied the thread test to his blood. However, in September 1873, Dr. Andrew Clark wrote him that his urine had uric acid and therefore he was "gouty."

Darwin came to believe that two causes for his illness were the ill effects of the *Beagle* cruise and heredity.

In the years 1857–60, when he was a patient at Moor Park, he told Dr. Lane that he "supposed" the *Beagle* seasickness caused his dyspepsia.[14] In 1864, he told his brother Erasmus that he did "not believe" his seasickness "was the cause of my subsequent ill health," and he stated the same belief to his son Francis.[15] In 1871 he said to a visitor that "some of his friends" thought that his illness "might be attributed to long-continued seasickness on his voyage years ago." He then abruptly changed the subject.[16] Francis, however, records that his father was "sometimes inclined to think that the breaking up of his health was to some extent due" to his September–November 1834 episode of Chilean fever.[17]

Darwin's most frequently stated opinion about the origins of his illness was that it was a form of gout that he had inherited. In 1868, in *The Variation of Animals and Plants under Domestication,* he published examples of the inheritance of illness, including gout: "With gout, fifty percent of the cases observed in hospital practice are according to Dr. Garrod, inherited, and a greater percentage in private practice." Near the end of the *Variation,* he published his theory of pangenesis: propounding that the body cells give off gemmules that become part of the reproductive cells and that "man carries in his constitution the seeds of an inherited disease."[18]

He applied his ideas about the inheritance of illness to himself in several ways. He observed that his family was gouty.[19] He believed that his father had had gout in January 1829 and August 1837.[20] When his grandfather, Dr. Erasmus Darwin, was forty-eight, he reported that he had an attack of acute gout "with much pain and tumour, and redness about the joint of the toe." He had two more attacks the following year. When he was fifty-six, he wrote that he

"had a little gout" and that "the top of the foot and right toe swell'd consider-
ably."[21] Erasmus described the health of his father-in-law, Charles Howard, as
follows: "The late Mr. Howard was never to my knowledge in the least insane,
he was a drunkard both in public and private—and when he went to London
he became connected with a woman and lived a deba[u]ched life in respect
to drink, hence he had always the Gout of which he died but without any the
least symptoms of either insanity or epilepsy, but from debility of digestion and
Gout as other drunkards die."[22]

Charles Darwin ascribed his illness to an inherited form of gout without
joint inflammation.[23] In 1859 he wrote a correspondent: "I am told that I suffer
from suppressed gout! Whatever it is, I am made wretched & almost useless."[24]
He also came to believe that several of his children had "inherited from me
feeble health."[25]

While the concept of "suppressed gout" explained Darwin's illness to several
of his doctors, and was accepted (with some reservation) by Darwin, it is a concept that is no longer held. Darwin's stomach symptoms and his "eczema" are
not part of the present clinical picture of gout. Although he sometimes complained of "rheumatism," he does not appear to have had the attacks of severe
joint pains and swelling that Dr. Erasmus Darwin had, which are characteristic
of gout.[26]

Several Different Theories

Soon after Darwin's death in 1882, a number of accounts of his life—obituaries in *Lancet* and the *Times*, short biographies by G. W. Bacon and L. C. Miall, and recollections by Darwin's *Beagle* companion John Lort Stokes, his physician Dr. Lane, and his biologist friend George J. Romanes—all stated that his illness resulted from *Beagle* seasickness.[1] In a Royal Society obituary on Darwin, Thomas Huxley also suggested that the 1834 Chilean fever "seems to have left its mark" on Darwin's constitution.[2] Huxley's son Leonard, in a short biography of Darwin, later agreed with this suggestion.[3]

The Huxleys offered no further explanation for their suggestions, and there is no hard evidence that seasickness can cause chronic flatulence. It is possible, however, that the years of *Beagle* seasickness accentuated his pre-*Beagle* tendency to sometimes react to strong emotions by having an upset stomach.

Five years after Darwin's death, in 1887, Francis Darwin published a three-volume edition of his father's *Life and Letters*. This book propounded (without any discussion) Darwin's thoughts that his illness was a form of gout, recounted the nature and course of many of his symptoms, and emphasized that his life was "one long struggle against the weariness and strain of sickness."[4] Although *Life and Letters* became, for ninety years, the main published source for information about Darwin's illness, it possessed several shortcomings. It omitted a number of facts about treatments, doctors, and symptoms, and when Darwin, in the course of describing his illness, had written *vomiting*, Francis Darwin had sometimes either deleted this word or substituted the word *sickness*. (*Sickness* was a word that had sometimes been used by Dr. Robert Darwin and Charles Darwin to denote vomiting.) Because of this editing, the severity of some of Darwin's gastric symptoms, and the exact nature of some of the exacerbations of his illness, were obscured. A fuller and more accurate account of the illness would only be provided in 1977, with the publication of *To Be an Invalid*.

Since the publication of *Life and Letters,* theories about the causes of Darwin's illness have proliferated. The proponents of these theories have been mostly English or American medical researchers, general practitioners, internists, parasitologists, ophthalmologists, psychiatrists, and psychoanalysts. They have studied Darwin's illness because of their admiration for his work and their professional interest in the nature of illness. Their theories of his illness have varied widely, reflecting different degrees of knowledge about Darwin, different periods of medical thought and knowledge, and different interests, predilections, and points of reference for viewing and studying illness. What follows will summarize and evaluate these theories.

The first article devoted solely to discussing the origins of Darwin's illness was written by Dr. William W. Johnston (1843–1902), who taught the theory and practice of medicine at Columbia University in Washington, D.C. It was entitled "The Ill Health of Charles Darwin: Its Nature and Its Relation to His Work" and was published in 1901 in the *American Anthropologist.* Dr. Johnston presented all of the *Life and Letters* evidences of illness, and then stated that Darwin was "suffering from chronic neurasthenia of a severe grade."[5]

The term *neurasthenia* originated in the United States in 1869 and was then used until about 1920. It is a clinical condition characterized by overwhelming weakness, weariness, and exhaustion; insomnia and diffuse anxiety; and a variety of somatic disturbances including cardiac arrhythmias, gastric and colonic upsets, and vasomotor instability so that the skin was sometimes flushed and sometimes sweating and cold. Neurasthenia was believed to be caused by a loss of nervous energy. It was thought that the nervous system had undergone an actual loss of energy, the way a partially discharged battery undergoes a loss of voltage.[6]

As Dr. Johnston described it, Darwin, because of his "intense and sustained" mental work, suffered from a "continued overstrain of exhausted nerve cells. They never, however, rendered the cerebrum incapable of the highest intellectual work, although making the accomplishment of his work both painful and difficult. . . . The chronic indigestion and disturbance in the action of the heart were the usual well-recognized accompaniments of the loss of the normal nerve supply to the digestive organs and the heart."[7]

Today neurasthenia is a diagnosis that is used with some frequency in Asia and Russia but not in the United States. Whether the nervous system undergoes a loss of energy remains unproved.[8] Dr. Johnston was correct in pointing out the relationship between Darwin's illness and work. Yet he does not recognize that combinations of family stresses and work were causes for illness, that certain kinds of work—such as writing the controversial *Origin of Species*—made Darwin quite ill, and that there were periods when Darwin worked hard and was not ill. Johnston quite wrongly has his subject's illness beginning during the *Beagle* voyage, the period when Darwin, aside from seasickness and infections, was in excellent health. And he does not mention that Darwin became ill following conversations with visitors.

In 1903 Dr. George Milbry Gould (1848–1922), an American physician who specialized in correcting errors of refraction of the eye, published a small book entitled *Biographic Clinics: The Origin of the Ill-Health of DeQuincy, Carlyle, Darwin, Huxley, and Browning*. Dr. Gould, respectfully disagreeing with Dr. Johnston, postulated that Darwin had a "refractive anomaly of the eyes," a failure to successfully adapt to near vision, which caused him to excessively strain his eyes when he read and, to a lesser extent, when he used a microscope. This excessive eyestrain caused his stomach upsets, headaches, apathy, exhaustion, and cardiac pain and palpitations. Dr. Gould asserted that these symptoms "are precisely those which the best American oculists find are the most common symptoms of this refractive anomaly of the eyes." Dr. Gould further believed that Darwin's *Beagle* seasickness was not due to the sea but due to his eyestrain when working with his microscope in his *Beagle* cabin, and that Darwin felt better during his last ten years because he became presbyopic and did not have to try to adapt to near vision.[9]

There are several serious objections to Dr. Gould's theory. It does not seem likely that uncorrected errors of refraction could produce such symptoms as Darwin's flatulence and vomiting and his episodes of eczema.[10] For most of his life, his vision appears to have been untroubled and excellent. His daughter Etty recollects that although "he had no special tastes for cats . . . he knew and remembered the individualities of many cats, and would talk about the habits and characters of the more remarkable ones years after they had died." In his "quiet prowls" about the grounds of his Down estate, he would identify less common species of birds, and up to the last years of his life he had "a special genius" for finding bird nests.[11] Dr. Lane recollected how at Moor Park, from 1857 to 1859, he was "all eyes": "Nothing escaped him. No object in nature, whether Flower, or bird, or Insect of any kind could avoid his loving recognition."[12] In 1859, he helped his sons give some names to the beetles they were collecting and rejoiced with them when he identified beetles that were rare.[13]

Only in his later years did Darwin use some visual aids. When he was fifty-three, in April 1862, his son William gave him a pince-nez, which he then put on "only for reading," and in carrying out some of his experiments. When he wanted to closely examine an object, he used a set of sectional glasses that he carried in a little portmanteau.[14]

In 1929, Darwin's son Leonard stated that his father's illness could have involved teeth and gums and been "pyorrhea" or some other form of auto-poisoning and that any excitement made the poison flow more freely."[15] While Darwin's teeth were influenced by vomiting, the influence occurred in a way he described as follows: "What I vomit intensely acid, slimy [sometimes bitter] corrodes teeth."[16] This indicates that Darwin's dental illness was a result of vomiting.[17] The illness consisted of teeth erosions and infections, which in June 1852 resulted in a toothache and then in the extraction of five teeth.[18] There is no evidence that it also consisted of pyorrhea, a discharge of pus from the gums.

18

Theories of Keith and Alvarez, and a Comparison of Darwin's Illness with the Illnesses of His Relatives and Children

After the publication of Leonard Darwin's theory of "auto-poisoning," two authors propounded psychiatric theories.

Sir Arthur Keith (1866–1955), an eminent English physician, anatomist, and champion of Darwinism, postulated that Darwin became ill because of mental overwork. In his 1955 book, *Darwin Revalued*, he wrote: "Darwin was familiar with the fact that when he overworked his stomach suffered. The puzzling aspect of his case, so it seems to me, is that notwithstanding he still continued to overwork his brain. . . . As we trace the development of Darwin's ill health, we find that when he gives up overworking his brain, his digestive organs at once assume their normal function."[1] However, Darwin's digestive organs did not become normal when he stopped overworking: he still had chronic flatulence. Additional shortcomings of *Darwin Revalued* are that Sir Arthur—like Johnston and Gould before him—does not discuss Darwin's other symptoms or other causes of illness.

In 1959 Dr. Walter Alvarez (1884–1978), a noted American physician and medical author, published "The Nature of Charles Darwin's Lifelong Ill-Health," in which he diagnosed his subject's illness as a "mild form of depression" that was inherited. Dr. Alvarez further describes the depression as "a minor 'equivalent' of the depressive psychosis," and he believes that Darwin's stomach symptoms were only the "manifestations" of depression, so that "Today a man with Darwin's type of abdominal discomfort usually has an operation on his abdomen in a futile search for a local cause for his pain and nausea and vomiting."[2] Dr. Alvarez's diagnosis has several shortcomings. He never explains what he means by a depression being "a minor 'equivalent'" of a "depressive psychosis," he does not mention Darwin's chronic flatulence or events that made Darwin both depressed and physically ill, and he omits instances where Darwin complained of being depressed because of the discomforts of physical illness.

Dr. Alvarez contends that Darwin's depression was inherited because it resembled the depressions of several of his Darwin and Wedgwood relations.[3] But was there a real resemblance between these illnesses? What follows will summarize what is known about the illnesses of seven of Darwin's relatives. (These seven are selected because of the availability of information about their health.)

1. When Mrs. Mary Darwin, first wife of Dr. Erasmus Darwin and grandmother of Charles Darwin, was in her late twenties, she had biliary tract disease secondary to gallstones, resulting in severe abdominal pains and transient episodes of psychosis (an "organic psychosis" due to the physiological effects of her biliary disease). She later had cirrhosis of the liver, caused by drinking great quantities of alcohol to relieve her pains, and also by her biliary disease ascending to the liver to produce biliary cirrhosis. She died of liver failure in 1770 at the age of 30.[4]

2. Mary's eldest son, Erasmus Darwin Jr., was a successful and respected lawyer, who was "gentle, ingenuous, and affectionate," yet with "a want of energy in his character," and "without any known or suspected attachment of the impassioned kind."[5] When he was forty, he retired from law practice and bought a small country estate near the town of Derby and the Derwent River. There, while worrying about finances, he drowned in the Derwent. It is not known whether his death was an accident or suicide.[6]

3. Mary's youngest son, Robert, who became the father of Charles Darwin, had stable health into his eighties except for episodes of illness that were described as "gout," from which he always soon recovered.[7]

4. Robert's wife, Susannah (first child of the potter Josiah Wedgwood), complained for years of feeling "never quite well, and never quite ill."[8] The cause and nature of her symptoms are not known, but her family came to regard her as an invalid.[9] In July 1817, she had what appears to have been a sudden onset of peritonitis, and she died after six days of acute prostration, vomiting, and abdominal pain.[10] At the time of her death she was fifty-two and her son Charles was eight.

5. Susannah's younger brother, Tom Wedgwood, was incapacitated by recurrent ill health that prevented him from completing pioneer work in pho-

tography. His early symptoms included depressions and restlessness, troubles with eyesight, "headaches so severe that he would sometimes throw himself to the ground screaming," and "an intestinal disorder diagnosed by one doctor as semi-paralysis of the colon, by another as chronic dysentery," and by Dr. Erasmus Darwin as "worms." He became addicted to opium, first prescribed for him in 1794 by Dr. Darwin. In the last three years of his life, he "suffered paranoid depressions and was at times psychotic."[11] In the summer of 1805, at the age of thirty-four, he committed suicide by taking an overdose of opium.[12]

6. Charles Darwin's paternal half cousin, Francis Galton, had a nervous breakdown when he was twenty-one and a student at Cambridge. He described it as consisting of an "intermittent pulse and a variety of brain symptoms of an alarming kind. A mill seemed to be working inside my head: I could not banish obsessing ideas; at times I could hardly read a book, and found it painful even to look at a printed page. Fortunately I did not suffer from sleeplessness, and my digestion failed but little . . . a brief interval of complete mental rest did me good. . . . I had been much too zealous, had worked too irregularly and in too many directions, and had done myself serious harm." After several months of mental rest, Galton recovered completely. From thirty-one up to about fifty-four, Galton had "giddiness and other maladies prejudicial to mental effort," and treated himself by changing his habits, traveling, and doing outdoor exercise. When he was forty-four, he had "a more serious breakdown than had happened . . . before," and treated himself by changing his "mode of life." When he was fifty-four, he had an episode of "irregular gout and influenza."[13]

7. Charles Darwin wrote that his older brother, Erasmus Alvey Darwin, had "weak" health as a boy and that "as a consequence he failed in energy." He added that Erasmus's "spirits were not high, sometimes low, more especially during early and middle manhood."[14] Erasmus was unable to work, never married, and lived to the age of seventy-seven. The nature of his inertia and "low spirits" is obscure. When he was fifty-three, Darwin reported to Fox: "but Eras. not so well with more frequent fever fits & a good deal debilitated."[15] Two years later, Erasmus wrote his brother: "My ague has left me in such a state of torpidity that I wish I had gone thro' the process of natural selection."[16] When Erasmus was fifty-six, Darwin told Fox: "Erasmus, I grieve to say, has not yet quite lost his ague."[17] This suggests that Erasmus suffered from a febrile illness, and there was a Darwin family belief that he had "tuberculous damage to one lung."[18]

Comparing the illnesses of Darwin's seven relatives, one is impressed by how each illness differed in its history and major symptoms and how none manifested Darwin's stomach or skin symptoms. One may conclude that when the youthful Darwin complained of "violent fatigues" and an affliction of his skin, he was manifesting two new Darwin-Wedgwood traits.

Dr. Alvarez also contends that Darwin's depression was "certainly" passed on to some of his ten children.[19] Let us now summarize what is known about their health.

Three children died young. Mary Eleanor died in October 1842, when she was three weeks old, from unknown causes. Annie died in 1851 at the age of ten from what her father believed was his inherited "wretched digestion" and what her doctor diagnosed as "bilious fever with typhoid character." Recently it has been suggested that she died from tuberculosis, then known as consumption. In June 1858, the Darwins' tenth and last child, Charles Waring, died of scarlet fever at the age of eighteen months. His father observed that he had been "backward in walking & talking," and it is now believed that he had Down's syndrome—a condition of mental retardation which had not yet been identified.[20]

The seven surviving children lived long lives. William was free of illness. Elizabeth, known as Bessy, was "nervous . . . not good at practical things" and "could not have managed her own life without a little help and direction."[21] She "had nervous tics and some strange ways of talking." Darwin felt a special closeness to her because he was aware of his own nervous tics, and believed Bessy had inherited these from him.[22] Etty had been greatly disturbed by Annie's death when she was a child, and during her adolescence she was severely ill from two protracted episodes of fever.[23] As an adult she became the most hypochondriacal of the children, so that it was said of her that "ill health became her profession and absorbing interest."[24] Despite her valetudinarian habits she was intelligent, perceptive, and well read, and her father trusted her to make corrections in the *Descent of Man* and some of his other books.

Francis, Leonard, Horace, and George had distinguished professional careers, along with symptoms of ill health. Francis had "fits of depression" and severe self-deprecatory thoughts.[25] Leonard "long suffered from incapacitating sick headaches."[26] Horace and George had gastrointestinal symptoms. When Horace was twelve, his father described him as "a regular invalid with severe indigestion, [which was] clearly inherited from me."[27] As an adult, Horace continued to suffer from "certain definite and serious illnesses," and when he was forty-two he had an appendectomy for "typhitis" (probably meaning appendicitis), after which his health improved.[28]

More is known about the illness of George Darwin. George "fell ill" when he was twenty-four and then became very ill when he was twenty-seven and twenty-eight and continued to be ill for years. According to Francis, George suffered from "digestive troubles, sickness [vomiting], and general discomfort and weakness." Sir Clifford Allbutt, Regius Professor of Physics at Cambridge, diagnosed George as having a "gastric neurosis," which was treated by emptying his stomach through a tube. Although George expected to die from some of his "attacks" of illness, his health gradually improved, and when he was forty-nine he underwent a "rest-cure," which produced a "permanent improvement, although his health remained a serious handicap throughout his life," and "his nerves [were] always as taut as fiddle strings."[29] Despite ill health, he accomplished important scientific work before his death at the age of sixty-seven.

Although there is much that is unknown about the nature and history of the illnesses of Horace and George, what is known suggests that their gastrointestinal symptoms were similar to their father's. This suggests that the illnesses of father and sons were related in two ways. First, Horace and George inherited their father's pre-*Beagle* tendency to have a stomach that was sensitive to various mental stresses—what became known as the "Darwin digestion."[30] Second, this tendency worsened in response to their father's frequent fretting over their health, his steady belief that he had transmitted his illness to them, and his sometimes becoming ill because of their discomfort.[31]

Thus Dr. Alvarez's contention that Darwin's illness was inherited lacks evidence, and his contention that this illness was passed on to the Darwin children requires much qualification.

Psychoanalytic Theories

In 1920 an American psychoanalyst, Dr. Edward Kempf, published a chapter in his book, *Psychopathology,* that was entitled "Charles Darwin: The Affective Sources of his Inspiration and Anxiety Neurosis." Kempf propounded that because Darwin experienced his father as a "repressive influence," he imposed on himself an "affective restraint," so that he "deprived himself of all channels of self-assertion in his relation with his father or anything that pertained to him."[1] As a result of his suppressing "all disconcerting affective reactions" he had the physical and mental symptoms of his illness, which Kempf diagnoses as a "serious anxiety neurosis."[2] Kempf's explanations and diagnosis need further evidences and discussion. They reflect an early period of psychoanalysis, when theoretical concepts were applied to the study of lives and illnesses in a simplistic and reductionist way.

A succession of psychoanalytically oriented psychiatrists then argued that Darwin had hostility for his father, which he repressed and never consciously acknowledged, but which influenced his manner of working and the nature of some of his psychiatric symptoms.

The English psychiatrist Douglas Hubble contended that Darwin needed to deny the occasion, recollected in his autobiography, when his father rebuked him for being idle and predicted that he would become a "disgrace" to himself and his family.[3]

> Charles Darwin's illness then arose from the suppression and non-recognition of a painful emotion. Such an emotion is always compounded of fear, guilt, or hate—and it is painful because it conflicts with the inner image of himself which each person carries. In the case of Charles Darwin, the emotion arose from the relationship with his father—the adored god who had unjustly condemned him for idleness—and thereby created the obsessional urge for work and achievement.[4]

In 1954, Dr. Rankine Good, another English psychiatrist, pictured a direct—although unconscious—struggle of a son revolting from his father:

> There is a wealth of evidence that unmistakably points to . . . [Darwin's] symptoms as distorted expression of the aggression, hate, and resentment felt at an unconscious level by Darwin towards his tyrannical father, although, at a conscious level, we find the reaction-formation of the reverence for his father which was boundless and most touching. At the same time, the symptoms represent, in part, the punishment Darwin suffered from harbouring such thoughts about his father. For Darwin *did* revolt against his father. He did so in a typical obsessional way (and like most revolutionaries) by transposing the unconscious emotional conflict to a conscious intellectual one—concerning evolution. Thus if Darwin did not slay his father in the flesh, then in his *The Origin of Species*, *The Descent of Man*, & c., he certainly slew the Heavenly Father in the realm of natural history.[5]

In 1963 American psychoanalyst Phyllis Greenacre wrote that Darwin had an "unusual capacity for neurotic denial," and that it was his need to deny his paternal aggression which contributed to his illness. "Nor did he [Darwin] really seem aware of his hostility to his personal father, which was betrayed, however, by the unfailingly exaggerated and superlative terms in which he spoke of Dr. Robert Darwin, except for a few timid complaints of the possible injustice of his father's derogation of him. . . . The massive aggression which had to be repressed contributed to the obsessional neurosis and the associated imposing array of somatic symptoms which so innocently incapacitated him, dominating his life and that of his whole household."[6]

Following the appearance of the views of Hubble, Good, and Greenacre, with their emphasis on Darwin's paternal hostility, several individuals questioned the validity of these views by putting them into a larger perspective. In 1988 R. G. Graber and L. P. Miles briefly evaluated the autobiography's memory of father rebuking son for being idle and a future family disgrace by commenting: "That a son should remember for life, with pain, a single reprimand for laziness suggests not a harsh but an indulgent father: the exceptional nature of the event is what would render it so traumatic."[7] A year later, Professor John Rosenberg, in the course of a more detailed analysis of the memory, expressed a similar opinion: "That Darwin retained his father's words with sufficient exactitude to put them in quotations after sixty years suggests something of the pain they inflicted. . . . Yet to appreciate the full force of the passage, we must recognize the fact of the father's kindness, the son's love of his memory, and his resentment of the indisputable cruelty and injustice of these particular words. They stand out so sharply in Charles's mind because they were so wrong in their prognostication and so *uncharacteristic* in their harshness and anger."[8]

In 1990 the English psychoanalyst, John Bowlby, in his biography of Darwin, delineated two kinds of father-son interactions. When son was a boy, he formed feelings for father consisting of a real reverence for the latter's opinions, an affection that was deep and reciprocated, and a "submissive and placatory attitude towards . . . father [that] became second nature" to him. On the unusual occasion of being rebuked by father, son was deeply mortified.[9]

When son was a man, while he experienced feelings of great pleasure in observing father's admiration for his scientific work, Bowlby contends that these happy feelings were "only half the story":

> Lurking always in the back of Charles's mind, ever ready to emerge, was a deep uncertainty. Was he the disgrace to his family his father had so angrily predicted, or had he perhaps made good? On this vital issue Charles oscillated. Again and again he knew he had made good—there was abundant evidence of it. Yet from time to time he was less sure; and occasionally his doubts became certainties.[10]

Bowlby believed that Darwin's main defense against his uncertainty was to work as hard as he could, "so that the unflagging industry and a horror of idleness were to dominate his life."[11] Bowlby's view that Darwin sometimes doubted his father's good opinion of his work seems more plausible than the view that he had conscious and unconscious paternal hostility.

20

The Possibility of Chagas' Disease

After many psychological reasons for Darwin's illness had been enunciated, infectious causes were considered.

In August 1958, Professor George Gaylord Simpson—an eminent American paleontologist, evolutionist, and Darwin scholar—wrote a review of Darwin's autobiography in which he suggested that, instead of a psychological illness, Darwin may have had chronic brucellosis,[1] an infection undiagnosed in Victorian times, endemic in some areas (such as Argentina) visited by the *Beagle*, and capable of producing Darwin's symptoms. Professor Simpson may have been influenced to think of brucellosis because he had suffered from this infection. He did not, however, press his suggestion or offer further proofs for brucellosis.

In September 1959, a medical writer stated that Darwin may have contracted the parasitic disease amebiasis during his *Beagle* travels.[2] Dr. Phyllis Greenacre, the psychoanalyst, later wrote that Darwin had "severe attacks of malaria while on the voyage of the *Beagle*."[3] There is no evidence for these assertions.

Then in October 1959, Professor Saul Adler, an Israeli parasitologist of world renown, published an article on "Darwin's Illness" in *Nature*: here, after saying that brucellosis infection could be neither proved nor disproved, he cited a previously unnoticed passage in the *Beagle* narrative, *Journal of Researches*, where Darwin described how on 25 March 1835, while in the village of Luxan, in the province of Mendoza, Argentina, he had been bitten by "the great black bug of the Pampas." Adler identified this "black bug" as *"Triatoma infestans"*—a frequent carrier of the protozoan *Trypanosoma cruzi*, which causes Chagas' disease. He reported that, according to South American physicians and scientists, in Mendoza province about 60 percent of the population gave a positive complement test for Chagas' disease, about 70 percent of *T. infestans* were infected with *T. cruzi*, and that in Chagas' disease the *Trypanosoma* frequently invade the heart muscle and destroy the nerves of the intestine, causing cardiac and intestinal disorders. In Chagas' disease there are also periods of latency. Adler concluded that Darwin's symptoms "fitted into the framework of Chagas' disease at least as well as into any psychogenic theory for their origin."[4] Since Chagas' disease would not be known until 1909, this would explain why no Victorian doctor was able to diagnose it.

Adler's theory of Chagas' disease met with a series of receptions: acceptance, rejection, again acceptance, and then controversy. At first, the theory was favorably mentioned by individuals with different trainings and viewpoints.[5] Sir Peter Medawar, director of the National Institute of Medical Research in Great Britain and winner of the Nobel Prize for medicine in 1960, and Dr. James Brussel, an American psychiatrist, each published articles that emphasized that Darwin had both Chagas' infection and a neurosis.[6]

However, A. W. Woodruff, an English parasitologist, published several articles in the 1960s in which he argued that there were six clinical and epidemiological objections to Chagas' disease.[7]

(1) The *Triatoma infestans* that bit Darwin may not have been a carrier of *T. cruzi,* and even if it was a carrier, its bite may not have transmitted an infection. The infection is transmitted indirectly, by the insect's contaminating its bite with excreta, and the majority of those who become infected have been exposed to triatomes not just for a few weeks but for years.

(2) There is no evidence in the Admiralty records for 1832–36 that other members of the *Beagle* crew had Chagas' disease.

(3) It is "very doubtful" that stomach symptoms occur in Chagas' in the absence of damage to the heart.

(4) Darwin demonstrated by his habit of daily walks and use of the stairs in Down House that his exercise tolerance was not severely impaired. Thus his fatigue could not have been caused by Chagas' disease of the heart.

(5) The worsening of his illness during times of stress and its improvement in the last ten years of his life are much more compatible with a psychosomatic disorder than with an organic illness.

(6) He had symptoms of flatulence "before he could have been infected" with Chagas' disease.[8] Woodruff concluded that the diagnosis of Chagas' does not explain "any significant proportion of the symptoms or course of [Darwin's] illness."[9] His diagnosis was that Darwin had "an anxiety state with obsessive features and psychosomatic manifestations."[10]

Adler replied to Woodruff's first article in a letter in which he briefly reaffirmed his belief in the diagnosis of Chagas',[11] but Adler died in January 1966 before he could write a more definitive reply. There was no further discussion of Chagas' until 1984, when it was suggested that Darwin may have had an asymptomatic form of the disease that could only be detected by present-day immunological tests.[12]

Then two physicians—David Adler in England and Jared Haft Goldstein in the United States—each published articles postulating that Darwin could have contracted Chagas' disease, and they assembled the following arguments against the objections of Woodruff: that while there was no certainty, there was the possibility that the triatome that bit Darwin in 1835 could have infected him with *T. cruzi*; that in his 1834–35 travels in Chile and Argentina, he could have been bitten by other similarly infected triatomes;[13] and that the period of four to five years between his exposures to these triatomes and the onset of his 1839–40 clinical symptoms is characteristic of the latent period for Chagas' disease. Because of this latent period, the 1832–36 Admiralty records on the health of the *Beagle* crew would have missed the evidence for Chagas' that occurred after 1836.[14]

Goldstein's contention that *T. cruzi* damaged Darwin's heart (along with his gastrointestinal tract) and that his heart then compensated for this damage is questionable.[15] It is more likely, as Adler propounded, that the *T. cruzi* involved only his gastrointestinal tract, as can occur in a number of cases of Chagas' disease.[16]

Adler and Goldstein contended that *T. cruzi* produced an "organic lesion" of Darwin's stomach and intestine, which then never progressed to the severe physical malformations of chronic Chagas' disease (megaesophagus and megacolon) but which became arrested, so as to produce a secondary Chagas' disease. Goldstein has vividly depicted how this secondary Chagas' consisted of a parasympathetically denervated gastrointestinal tract that had become more sensitive to sympathetic stimulation and that was organically disturbed in its movements and secretory functions.[17]

Two clinical manifestations of secondary Chagas' were Darwin's tendency to have an upset stomach after he had conversed with individuals and his flatulence. The first, beginning in 1842, soon after the onset of secondary Chagas', was from his increased sensitivity to sympathetic stimulation. The second began in 1840, simultaneously with the beginning of Chagas', and was caused by organic disturbance in the stomach. There is no evidence (despite the assertion of Professor Woodruff) that flatulence was among the various stomach symptoms that Darwin had before the *Beagle* voyage. During the voyage, flatulence was not a component of his severe seasickness, and it does not appear to have been present in the stomach complaints he had in the several years after the voyage. It was only in 1840 that he first had extreme spasmodic flatulence, day and night, and he continued to have flatulence for the rest of his life.[18]

Since I published the theory of secondary Chagas' disease in my 1998 essay, "*To Be an Invalid*, Redux," about half the individuals with whom I have discussed Darwin's illness have thought that he could have had Chagas'. The theory has become the object of an ongoing controversy that does not appear to be near any sort of resolution.[19]

In 2003, Icon Films in England produced *Diagnosing Darwin*. In this documentary, zoologist Robert McCall reported failing to find *T. cruzi* antibodies in envelopes that Darwin may have licked and that would have contained his saliva. Dr. Robert Fleischer, a geneticist, reported finding no evidences of *T. cruzi* antigens in what may have been a blood stain in one of Darwin's *Beagle* notebooks. Dr. Fleischer comments that these negative results are not that meaningful, and because of the degraded and uncertain nature of the materials he and Dr. McCall examined, it would have been possible for Chagas' disease to have been missed even when it was present.

Conclusive evidence for Chagas' could only be obtained if a coroner issued a warrant for Darwin's body to be exhumed from its Westminster Abby grave and if the body were then tested for *T. cruzi* antibodies and antigens. In *Diagnosing Darwin,* however, a coroner explains that warrants to exhume a dead person are only issued in cases where the person is thought to have been the victim of a crime. And since there is no reason to believe that Darwin was such a victim, there is at present no valid reason for a coroner to issue a warrant to exhume him.

21

Medical Theories

Since Darwin had severe episodes of vomiting and abdominal pains, it has been suggested that he may have had appendicitis, gastroduodenal ulcer, or cholecystitis.[1] However, although his mother and paternal grandmother died from acute abdominal diseases, the patterns and course of his vomiting and abdominal pains do not appear to be similar to any of these diseases.[2]

Whether Darwin was ever "yellow" as a result of his becoming jaundiced is questionable. The sole source for this is an observation that was made by the poet William Allingham on 11 August 1868, when Darwin was convalescing from an exacerbation of illness on the Isle of Wight. This was Allingham's first and only contact with Darwin. They did not formally meet or converse, and it is not known from what distance or for how long the poet observed the scientist. Five years later, Darwin would describe his appearance as "rather sallow" (a term meaning yellow or brownish yellow color), and Allingham may have perceived this appearance as being yellow without intending to mean that Darwin was jaundiced.[3] At this time the manifestations of jaundice were well known and feared. During his stay on the Isle of Wight, Darwin did not mention having these manifestations, nor were they mentioned by those individuals he was in contact with, who included Emma, Etty, Hooker, and the poets Tennyson and Longfellow.[4]

Darwin scholar David Kohn has suggested that Darwin may have had a diaphragmatic hernia: "He had to eat simply. . . . He apparently improved when . . . put . . . on strict diets . . . a plan of small meals. . . . Repeatedly he is described as having to sit up at night in bed or in a chair because of indigestion, and this is a characteristic of a hiatus hernia. Flatulence accompanied these nights, and this is usually associated with large bowel distension, but the term has been used to include belching."[5] There are several evidences against this diagnosis. Darwin did get better when Dr. Bence Jones put him on small feedings and when Dr. Andrew Clark put him on a strict diet that may have consisted of small feedings. However, during the latter part of his sojourn at Malvern, his eating increased with no ill effects to his stomach. He seems to have eaten well at Moor Park when he was recovering from his illness.

Every day, immediately after lunch, he lay on the sofa reading the *Times* and seemed to suffer no illness from this reclining. When he had severe vomiting, he sometimes was relieved by reclining. His flatulence does not seem to have become appreciably worse at night, when he was lying in his bed. He seems to have sat erect in a high chair mainly (if not only) in the evening, several hours after a small supper, and his erect sitting seems to have been more of a compulsion than a way of aiding the emptying of his stomach.[6]

Two metabolic diseases were considered as possible causes for Darwin's illness. In 1959 Dr. DeWitt Stetten Jr., an American physician then associated with the National Institute of Metabolic Diseases, stated that Darwin had gout (not to be confused with the Victorian diagnosis of "suppressed gout").[7] No evidence was offered for this, and as has been noted, Darwin did not present a history of acute joint pains characteristic of gout.

In 1966 and 1967, Dr. Hyman J. Roberts, an American internist, suggested that Darwin may have had an illness that he called the "syndrome of narcolepsy and diabetogenic ('functional') hyperinsulinism."[8] This syndrome consists of narcolepsy—meaning episodes of "irresistible drowsiness and actual sleep" in a subject who is well rested and not physically fatigued—and a variety of symptoms—headache, abdominal pain, cardiac arrhythmias, peripheral neuropathies—all occurring several hours after meals and believed to be, largely caused by hypoglycemia.

Let us see how this syndrome applies to Darwin. When he was not doing scientific work, he spent most of his time in other kinds of mental activity: reading or listening to Emma read aloud, writing letters, examining his plants, making financial investments, and playing backgammon with his wife. Sometimes around 3 p.m., while his wife was reading to him, he would fall asleep. He would then always wake up shortly before 4 p.m. Aside from this afternoon nap he does not seem to have had any other daily episodes of sleep or drowsiness.[9]

Certainly this is not the picture of narcolepsy. Although he had a craving for sweets, there is no evidence that this was caused by hypoglycemia.[10] He was very punctual about eating his meals, and if he had to wait, he would eat something. However, if he knew several hours beforehand that this meal would be late, "he could manage to wait much more easily."[11] This suggests that his meal punctuality was due to a psychological compulsion, rather than to a low blood sugar level.

The Possibility of Toxicity from Arsenic, and from Other Medicines

In October 1971, John H. Winslow from the Department of Geography-Anthropology at California State College wrote a brochure entitled *Darwin's Victorian Malady: Evidence for Its Medically Induced Origin*. Published as one of the Memoirs of the American Philosophical Society, this was the first book length explanation for Darwin's illness. In it Dr. Winslow rejected all previous explanations and held that his subject suffered from chronic arsenic poisoning, a cause that had already been discounted.[1] Dr. Winslow presented two main arguments: that twenty-one manifestations of Darwin's illness and of arsenic poisoning form a "very close match," and that Darwin took arsenic throughout his life, probably in the form of Fowler's solution, beginning in his teens, or that he "either ceased to take arsenic or significantly lessened the amount he was taking sometime during his late middle years."[2]

Let us consider these arguments. Both the illness of Darwin and chronic arsenic poisoning manifested erythema, eczema, paresthesia, and headaches, as well as cardiac palpitations, weakness, and depression. These manifestations, however, lack specificity and may be similar only in name. There is no evidence that Darwin's erythema (which was never described), his fluctuating episodes of facial "eczema," his paresthesia, and his headaches (variable in character and duration) were similar to the erythema, eczema, paresthesia, and headaches of arsenic poisoning. Cardiac "palpitations" vary greatly in nature and intensity and are present in many illnesses. Depression and weakness are, of course, tendencies that are part of most illnesses.

There are definite differences between Darwin's gastrointestinal upsets and those of arsenic poisoning. Darwin's acute nausea and vomiting would sometimes abruptly cease, and his stomach would return to its state of discomfort from chronic flatulence. In the acute gastroenteritis of arsenic poisoning, where there was "intense irritation, congestion, intestinal capillary hemorrhage, and a swollen and thickened appearance of the gastrointestinal tract," such abrupt reversals are unusual.[3] The gastrointestinal upsets of arsenic poisoning are usually characterized by nausea and vomiting, disturbances of the lower bowel, and anorexia followed by weight loss. Darwin never complained of serious colonic disease. In May 1865, when he was vomiting daily, he wrote: "Evacuation regular & good."[4] How much he suffered from anorexia is uncertain. In 1849, he wrote that he had been "oppressed" by his food.[5] In 1857 he commented that, because his illness had improved, he could "eat like a hearty Christian."[6] In 1863 and 1865, despite severe vomiting, he ate regularly and his appetite remained good, and throughout each of his four major periods of vomiting he did not complain of significant weight loss. It was when he was recovering from his vomiting, and under the care of a physician, that he had large changes in weight.

Dr. Winslow contends that Darwin had two physical signs that were especially indicative of arsenic poisoning: horny keratoses and "a brown or coppery complexion." The evidence for the first is a photograph of Darwin at the age of fifty-one (reproduced in Barlow's edition of Darwin's autobiography), which is said to reveal "multiple corn-like elevations" on Darwin's hands, and a photograph of Darwin as an old man showing a "wart-like feature on his right cheek."[7] After studying both photographs, I could not ascertain the "corn-like elevations" on the hands.[8] I could confirm the "wart" on the cheek (it is also apparent in the 1881 painting of Darwin by John Collier); however, warts are not specific for any particular skin condition. As for Darwin's complexion, observers described it as follows: "brown out-of-door looking complexion" (Emma), "ruddy" (Francis), "very ruddy" (Henry Fairfield Osborn), or "yellow" (William Allingham).[9] Darwin described himself as "ruddy" in 1849; in 1873 he described his complexion as "rather sallow" and the complexion of his father as "ruddy."[10] His facial coloring thus may have varied; at times it may not have been prominent. Descriptions of Darwin's features by some of his supporters, such as John Fiske, Ernst Haeckel, and Ferdinand Cohn, omit any mention of his facial colors.[11] Sir William Osler, in a 1915 recollection of an 1874 meeting with Darwin, wrote: "A most kindly old man, of large frame, with great bushy beard and eyebrows."[12] One would expect that Osler, an eminent physician and thus a sharp observer of physical signs, would have remarked on Darwin's complexion if it had been unusually colored. Dr. W. D. Foster, after studying an oil painting of Darwin at Down House, thought that Darwin's complexion was "within normal limits."[13] In view of the above conflicting evidences about Darwin's complexion, one cannot say that this complexion had any consistent color.

In the course of trying to demonstrate that Darwin's illness resulted from arsenic poisoning, Dr. Winslow makes a series of statements about Darwin's health that are either untrue or only partially true.

Winslow says that Darwin had "catarrhal dyspepsia" and "a bout of pleurisy, and pleurisy and fever." He then compares catarrhal dyspepsia with "a catarrhal state of the exposed mucous membrane of the nose, larynx, pharynx, trachea, and bronchi . . . quite common in cases of chronic arsenic poisoning."[14] This comparison is not valid. The diagnosis "catarrhal dyspepsia" (applied to Darwin by the *British Medical Journal*) was a Victorian medical non sequitur because it was not supported by any direct examination of Darwin's stomach.[15] As far as can be determined, Darwin only once had what he called a "very short but sharpish touch . . . of pleurisy" that "came on like a lion, but went off like a lamb." He complained of many "colds," but he does not describe what he meant by a cold.[16] He only occasionally complained seriously of coughing, which is a pathogenic symptom of catarrhal states of the larynx, trachea, and bronchi.

Dr. Winslow notes that Darwin "mentioned growing bald at the age of twenty-eight," that he was "predominantly bald at thirty-three," and that he was "very bald except for the side of his head and perhaps a fringe in back a few year later." He then states, "There is a tendency for hair to fall out in cases of arsenic poisoning. . . . Alternatively, Darwin may have inherited the trait."[17] Darwin never mentioned growing bald at twenty-eight.[18] A portrait of him at thirty-one shows that he had a full head of hair.[19] He was certainly not "predominantly bald at thirty-three," though at this time his hair had probably begun to recede. His hair can be seen steadily receding in pictures of him at forty, forty-three, and forty-four, and by fifty-one he was entirely bald on top.[20]

It is asserted that Darwin had "tooth and gum problems; five molars out at once at the age of forty-three; fairly early loss of all teeth; pyorrhea; sore gums" and that "gums are sometimes sore and swollen in cases of chronic arsenic poisoning."[21] While Darwin's vomiting may have corroded some of his teeth, resulting in "toothache" and the extraction of five teeth when he was forty-three years old, there is no evidence that he had pyorrhea, complained of sore or swollen gums, or was edentulous.[22] He may, however, have thought that he transmitted his tooth defects to his son George.[23]

Since Dr. Winslow apparently has not directly studied Darwin's health diary, he has relied on the opinions of those who have written about it. Influenced by the surgeon Buckston Browne, who has reported that in the diary Darwin "mentions lumbago and arthritis,"[24] Dr. Winslow states that Darwin had "arthritis; lumbago; gout; suppressed gout; gouty constitution." This is then compared to the arthralgia—"usually located around the knee, ankle or foot, and less frequently in the wrist or hand"—of those who have chronic arsenic poisoning.[25] The health diary contains the following mentions of "rheumatism" and "lumbago": 14 August 1851: "rheumatics"; 15 August 1851: "Little rheumatism"; 6–10 August 1854: "Bad boil. Lumbago: very poorly." In March 1855, Darwin reported to Fox that he and Emma had a month of "coughs & colds & rheumatism."[26] In October 1856, he told Fox that he had recently experienced "just a touch" of "my back feeling locked and rigid! I never felt such a thing before."[27] In January 1864, he told Hooker of a "slight attack of rheumatism in my back," which stimulated him to walk.[28] We do not know what he meant by "rheumatism" and "lumbago." It seems evident, however, that these occurred less frequently than his stomach and head symptoms and that they were not incapacitating. He did not complain of pains in his extremities, such as occur in arsenic poisoning and in gout.

Dr. W. D. Foster, in his study of Darwin's health diary, has written that it is "not clear" what Darwin meant by the "fits" that he frequently records in the diary. Dr. Foster then suggests that these "fits" were probably "of psychogenic origin."[29] Dr. Winslow, after quoting this opinion of Dr. Foster, states that these "fits" may be related to the "epilepsy-like seizures" of Darwin's maternal grandmother, Mary Darwin, or that the "fits" may have been caused by arsenical neuritis. The symptoms of arsenical neuritis are described as "motor and sensory sensations (sometimes pains) which may be violent in character. They are usually located initially in the hands and feet, and they then soon rise slowly up the trunk."[30] Since we now know that the health diary "fits" were episodes of gastrointestinal flatulence, they certainly do not resemble the symptoms of Mary Darwin or of arsenical neuritis. Nor is there any evidence that Darwin ever had "epilepsy-like seizures" or symptoms that resembled the motor or sensory sensations of arsenical neuritis.

Let us now review what is known about Darwin's taking of arsenic. According to the "Recollections" of J. M. Herbert, he took "small doses" of arsenic in 1828–31 for his "bad" lips and presumably benefited by this, and he was also impressed by his father's warning about arsenic's toxicity. In September 1831, he was first tempted to take arsenic for his hands being "not quite well," but then desisted. Following this, for the remaining fifty-one years of his life, he made no mention of taking arsenic in his correspondence, receipts and memoranda book, health diary, or private diary. During these years Emma makes only one mention, in her diary of her using arsenic: 13 March 1873, "began Arsenic;" 5 April, "Left off arsenic."

In conclusion, it may be said that there is no evidence that Darwin took arsenic after age twenty-two.

In a footnote at the end of his brochure, Dr. Winslow raises the possibility that, in addition to suffering from arsenic, Darwin may have become ill from the "prolonged and liberal use of calomel and . . . closely related inorganic mercurial preparations."[31]

When he was suffering from Chilean fever in 1834, Darwin was treated with calomel by the *Beagle* surgeon, Benjamin Bynoe. In 1840, in the beginning of his vomiting, he consulted with Dr. Holland, who favored the use of calomel, and with his father, who said he "may often take Calomel."

Emma's diary for 1840 records "calomel" on 22 and 23 September without identifying who it was intended for. While her husband was very sick, she was in the first trimester of her second pregnancy and may have taken calomel for nausea and vomiting, or they both may have taken it. In 1841, her diary records that her husband took calomel on 22 March and 27 April. In 1846 he sometimes took "blue pills" (mercuride chloride) for accentuations of flatulence, and he may have continued to take these pills for most of the 1840s. From 1849 through 1860, he was often under the care of Gully and Lane, who were against the use of mercurial medicines.[32] On the following occasions in the 1860s, Emma's diary records mercurial medicines, without recipient identification, that were probably intended for her husband: "grey powder," a mixture of mercury and chalk (often taken by Emma), on 19 and 28 July 1862; "blue pills," on 29 December 1863; "blue pill," on 9 January 1864, "pills" (without being named) on 2 March 1864, "grey powder" on 3 and 4 June 1864; and "blue pills" on 29 April, 12 and 14 May, and 13 July 1865. After 1865, Darwin appears to have stopped using mercurials.

In retrospect, while much about his use of mercurials is unknown (the references to using them in his letters and in Emma's diary often lack dosage and duration of use), what is known indicates that when he used them for his illness it was only occasionally and in small doses. So if this use induced vomiting or other toxic effects, these effects may have been of brief duration. His occasional use contrasts with Emma's frequent use of grey powder and with Etty's being given "loads of calomel" for her febrile illness in 1861.[33]

Some of the more frequently used of these medicines included bismuth, acids (weak solutions of hydrochloric nitric or sulphuric acids), alkaline compounds, podophyllin, taraxacum, colchichine, and iron compounds, quinine, opium, and pepsine.[34] In retrospect, of all the many different nonmercurial medicines that Darwin used, only the alkaline compounds were therapeutically effective in checking his vomiting in 1864, but not at other times. From the available information, which is sparse, the therapeutic effects of the other medicines do not appear to have been great, because Darwin limited his use of them. Whether any of these medicines caused toxic reactions in the limited time that Darwin used them cannot be determined.

The Possibility of Illness from Pigeon Allergens

In 1974 Dr. Howard Gruber, professor of psychology at Rutgers University, and Dr. Paul H. Barrett, professor of natural science at Michigan State University, published *Darwin on Man,* a transcription of Darwin's 1838–39 evolutionary thought. In a footnote in this book it was suggested that Darwin may have become ill because of "a severe allergy, possibly to pigeons, with which Darwin associated much."[1] It is possible that Darwin was allergic to some of the objects he lived with and worked with.[2] There is, however, no evidence that he was allergic to pigeons. When he was a small boy, growing up at the Mount, his mother was breeding pigeons,[3] yet, as far as can be ascertained, he was not ill. In the early 1850s he began examining and dissecting dead pigeons; he then built a large aviary (near where his hydropathy douche was located), and here he experimented in crossing and breeding different strains of pigeons. Every day, from 1856 through 1858, he would go to the aviary and closely examine the pigeons.[4] Yet his illness was subacute and did not become especially severe. He does not seem to have been exposed to pigeons during the very severe exacerbations of his illness (1839–42, 1848–49, 1863–64, and 1865). The main symptoms of his illness were not similar to the symptoms of pigeon allergy.[5]

Two Psychosomatic Theories

In 1974 two English doctors—Sir Hedley Atkins and Professor George Picker-ing—published books containing chapters on the symptoms and causations of Darwin's illness, stating that Darwin had a psychosomatic illness caused by his evolutionary theory.

Sir Hedley depicted Darwin's interaction with his theory as follows:

> Poor Darwin! He had so many real worries—the opprobrium which he incurred when his views on evolution were made known in *The Origin* and particularly in the *Descent of Man*, the knowledge that his wife, whom he loved dearly, could not but disapprove of the consequences of the revelation of his ideas and the fact that he had so few friends and allies in the battle for what he believed to be the truth. These worries playing upon a naturally reserved and sensitive nature would be likely to affect far more insensitive men than he.[1]

Professor Pickering believed that Darwin was afraid of putting forward a hypothesis that he knew was right but that lacked scientific proof.[2] He postulated that "the cause of Darwin's psychoneurosis was the conflict between his passionate desire to collect convincing evidence for his hypothesis and the threat imposed on his work by social intercourse."[3]

Although I believe that Darwin may have had Chagas' disease, I also believe that the contentions of Sir Hedley and Professor Pickering are plausible as an alternative theory. Darwin's mental conflicts and the controversial nature of the subject he was working on could have resulted in his becoming ill without Chagas', but such an illness may have been less severe than the illness he had.

Psychiatric Theories of Bowlby,
and of Barloon and Noyes

In studying Darwin's illness, John Bowlby, Thomas Barloon and Russell Noyes drew on information about the illness given in *To Be an Invalid*, the volumes of Darwin's *Correspondence* and the *Calendar of the Correspondence*, and advances in adult and child psychiatry.

In his 1990 biography of Darwin, Bowlby contended that his subject suffered from the hyperventilation syndrome. This develops when hyperventilating in an anxious individual results in a fall in blood carbon dioxide, which then produces many of the symptoms that Darwin complained of. When hyperventilating becomes persistent, yet so slight as to be imperceptible to the individual, there occurs a blood condition, which Bowlby describes as follows: "The carbon dioxide in the blood comes to be maintained continuously at a level only just above that at which symptoms are produced. As a result, any situation, however commonplace, that increases arousal and lowers the level still further will produce symptoms. It is thus that situations that are seemingly trivial such as animated conversation that Darwin liked to engage in, or even a heavy sigh can bring them on."[1]

Bowlby further contends that the silence of Darwin's family about the death of his mother, when he was eight, "made him intensely sensitive to any illness or possible death in the family."[2] His failure to grieve for his mother may have resulted in his becoming depressed and vulnerable to having psychosomatic symptoms.[3] Bowlby states that there is a "significantly increased incidence of depressive and related disorders in those who have lost their mother during childhood," and to support this he cites the 1985 research led by the London medical sociologists George Brown and Tirril Harris.[4]

The above contentions about the hyperventilation syndrome and the impact on Darwin's health of his mother's death raise various difficulties. While Bowlby believes that the hyperventilation syndrome and panic disorder are the same disease,[5] recent research has tended to indicate that patients with panic disorder appear no more likely to panic when they hyperventilate than any other group of people. It now seems likely that, although hyperventilation often occurs during panic attacks, it is a secondary phenomenon, driven by the same processes that started the attacks in general. Thus, while some of Darwin's symptoms may have been caused by hyperventilation, the same symptoms may also have been caused by panic attacks (with or without hyperventilation).[6]

Bowlby's assertion that Darwin's inhibition of grief over the death of his mother made him sensitive to illness and death in his family partly explains the severity of his 1848–49 illness when he was unable to grieve over the death of his father.[7] However, in the opinion of his recent biographer, Janet Browne, there is no evidence that in the years after his mother's death there was "any discernable or long-lasting crisis in Darwin's emotional life."[8] The origins of his violent fatigues and bad lips remain unexplained. While he was sometimes depressed, depression was not a significant psychological force in his childhood or in his youth up to the voyage of the *Beagle*.[9]

The main family event in Darwin's life after the death of his mother was his education by his sister Caroline. Although Bowlby notes that Caroline's methods were "well-intentioned" but produced "undesirable effects" on him,[10] more could have been said about the details of these undesirable effects and how they included his feelings of being ugly. Darwin's daughter Henrietta has the following recollection of her father: "Late in his school life he was very sensitive as to his appearance. As to his feet especially, which were large & with bunions. He used to think himself so painfully ugly that he walked through the back streets of Shrewsbury habitually. I have a dim fancy Aunt Caroline had told him he was ugly."[11]

While Darwin felt inferior because of Caroline's criticisms of him, he also became (as he later recollected) "dogged so as not to care what she might say."[12] Frank Sulloway has commented that doggedness toward Caroline was the beginning of Darwin's "tenaciousness, which included a strong element of indifference to the opinions of others, [and which was] central to his success."[13] Being dogged also meant continuing to work despite illness, as well as exacerbating his illness by working too hard. Because Darwin was dogged for most of his life, and because this was an attitude that was both an adaptation to and a cause of his illness, becoming dogged may have been the most important childhood influence on his illness.

Seven years after the publication of Bowlby's contentions two American physicians—Thomas Barloon, a radiologist, and Russell Noyes Jr., a psychiatrist—postulated that Darwin's illness resembled panic disorder.[14] This was a psychiatric illness that in 1980, in the third edition of the *Diagnostic and Statistical Manual of Mental Disorders* (DSM-III) of the American Psychiatric Association, had been classified as a separate category of anxiety. In 1994, in the fourth edition of the *Diagnostic and Statistical Manual* (DSM-IV), panic disorder has been described as sudden attacks of intense discomfort and fear that can occur with some frequency and that show four (or more) of the following cognitive or somatic symptoms: (1) palpitations, pounding heart, or accelerated heart rate; (2) sweating; (3) trembling or shaking; (4) sensations of shortness of breath or smothering; (5) feeling of choking; (6) chest pain or discomfort; (7) nausea or abdominal distress; (8) feeling dizzy, unsteady, lightheaded, or faint; (9) derealization (being detached from oneself); (10) fear of losing control or going crazy; (11) fear of dying; (12) paresthesia (numbness or tingling sensation); (13) chills or hot flushes. These attacks may be psychologically caused by disturbing thoughts or situations or may occur in the absence of any known cause. They may be followed by several hours of fatigue after the attack has subsided.[15]

While in the course of his illness Darwin experienced ten of the above symptoms of panic disorder—(1), (3), (6), (7), (8), (9), (10), (11), (12), and (13)—he only experienced four symptoms at the same time on the one occasion of his "miserable" pre-*Beagle* illness—(1), (6), (7), (11)—and on the other occasions he had fewer than four symptoms that occurred in varying combinations with each other. Thus, having only one recorded attack of panic disorder early in his life, he does not strongly qualify for the American Psychiatric Association's diagnosis of panic disorder. It should also be remembered that, in addition to panic disorder symptoms, he also had other symptoms such as eczema; headaches that varied greatly in character, intensity, and duration; "rocking"; a tendency to worry over great and small issues; acute and subacute obsessional thoughts; and chronic flatulence.

Barloon and Noyes further believe that, concomitant with panic disorder, Darwin had features of agoraphobia, which the DSM-IV defines as "anxiety about being in places or situations from which escape might be difficult (or embarrassing) or in which help may not be available in the event of having a

Panic Attack . . . or panic-like symptoms. . . . The anxiety typically leads to a pervasive avoidance of a variety of situations."[16]

Barloon and Noyes support their belief that Darwin had "panic disorder with agoraphobia" by stating that he lived "a secluded lifestyle," had difficulties in speaking to his colleagues and in attending scientific meetings, and that he "only infrequently" left his Down home.[17] However, although Darwin found that conversing with colleagues could severely upset his health, he also found that by limiting the duration of these conversations he could often converse without becoming ill.[18] He could sometimes attend meetings of the British Association for Advancement of Science by avoiding having social contacts with participants at these meetings.[19]

It has been observed that when Darwin was a member of the Council of the Royal Society in 1855–56, he attended meetings "on 16 occasions," and that he "was away from home for about 2000 days" between 1842 and his death in 1882.[20] This pattern of activities shows that, while Darwin had a tendency for agoraphobia, he was sometimes able to modify and manage this tendency so as to meet the needs of his scientific work. Thus "panic disorder with agoraphobia" is a diagnosis that only partly explains the manifestations of Darwin's illness.

The Theory of Dysfunction of the Immune System

Fabienne Smith, a Scottish medical writer, believes that all of Darwin's variform symptoms, from youth through old age, were due to a dysfunction of his immune system. In two essays, published in 1990 and 1992, she argues that this dysfunction was an inherited genetic trait and that because of "physical distress," Darwin showed signs of it before the *Beagle* voyage. According to her, his health became worse during the voyage in 1834, while he was exploring in Chile: first, when the combination of physical stress, a highly allergenic diet, and an acid drink caused a collapse of his immune system, which was manifested by his September/October fever, and then when the fever was treated by having him ingest "a great deal of calomel," a mercurial medicine that can depress the functions of the immune system. She also believes that he may have suffered further immunological damage by ingesting lead that was used to seal the canned *Beagle* food that he ate. Thus, possibly by 1834, and probably by the end of the *Beagle* voyage, Darwin had become "permanently vulnerable to all forms of immunosuppression," so "that the slightest addition to his total stress load—whether from allergens or from physical or psychological stress—gave him fearful trouble."[1] The illness that he had after his return to England resulted mainly from the effects of various toxins, allergens, and infections acting on his already weakened immune system.

I believe that the diagnosis of immune deficiency by the available evidences is only supported partially. Let us first consider the possible genetic nature of Darwin's illness. Smith contends that Darwin's maternal uncle Tom Wedgwood provided a "gene pool" for his immune dysfunction,[2] that he and his brother Erasmus had similar illnesses,[3] and that his daughter Annie died from a collapse of her immune system.[4] But it has been shown that there were marked dissimilarities between the illnesses of Darwin and Tom Wedgwood, that very little is known about Erasmus's symptoms, and that Annie may have died from tuberculosis.[5]

To support her contention that the pre-*Beagle* Darwin became ill from physical stress, Smith quotes Darwin's account of his October 1829 sojourn in Birmingham when, while visiting relatives and attending concerts, he became "knocked up."[6] Since I have discussed this 1829 account previously, I will now only say that I believe that, instead of showing the effects of physical distress, it showed that Darwin became psychologically disturbed when listening to certain kinds of music at the concert. There is no evidence that any of his pre-*Beagle* health disturbances resulted from physical stresses, and there is much evidence that he could withstand such stresses.[7]

The contention that Darwin, between recovering from the 1834 fever and returning to England in 1836, became vulnerable to the "slightest . . . physical or psychological stress"[8] is incongruous with the following facts. After recovering from the fever and its mercury treatments, Darwin carried on with *Beagle* work that involved exploring the Andean Mountains. During the first two years and three months after returning to England he experienced his "most active" period of scientific work, which involved exploring the geological site of Glen Roy in Scotland and was not seriously interrupted by his having "occasional" illnesses.[9] That he was able to do this work makes it unlikely that he suffered from lead toxicity, at least from its neuromuscular effects.[10]

I shall now discuss Smith's other contention about Darwin's contacts with various allergens and toxins that were in the air he breathed, the objects with which he experimented, and the foods and medicines he ingested. The nature and history of his infections will then be considered.

Illuminating Gas

Smith contends that the onset of Darwin's 1839–40 London illness may have been influenced by his being exposed to illuminating gas, which at the time was unpurified and conducted in leaky service pipes.[11] (Illuminating gas mainly caused respiratory symptoms, but it also caused nausea and what an American physician described as "catarrhal dyspepsia.")[12] Darwin did complain of London's bad air and "smoke," and in June 1840, when he was recovering from his first exacerbation of vomiting, he moved from London to Maer, where he enjoyed "the delightful smell of the damp earth & plants." However, from July to November, while he continued to reside at Maer and was away from London's gas, he had his second exacerbation of illness.[13] Thus, while gas may have aggravated his illness when he was in London, it does not seem likely that it was a major cause of the illness.

Barnacle Preservatives

Inhaling the alcoholic preservatives of the barnacles he dissected is held to have been a predominant cause for his illness.[14] Although work on barnacles often caused him mental stresses, it is doubtful whether being exposed to small amounts of barnacle preservatives produced chemical injuries. His barnacles were often very small, sometimes the size of the head of a pin.

Some information on how his 1850–53 work on barnacles influenced his health is contained in his health diary, with its record of double underlinings when he felt somewhat improved in his chronic illness. In 1850, when Darwin was mainly working on contemporary living barnacles that contained preservatives, he recorded 130 double underlinings; in 1851, when he was mainly studying and writing up extant fossil barnacles containing no preservatives, he had recorded 111 double underlinings; in 1852, when he was again working on preservative containing living barnacles, he had 193 double underlinings; and in 1853 when he was preparing a manuscript on these barnacles, he had 171 double underlinings. This rough comparison of alternating exposures and nonexposures to preservatives shows that he felt best for one year when he was exposed; next best in a year when he was not exposed; worst in a year when he was not exposed; and next worse when exposed. There thus appears to be no relationship between his inhaling barnacle preservatives and his not feeling well. (This comparison obviously excludes a consideration of other factors that could have influenced his health in these years.)[15]

Although Francis Darwin states that his father was "perhaps" more ill "than at any other time of his life" in the years 1842–54—years that were mainly occupied with work on barnacles—no substantial evidence is offered to support this statement.[16]

Bird "Spirits"

Smith believes that Darwin's 1863 exacerbation of illness resulted from his inhaling the allergenic "spirits" that were given off by his boiling the corpses of birds so as to obtain their skeletons.[17] Her belief is based on Adridon Desmond and James Moore's *Darwin,* which gives an account of an October 1862 visit to Down by three former *Beagle* officers—James Sullivan, John Clements Wickham, and Arthur Mellersh—who are described as finding Darwin occupied with dead birds that were "brewing in foul-smelling spirits."[18] This description is a reconstruction by the authors of *Darwin* that draws on several 1854–55 letters that Darwin wrote his friends Hooker, Fox, and Thomas Eyton, in which he reported how he prepared bird skeletons by boiling the bodies of the birds "in water with caustic soda [potash]." The "foul smell" was produced not by allergenic spirits but by putrid flesh adhering to the bones of the birds. It seems unlikely that Darwin was boiling birds in Down in 1862–63 because beginning in 1856, he sent the specimens out of his home to have the skeletons prepared. Also, there is no mention of these boilings in his published volumes of *Correspondence* for 1862 and 1863.[19]

Food

Smith's suggestion that Darwin may have become ill from allergens in the many eggs Emma used in preparing his puddings and other foods,[20] has largely been superseded by the recent theory that he may have been ill because of being intolerant to the lactose in his food.[21]

Mercury Medications

While Smith has stated that mercurial medicines can induce vomiting, and that Emma's diary showed Darwin's "frequent use" of these medicines,[22] I have argued that his use appears to have been infrequent and in low doses and thus unlikely to have caused serious vomiting.

Infections

Smith's contention that Darwin's episodes of boils in the 1840s indicated "a clear sign of immune system dysfunction" needs to be evaluated by considering what is known about his post-*Beagle* susceptibility to infections in himself, and when he was in contact with individuals who had febrile illnesses.[23] During the 1840s and 1850s, he had episodes of boils that often correlated with his upset stomach and that abated after 1862. He also had (what appears to have been) a resistance to the spread of infection from boils into his blood, so that boils alone did not seriously interrupt his schedule of work. (Except for early April 1847, when he "lost several weeks by Boils & unwellness.")[24]

There were many occasions when Darwin was exposed to febrile illnesses in his family. When his young children were sick, he sometimes watched over them in his study; in 1851 he cared for his daughter Annie when she may have had advanced tuberculosis; he had much contact with his daughter Etty when she had diphtheria in 1858 (which was especially dangerous because it was new and epidemic) and "Typhus fever" in 1860; and in the early 1860s he was exposed to fevers in Etty, his son Leonard, and in Emma. On none of these occasions does he seem to have contracted a serious fever.[25]

The above record suggests that, because of unknown causes, Darwin had a temporary susceptibility to outbreaks of boils and a prolonged resistance to contracting infectious illnesses (which were sometimes contagious) from others. It is not a record that suggests he had a permanent sensitivity to infections.

In conclusion, although Fabienne Smith has raised some important questions about the impact on Darwin's health of toxins in the air, in his foods and medicines, and in the preservatives of animals he studied, I do not believe she has presented convincing evidence that these toxins were significant causes of the onset of illness in 1839–40 and his subsequent major periods of illness.

The Possibility of Adrenal Disease

Betsy King has suggested that Darwin was ill because of a diminished function of the cortex of his adrenal gland, caused by his 1834 Chilean fever and its treatment with calomel and manifested by symptoms of hypoadrenalism, including hypoglycemia (low blood sugar).[1]

There are several serious medical objections to this diagnosis. (1) The adrenal gland supports the body in situations of acute stress. Darwin experienced such a situation in his 1834 illness, which affected "every secretion" of his body.[2] If his adrenal had been only partly available, his chances of surviving the illness would have been small. (2) If he survived with damaged adrenals, he would have had weakness and fatigue (major symptoms of hypoadrenalism), and he would not have been able to participate in the strenuous explorations of the Andean Mountains. (3) After his return to England he often recovered rapidly from his periods of fatigue and weakness, whereas if his adrenals had been impaired, his recovery would have been much slower. (4) Even in his most severe episodes of vomiting, he does not appear to have gone into shock—a physical state of low blood pressure, with cold extremities, disturbances of consciousness, and somnolence—whereas individuals with adrenal insufficiency, who also have vomiting, have a high risk of going into shock. (5) If his symptoms were caused by an organic deficiency of his adrenals, it does not seem likely that they would have improved in his later years.[3]

The role of hypoglycemia in his illness may never have been known because the occurrence of low blood sugar can be diagnosed only by chemical tests that were not available in Victorian times.

The Possibility of Systemic Lupus Erythematosus

In 1997 D.A.B. Young published an article suggesting that Darwin's illness was caused by systemic lupus erythematosus. SLE is a chronic inflammatory disease of unknown origins, occurring predominantly in women, manifested by a variety of symptoms affecting many parts of the body, and often ending in death. As evidence for this suggestion, Young gave a table that divided more than thirty of Darwin's symptoms into the categories "Gastrointestinal," "Cutaneous," and "Other." On comparing these symptoms with corresponding ones in SLE patients, Young argued that the two illnesses were similar in practically all ways.

I question the validity of many of these similarities, and in what follows I will discuss and evaluate some of Young's arguments. To facilitate this discussion, I will divide the symptoms of the illnesses into the categories used by Young and then briefly indicate and compare their individual clinical characteristics and their congruities and incongruities.

Gastrointestinal Symptoms

Both Darwin and SLE patients have episodes of nausea, retching, vomiting, and abdominal pain. Although 49–82 percent of SLE patients complain of anorexia, this symptom appears to have been rare with Darwin. In none of the several accounts of the gastrointestinal symptoms of SLE patients is it recorded that any of these had flatulence, especially the daily protracted form that Darwin had for most of his life. Young suggests that lupus injuries to the esophagus may (questionably) have caused Darwin's flatulence, but he does not comment on the absence of flatulence among lupus patients.[1]

Cutaneous Symptoms

Young's contentions that Darwin's 1828–1829 lip eruption was a form of "discoid lupus" and that the lesions of his hands and face were manifestations of SLE are questionable for several reasons. His lip lesions do not appear to have formed plaques or caused the scarring that is typical of discoid lupus.[2] His facial eruptions of the 1840s, 1859, and the 1860s appear to have occurred indoors (inside Down House or the hydropathy establishment at Ilkley) and away from sunlight and to have been caused by mental stresses. The facial eruptions of SLE were often precipitated by exposure to sun, and the role of mental stress in producing these eruptions has not been clinically evaluated.[3] Whereas hand lesions with erythema are "common" in SLE, Darwin complained about what appear to have been sensory changes in his hands.[4]

To evaluate Young's suggestion that Darwin's "boils" were painful lupus nodules situated deep in the dermal part of his skin, more information would have to be known about the clinical-pathological nature of these boils—whether they appeared to be located superficially or deep in the skin and how they looked. This information is not available.[5]

One of Young's most strongly argued beliefs is that Darwin was photosensitive (as is typical of SLE patients) and that during the *Beagle* voyage there were times when he became ill after experiencing conditions of strong sunlight and heat or ultraviolet light as he climbed high mountains. However, there were other times when he experienced these conditions without becoming ill.[6] Soon after his return to England, he went on a geological trip where, after enjoying "five days of the most beautiful weather, with gorgeous sunsets," he felt happy in being successful in his scientific work and in having good health.[7] Several months later, he first noted the onset of serious illness when he was inside a church with his wife, attending a religious service. During the next thirty-four years, although he became ill from several causes, none of these appear to have included exposures to light. His daily way of relaxing from work when the weather was good was to walk or sit outdoors on the grounds of his Down estate. His daughter Henrietta has "happy" last memories of how, several months before his death, he sat with his wife in Down's "orchard, with the crocus eyes wide open and the birds singing in the spring sunshine."[8]

Other Symptoms

Young explains three of Darwin's other symptoms as follows. (1) Darwin's first complaining of fatigue and being unable to walk more than a short distance and then, after a few weeks, being able to walk several miles is ascribed to his having a moderate anemia from which he was soon able to recover. (Moderate anemia occurs in 57 percent of SLE cases.) (2) His appearing "yellow" in 1868 is diagnosed as his being jaundiced as a result of having an attack of acute hemolytic anemia. (Such jaundice-producing attacks occur in 4 percent of SLE cases.) (3) His 1843 complaint of "numbness" in his fingertips and his many years of feeling coldness in his feet are interpreted as being Raynaud's phenomenon—an illness manifested by changes in skin color, temperature, and sensation, and caused by a vasoconstriction of the arteries supplying blood to these extremities. (This is present in 18 percent of SLE cases.)[9]

I believe that there are alternative explanations for the above symptoms that better fit what is known about Darwin's illness and the facts of his life. (1) The most apparent reason for a decrease of Darwin's fatigue and an increase in his ability to walk was a diminution in the pain and discomfort of his flatulence and an absence of vomiting. (2) Whether he was ever "yellow" from being jaundiced is unlikely. (3) His 1843 sensation of "numbness" in his fingers was most likely a paresthesia (disturbance of sensation) caused by anxiety. His feeling of coldness in his feet may have been an obsessional concern about trying to find a temperature that best suited him and being unable to find this temperature. Francis Darwin observed that "it was as if he could not hit a balance between too hot and too cold."[10]

Two other groups of symptoms—involving the lungs and joints—showed the differences between lupus and Darwin's illness. Although about 45 percent of SLE patients had recurrent episodes of pleurisy, often lasting for days (with pleuristic pain that sometimes persisted for weeks),[11] Darwin recorded only two brief episodes of pleurisy: 19 April 1853 and 28 February–2 March 1860, from which he made complete recoveries. While 53–93 percent of lupus patients had lesions involving their joints, which were often manifested by a recurrent pattern of arthritis,[12] Darwin only mentioned occasionally having "rheumatism" and "lumbago" (much less frequently than his stomach and skin problems), and they do not appear to have been seriously incapacitating.

The above comparisons of the symptoms of Darwin's illness with those of SLE may be summarized as follows. While much is unknown about Darwin's skin lesions, what is known suggests that they were not caused by exposure to light as is characteristic with SLE.[13] A comparison of Darwin's prominent other symptoms with the prominent symptoms of SLE indicate that there are many qualitative and quantitative differences between these two groups of symptoms and therefore that Darwin's illness and SLE are two separate diseases.

A Dermatological Diagnosis

In the year 2000, Gordon Sauer, an American dermatologist, published an article, "Charles Darwin Consults a Dermatologist," in which he diagnosed Darwin's skin disease as being atopic eczema. This was the first time in nearly 120 years of comments on Darwin's illness that anyone had proposed a diagnosis for his dermatological symptoms.

Sauer explained that, whereas the term *eczema* means a group of skin symptoms of unrelated causation, if the term is preceded by the adjective *atopic,* a rather definitive disease is indicated. The term *atopy* or *atopic* means that the body's capacity to act or respond has been altered because it is in an allergic state. While Dr. Sauer believes that this allergic state is a cause for Darwin's skin symptoms, he does not believe that allergy can account for the other symptoms of Darwin's illness, as has been proposed by Fabienne Smith (see chapter 26).

In presenting the evidence for his dermatological diagnosis, Sauer draws on a 1980 article by J. M. Hanifin and C. Rajka, "Diagnostic Features of Atopic Dermatitis," which lists four basic features and twenty-three minor or less characteristic features. Of the basic features (three of which an individual must have for a diagnosis), Darwin had skin lesions seen in a particular body location, chronicity of these lesions, and (perhaps) pruritis, or itchiness, from them.[1] The fourth feature is heredity, which Sauer notes "cannot be proved one way or another for Darwin."[2]

Of the minor features (three of which are needed for a diagnosis), Darwin had an early age of onset, cutaneous infections, and a "course influenced by environmental and emotional factors." "Recurrent conjunctivitis," with "lymphoid infiltration [causing] considerable corneal discomfort," may explain his "eyes [becoming] almost closed up" when he was at Ilkley in October 1859. His having what he called "stars in the eyes," when he argued evolutionary ideas with Hooker, may have been an example of what Hanifin and Rajka explained as "orbital darkening," with "so-called allergic shiners."[3]

"From personal experience," writes Sauer, "I have had many patients with a similar history and symptoms to Darwin's eczema (dermatitis). It is typical to have flare-ups of dermatitis for no apparent reason or, on some occasions, foods, pollen, or molds can be incriminated. One major factor in most flare-ups of dermatitis is stress."[4]

Whether or not Darwin had atopic dermatitis can only be confirmed by allergen tests that have been developed since his death, and he may occasionally have had other kinds of skin disorders.[5] But the diagnosis of atopic dermatitis fits what is known about the nature and history of his dermatitis better than any other diagnosis.

The Possibility of Systemic Lactose Intolerance

Anthony Campbell, a professor of medical biochemistry at the University of Wales and his wife, Dr. Stephanie Matthews, contend that Darwin's illness fits the syndrome of systemic lactose intolerance (SLI), a new syndrome that they have defined, researched in patients, and written about in articles and a brochure but that has not yet been evaluated in double-blind studies. It occurs when an individual lacking the lactase enzyme eats foods containing lactose. Normally, when these foods reach the small intestine, which contains the lactase enzyme, the enzyme splits the lactose into sugars that are absorbed into the blood without resulting in any disturbance. If lactase is lacking, the unsplit lactose reaches the colon, where it becomes a toxic substance, which causes reflux vomiting, and then when absorbed into the blood results in a variety of systemic symptoms.[1]

I shall consider the contention of Campbell and Matthews first by summarizing what is known about Darwin's consumption of lactose after he married Emma and became seriously ill and how this consumption may have influenced his illness, and then by comparing his symptoms to those of SLI.

Emma kept recipes for many puddings made with milk, cream, butter, eggs, and sugar.[2] These ingredients are rich in lactose, which occurs in milk (its only natural source) and milk derivatives and can also be present (without being identified) in some sugars and sweets.[3] Since childhood, Darwin had a craving for sweets that was especially intense and that he described often by saying that "the meat of dinner was very dull & the sweets the only part worth."[4] Early in his marriage, when he described Emma's dinners as being "very good," he may have been referring to the sweetness of her puddings,[5] and throughout his marriage he (doubtless) often enjoyed eating these puddings.

Explaining how these meals influenced his health is problematic. The causes for illness that Darwin mentioned most frequently were mental pressures, boils, and colds. When in the months of October–December 1862 he had three episodes of illness, each after eating an evening meal in the company of visitors, he believed the illness resulted not from what he ate but from the mental pressures of conversing with the visitors. During these months he never had any illness after eating meals with Emma, with whom he could always converse without becoming ill.

Although he did not complain that Emma's sugar-sweetened puddings may have sometimes made him ill, there were occasions when, on the orders of doctors, he at first had an improvement in health after he restricted sweets. In 1844 he reported to his father that, following the latter's advice, he was feeling "very well" from eating a "non-sugar" diet. In January 1860, under the direction of Dr. Headland, he limited sweets, and in March he reported having no change in health, but in May he became "inclined" to believe his health had improved.[6] In August 1865, Dr. Bence Jones placed him on a near starvation diet that still contained some sugar, and by September he was much better.[7] In December he stopped eating sugar. In January 1866 he reported to Bence Jones that he had successfully treated episodes of headaches and flatulence by taking coffee without sugar, and then he made no further mention of these treatments. At this time he also told Bence Jones that he had become fond of eating cheese (a food he had previously disliked), which was a source of lactose. It is not known how eating cheese influenced his health.[8]

There is no mention in the writings of Darwin and Emma that restrictions of sweets became a long-term form of treatment for his illness. One reason may have been that the treatments became ineffective after a time, as happened with practically all of the treatments Darwin took. Another reason was that Darwin disliked very much having to curb sugar, and sometimes he playfully refused these restrictions. In the last years of his life he would make "vows" not to eat sweets. As Francis Darwin recollected, he was not particularly successful in keeping such vows. Francis does not record how his health was affected on the days he ate sweets.[9]

Campbell has published a table comparing the symptoms of 157 SLI patients (symptoms produced by giving these patients lactose) with Darwin's symptoms, explaining the similarities, questionable similarities, and differences. Both the patients and Darwin had headaches, lightheadedness, tiredness, and chronic fatigue. However, while the SLI patients had symptoms of flatulence and eczema, more information is needed to determine whether these symptoms were similar to Darwin's flatulence and to his head and hand eczema. While 84 percent of the SLI patients had large bowel complaints of diarrhea and farting, Darwin had few large bowel complaints.

Campbell emphasizes that because SLI patients' vomiting is caused by unsplit lactose becoming toxic when it reaches the colon, there is a delay of several hours between eating food containing lactose and the onset of vomiting. He then observes that Darwin's 1863–65 period of vomiting showed the same kind of delay, and he concludes that this is evidence for Darwin's vomiting being similar to the vomiting of SLI.[10]

However, in first reporting her husband's 1863 delay in vomiting, Emma comments that it was "surprizing," suggesting that the delay was a new kind of vomiting differing from previous vomiting.[11] Thus the accounts of Darwin's 1840 and 1848–49 vomiting do not mention any delays between eating and vomiting. During his 1840 illness, Maria Edgeworth, a visitor to his home, reported: "His stomach rejects food continually; and the least agitation or excitation brings on the sickness directly so that he must be kept as quiet as is possible and cannot see any body."[12] Why the pattern of vomiting changed from vomiting soon after eating to a delay in vomiting is not known.

From the information that is presently available, I believe it is not possible to form a definite opinion on whether Darwin's illness resembled the illness of SLI. The effects on his health of eating the foods containing lactose and of restricting these foods can only be evaluated sporadically and partially. While his pattern of vomiting was sometimes similar to the pattern of SLI vomiting, at other times it appeared to differ. His flatulence was practically always located in the stomach, and it spared the colon, while the flatulence of SLI was frequently in the colon and manifested by farting (a symptom he never seems to have reported). It is not known how his eczema compared to the eczema of SLI.

Perhaps after more information has been accumulated on the history and clinical nature of the main symptoms of SLI, it may be possible to form a more definitive opinion on whether Darwin's illness resembled or differed from SLI.

The Possibility of Crohn's Disease

In 2007, two Chilean physicians, Fernando Orrego and Carlos Quintana, published an article criticizing all previous diagnoses of Darwin's illness, including my own of Chagas' disease. They argued that the illness was Crohn's disease, which is an inflammatory gastrointestinal disease, located mainly in the upper small intestine and manifesting symptoms of abdominal pain, diarrhea, and fatigue.

In their opinion, the diagnosis of Chagas' disease can be "easily discarded" because Darwin did not show the acute symptoms of early Chagas' and its later chronic symptoms of myorcarditis, megaesophagus, and megacolon. I think this is an opinion that much too easily ignores the possibility that Darwin could have had Chagas' of the stomach and small intestine that became inactive. I have elaborated on this possibility in this book and mentioned it in my essays, Colp 1998 (which Orrego and Quintana refer to) and Colp 2000.[1]

I believe that the case for Crohn's disease frequently consists of questionable connections between contentions advanced by Orrego and Quintana and the evidences they give to support these contentions.

They suggest that when Darwin had his severe 1834 fever in Chile, this led to a bacterial infection of his small intestine, which was the beginning of an "inductive phase" of Crohn's disease, which would later result in clinical signs of the disease. They then state that when the Chilean fever was treated with calomel, a medicine sometimes used as a purgative, this was evidence that Darwin did not have colitis and that his infection was confined to the upper intestine.[2] However, all that is known about Darwin's clinical symptoms is his later recollection that during the fever "every secretion of the body was affected." When he described these symptoms to his father, Dr. Darwin "could make no guess as to the nature of the disease."[3] Since every secretion of his body was affected by his fever, it does not seem likely that his use of calomel, one of the most widely used medicines in all kinds of fevers, indicated that he did not have colitis.

Orrego and Quintana write that by September 1839, almost three years after Darwin's return to England from the *Beagle,* he had the symptoms of the illness that would afflict him for the rest of his life.[4] This is not true. He did not have two of his major symptoms—flatulence and vomiting—until late December 1839 and early January 1840.[5]

In giving a history of Darwin's symptoms of flatulence and vomiting, Orrego and Quintana are often vague as to when these symptoms have a specific relation to Crohn's disease (vomiting is not a frequent symptom of Crohn's) and when they result from overwork, prolonged conversation, and other mental stresses Darwin was under, or other causes.

They write that, although Darwin's "evolutionary ideas and the mental conflicts derived from them did influence his disease, a causal relationship is unwarranted." As evidence for this, they cite Darwin's eight years of work on barnacles, "a non-conflicting subject," when he lost two years to illness. This ignores the fact that during those eight years Darwin continued to work on his evolutionary ideas and to experience mental conflicts over them. As he wrote in his autobiography, after July 1837 he "never ceased working" on the subject of evolution," and he "could sometimes do this when [he] could do nothing else from illness." Orrego and Quintana further write that Darwin "had no special troubles when writing the first volume of his *Natural Selections* book on the transmutation of species." At first when he was doing this work Darwin was in relatively stable health. But as his work progressed, he began feeling "very much below par," and he went for hydropathy treatment at Moor Park. There, as he continued to work on *Natural Selections,* he had a return of his "old vomiting," which caused him to describe himself as a "wretched contemptible invalid." He was at Moor Park, under the care of Dr. Lane, when he changed from writing *Natural* Selections to writing *On the Origin of Species.* This change greatly exacerbated his illness.[6]

Orrego and Quintana write that during Darwin's life "the most accurate diagnosis" of his illness was made by Dr. Lane, who said he suffered from "dyspepsia of an aggravated character." They then comment that at the time this diagnosis "was the closest he [Lane] could get to Crohn's disease."[7] However, Lane's diagnosis was evidence not for Crohn's disease but for the impact on Darwin's health of his working intensely on *Natural Selections* and *On the Origin of Species.* Lane saw Darwin only during the period when he was writing these books.

In addition to comparing Darwin's dyspepsia with the dyspepsia of Crohn's disease, Ortega and Quintana compare several other nongastrointestinal symptoms of the two illnesses that have been less considered by others. They list some of Darwin's parasthesias (disorders of sensation), which mainly involved his hands—numbness in his fingers and burning in his hands—and an episode of feeling the sensation of "pins and needles" when he was writing *The Descent of Man.* They believe that these parasthesias correspond to a "peripheral neuropathey . . . common in Crohn's disease and usually attributed to vitamin B$_{12}$ deficiency, either as a result of defective absorption or, more frequently, bacterial overgrowth syndrome."[8] However, this list omits mention of Darwin's 1831 pre-*Beagle* letter to Susan, in which he first complained of having hand parasthesias. After this he complained of these parasthesias for most of his life. Thus his hand parasthesias occurred before the voyage of the *Beagle,* and was probably independent of any post-*Beagle* changes in his health.[9] Nothing more is known about his "pins and needles" sensation.

Orrego and Quintana believe that other symptoms of Crohn's disease, less known yet worth considering, are its articular manifestations, which they infer resemble the articular manifestations of Darwin. They summarize this as "non-deforming migratory arthritis of large joints or, in the spine, sacroiliitis or ankylylosing spondylitis." Let us see how these manifestations compare to what is known about Darwin's articular symptoms. Over a span of twelve years he complained of the following back afflictions: November 1853, "poorly from sorry back"; August 1854, "bad boil, lumbago; very poorly"; October 1856, "just a touch" of "my back feeling locked & rigid! I never felt such a thing before"; January 1864, "a slight attack of rheumatism in my back"; and in May 1865 he recorded "(now constant) lumbago."[10] Since no additional information is given on any of these episodes of lumbago, it is not known how they compared to the lumbago of Crohn's disease. On occasions Darwin complained of what he called "rheumatism" without giving its location, so that it cannot be compared to the joint symptoms of Crohn's disease.[11] "Rheumatism" is one of his most infrequent and least understood symptoms.

And while they contend that Darwin's decrease in illness in his old age resulted from a decrease in the symptoms of Crohn's disease, they say nothing about apparent causes in Darwin's life for this decrease. These causes, as has been shown in this book, included Darwin's being happy in work and family life, not becoming involved in intense controversies, curtailing work by taking holidays with Emma, and (for unknown reasons) no longer suffering from boils.

To summarize two of my main criticisms of the arguments of Orrego and Quintana, I think that their discussion of Darwin's gastrointestinal symptoms gives a picture of Crohn's disease that is vague and inchoate, and I believe that they largely ignore the stresses on Darwin's health of his working on his controversial theory of natural selection.

In contrast to the diagnosis of Crohn's disease, the diagnosis of Chagas' disease postulates that Darwin had an active infection of his stomach and intestine that became arrested after inflicting permanent injuries. As a result of these injuries, his sensitivity to becoming ill from various mental stresses, including stresses from his evolutionary ideas, was greatly increased.

Summary

This last chapter will draw on the information given in this book (while occasionally adding some new information) so as to offer reviews and overviews on the following aspects of Darwin's illness: the clinical nature of his main symptoms and their causes, how he responded to various treatments, and how illness influenced his work, moods, and relationships.

When he was growing up, he experienced three kinds of disturbances to his health: "violent fatigues" caused by mental stresses, parasthesias of his hands resulting from unknown stresses in his manner of living, and skin disorders of his lips that may have resulted from mental stresses and/or allergies.

Most of these disturbances were of brief duration and did not seriously interfere with his patterns of living and working. Only when he was twenty years old in 1829, because of "bad" lips that persisted for several months, did he become so depressed that he stopped collecting beetles and meeting with friends. When his lips became better, he regained his "high" spirits for doing scientific work, and for socializing with a group of friends, among whom he "kept up the closest conversation . . . [and] was ever one of the most cheerful, the most popular & the most welcome"[1]

There is no evidence that any of Darwin's relatives complained of violent fatigues, parasthesias of the hands, or skin disorders. He thus appears to have been the first member of his family to have had these symptoms.

In 1831, after accepting the position of being a naturalist on the *Beagle,* he became "miserable" for two months from symptoms of depression, heart palpitations, and fears of heart disease. But he never seriously considered not going on the voyage, and as he waited for the *Beagle* to sail, he wrote his friend Whitley: "All is finally settled & I have sealed away about half a chance of life.—If one lived merely to see how long one could spin out life.—I should repent of my choice. As it is I do not."[2]

For most of the five years of the voyage, he adapted to dangers and hard-ships. He suffered from seasickness and homesickness. In 1834 in Chile, he had a severe fever that confined him to bed for over a month. In March 1835 in Argentina, he was bitten by a number of *Triatoma infestans* bugs, which can be carriers of the *Trypanosoma cruzi* protozoa that causes Chagas' disease, and then he may have had an episode of subclinical Chagas' disease that subsided.

During the voyage he determined to have a career in which he would add to scientific knowledge, and he developed a habit of regularly doing hard scientific work—sometimes while being seasick—in which he discovered that "the golden rule for saving time" was "taking care of the minutes."[3] In the last year of the voyage, his seasickness and homesickness increased.

After he returned to England in October 1836, he settled in London and engaged in the "most active" period of his scientific career. He formed close social and professional relationships, participated in the affairs of the London Geological Society and other scientific societies, prepared manuscripts for pub-lication, and formed his theory of evolution by natural selection and other new theories. He complained of "uncomfortable palpitation of the heart," head-aches, and an undefined stomach disorder without vomiting. When he read papers aloud to meetings of the Geological Society, he sometimes felt "as if my body was gone, & only my head left." Although he observed that "it is very bad for one's health to work too much," and although doctors urged him to take a holiday, he continued to work hard and to progress in his work.[4]

In January 1839, when he was almost thirty, he married Emma Wedgwood, and then he did less work than at any other comparable period of his life, al-though he tried to work as hard as he could. This was because of a severe wors-ening of illness. First there were many months of malaise, languor, and fatigue from socializing with friends, then "periodical vomiting" (the first vomiting since the *Beagle* seasickness), and flatulence (the first time he had this symp-tom), and then several months of "great flatulence," day and night vomiting, and weakness. In 1841–42 the vomiting decreased, and he regained some capac-ity for work. But for the rest of his life he would have physical weakness, fatigue from doing work, and flatulence.

Some of the causes for this illness were his distress over Emma's sufferings in her pregnancies, stress over writing up his *Beagle* geological and zoological work for publication, and anxiety over secretly beginning to develop the theory of natural selection, which he knew would encounter "prejudice." He may have experienced the onset of Chagas' disease, which produced vomiting and flatu-lence by injuring the stomach and its parasympathetic nerves. Although the

Chagas' would become arrested, its injuries to the stomach and parasympathetics increased Darwin's sensitivity to stress.[5]

In the course of this illness, he became depressed and self-punitive, and in 1841 he wrote his old friend Fox: "I am grown a dull old spiritless dog to what I used to be. One gets stupider as one grows older I think." In 1842, he and his family moved from London to Down because of a need to preserve health by limiting contacts with London society, while still having some contacts with London's scientific organizations and men.

Over the following three decades, his illness largely consisted of "extreme spasmodic daily & nightly flatulence," episodes of vomiting, sometimes becoming prolonged, and episodes of a "swimming head," trembling, and seeing black spots. He also had cardiac palpitations, paresthesia in his hands, headaches, "rocking," depressions and obsessions, and "eczema" of his face.

The main causes for these illnesses were various mental pressures. In 1851 Emma told a relative that his health was "always affected by his mind," and in 1854 he summed up the psychosomatic sensitivities of his stomach by writing Hooker: "Be careful of your stomach, within which as I know full well, lie intellect, conscience, temper & the affections."[6]

Some of the stresses that he said resulted in his having short periods of increased illness were travels and visiting new places that mentally disturbed him, overworking, seeing his son George having teeth extracted under chloroform anesthesia, presiding over scientific meetings, and speaking before audiences. In 1847 he told Hooker that criticisms by David Milne of his theory of Glen Roy caused him to vomit for several days. Several illnesses where he did not mention a particular cause may have resulted from working on his evolutionary theory, work which he often kept secret from his friends.

In 1859 he wrote Fox that his frequent months of "old severe vomiting" resulted from writing *On the Origin of Species*. However when he had months of vomiting in 1848–49 and 1863–64, that were caused by grief over the death of his father and then by anger over the failure of his friend Lyell to fully support natural selection, although he mentioned his disturbed feelings about father and Lyell in letters to Fox and Hooker, he held back from writing that these feelings were a cause for his vomiting. He never mentioned any possible causes for his months of prolonged vomiting in 1865, although during these months he suffered from stresses over not finishing *The Variation of Animals and Plants* and not writing about human evolution.

Although psychologically disturbing events often made him ill, on two occasions he confronted events that were mentally severely disturbing: the death of his daughter Annie in 1851, and being forestalled by Alfred Wallace's discovery of natural selection in 1858. On each of these occasions he did not have a serious increase in vomiting or flatulence. This was because in 1851 he was able to mourn for Annie by weeping with Fanny Wedgwood and Emma, and in 1858 Lyell and Hooker arranged for a joint public presentation of his ideas and those of Wallace.

Two physical causes of illness were the pains and discomforts of boils and colds.

Darwin's frequent episodes of facial eczema may have been a form of "atopic dermatitis," resulting either from allergic reactions to a variety of substances in his environment or from emotional stress, or both. It is not known what caused what he called "rash," "erythema," or "eruptions."

When illness forced him to diminish or stop work, he would become so depressed that in June 1863 he reported to Whitley: "I have become that most wretched and despicable object, a confirmed valetudinarian." At this time he described himself to Hooker as being "languid & bedeviled," and having "hate for everybody." Months later he wrote Hooker: "Unless I can . . . work a little I hope my life will be very short."[7]

However, he was always able to return to work and to experience this return as making a "wonderful difference" in his life, so that his desire to do work never seriously faltered. He expressed this desire after seventeen years of illness when he wrote Hooker: "I would sooner be the wretched contemptible invalid, which I am than live the life of an idle squire." After twenty-four years of illness, he wrote Fox that working two or three hours a day was "the only thing which makes life endurable to me." Several years later, he wrote an acquaintance he had known as a youth that doing scientific work had always been his "passion."[8]

His passion to persevere in this work despite being ill was aided by his receiving different kinds of help from friends, doctors, and his wife. From friendship with Hooker he received both support for his work and sympathy for his illness. Early in his friendship, after he told Hooker, "I have not had one whole day or rather night, without my stomach having been greatly disordered," Hooker replied, "I would willingly take a little bad health (temporarily only) to let you work in comfort, you do so richly deserve a little peaceful working." (The day and night chronicity of his flatulence was one of the main differences between his illness and the illnesses of Hooker and other friends.) In 1849 when he was recovering from prolonged vomiting, Hooker wrote him: "Your bettered health rejoices me greatly. . . . I . . . court all the medical details you send, & beg you to continue to me particulars of your case. I read that part of your letter with as much interest as any other."

After *Origin* was published and had received the approbation of three judges—Lyell, Hooker, and Huxley—he felt "splendidly well" and "as bold as a Lion" when he anticipated confronting the controversy that he knew would follow the publication of his book. Although Lyell's subsequent lack of support then made him ill, he was cheered and moved to tears when Hooker and Huxley publicly advocated and advanced *Origin*'s ideas in ways he could not do by himself because of his illness. Hooker continued to be his medical confidant who became "extremely" concerned about increases in his illness, while also predicting that he would recover from these increases. Darwin wrote Hooker that "grumbling" about his moods and illness to the latter "does one good," and after writing Hooker that he hated "everybody" he at once added: "No, that is not true for in my worst state I do not hate you." In his autobiography, he recollected: "I have known hardly any men more lovable than Hooker."[9]

But when meeting and conversing with Hooker, Huxley, and other friends, Darwin always needed to take the precaution of limiting the time he talked with them, so as to protect himself from too much excitement. Thus he wrote his friend Hugh Falconer: "Instead of your coming here [Down] I should prefer coming to you.... *I know* I may speak truth to you; I prefer it, because I feel if my head is swimming I can go away at once; but if you were here I could not send you away."[10] However, there were occasions when, even though he controlled the length of his conversations with friends, he became "worked ... up to that degree I wished myself dead."[11]

Whenever he had prolonged vomiting, he stopped meeting all his friends and largely isolated himself and his family from neighbors so that his children "had rather a desolate feeling that [they] were aliens."[12] On three of these occasions he was treated by a doctor with a new medical regimen—Gully in 1849 with hydropathy, Jenner in 1864 with alkaline medicines, and Bence Jones in 1865 with a "scanty" diet of "toast & meat." Each of these regimens checked vomiting and enabled him to resume work. However, none became a permanently effective treatment for vomiting (although he would have continued to use hydropathy if he had been strong enough to bear the physical effects of this treatment) or flatulence, which he once described as "incessant discomfort, I may say misery."

He often tried treating his flatulence by applying electric currents (first from a voltaic battery—galvanism—and then from hydroelectric chains), visiting relatives, riding horses, changing his diet, eating lemons, taking his coffee without sugar, playing billiards, and experimenting with logwood, "bitters," mercury compounds, acids, alkaline preparations, iron preparations, Condy's Ozonised Water, pepsine, bismuth, podophyllin, taraxacum, colchicine, opium, and croton.

None of these treatments (which he sometimes repeated) stopped the flatulence for long. Near the end of his life, he stated that he had "very little faith" in adhering to a medical regimen, and he came to believe only in the temporary effectiveness of different changes. "Changes of all kinds," he told Huxley, "are at first highly beneficial to me."

In the beginning of his acute and chronic illness, which was also the beginning of marriage, he was nursed by Emma, who continued to nurse him for the rest of their marriage. In the periods of prolonged vomiting, when he withdrew from friends and neighbors, he needed to be physically and emotionally close to Emma and would talk to her in a sustained and "warmly affectionate" manner about how he was experiencing his symptoms. (At the same time, he would briefly see his children and relatives.) He painfully expressed the need for Emma in May 1848, when he was away from her, visiting his father and sisters Susan and Catherine at Shrewsbury. He wrote her a letter reporting an acute attack of illness, and then commented: "Susan was very kind to me, but I did yearn for you. Without you when sick I feel most desolate." Near the end of the letter he repeated: "Oh Mammy I do long to be with you & under your protection for then I feel safe." In March 1849, when he was still acutely ill, he wrote Susan: "Emma, bless her old soul, thinks as much about me as I do even myself."

When illness was chronic, he followed a daily routine of doing periods of scientific work that alternated with periods when he and Emma talked, walked, read books, and played backgammon, and he listened to her play the piano. Such activities often eased his discomfort, so that in his autobiography he called her his "cheerful comforter."[13] while she commented after thirty-two years of marriage that "nothing marries one so completely as sickness."[14]

In the last decade of his life, he continued to suffer from flatulence and fatigue and to live in what he described as a "perpetually half knocked-up condition." However, as the stresses from work and family lessened, and as Emma insisted that he go on holidays with her when she saw he was overworking, he was able to work without having serious increases of illness.

Appendix

Darwin's Diary of Health

The <u>Diary of Health</u>

Jan 1 +[1]	Feb 1 +	March 1
2	2 +	2 +
3 + +	3	3 +
4	4	4 +
5	5	5
6 +	6 very poorly	6
7 + +	7	7
8	8	8
9	9	9
10 poorly very	10 +	10 + Malvern
11	11	11
12	12 +	12 10. 7. 12 [5]
13	13 + +	13 +
14 – poorly very	14 + <u>Boil</u>	14
15	15	15
16	16	16 +
17 7 Days [2]	17	17 +
18	18 9 Days [4]	18 +
19	19	19
20 +	20	20
21 + +	21	21
22 + +	22	22
23	23	23
24 +	24 + +	24
25	25 +	25 st. lb. oz.
26	26 +	26 10. 7. 2.
27 +	27 + +	27
28	28 +	28
29		29
30		30
31 [3]		31 poorly

	April		May		June.
	1 poorly		1 well nearly		1 well
	2 do		2 well		2 well
	3 no more snuff		3 do		3 well
	not very well	+ +	4 poorly ["perhaps	10.12.7	4 well
	4		from walk" del.]	compress off	5 well not quite
	5		5 poorly		6 well almost very
	6 poorly		6 well		7 well
	7 do	10.11.13	7 well		8 well very
	8 well		8 well very		9 well very
10.8.8	9 well		9 do do	11. 0. 0	10 well very
	10 well		10 do (nearly		11 well very (in evening
	11 well		11 well		not quite)
	12 well		12 well		12 well
	13 well		13 well		13 well almost very
	14 well, not quite .	(10.12.3)	14 well		14 well very 2*
	15 poorly	[with Fl.	15 well very		15 well very
10.9.10	16 well	W is 4 oz][7]	16 well		16 poorly in evening
	17 do		17 poorly		17 poorly
	18 do		18 poorly in Bed	st. lb oz	18 poorly rather
	19 do		19 poorly rather	10 13 15	19 poorly a little
	20 poorly little		20 well nearly		20 well nearly
	21 do do		21 well		21 well
st. lb	22 well		22 well not quite		22 well
10.10.12	23 poorly, rather		23 well		23 well
	24 well		24 well		24 well
	25 do		25 well	st lb oz	25 poorly little
	26 do		26 well not very	11 0 4	26 well
	27 poorly		27 well: in evening		27 well
	28 do. slight sinking[6]		poorly		28 well
	29 do – trace of	10.12.10	28 well do		29 well
10.11.12	30 do		29 well		30 well
			30 well very		travelling treatment interrupted
			31 well very		* very little flatulence
					*2 do except early at night

<u>July</u> 1849

Temp. 54°.

1 Sunday. Shallow Bath 5' 8	2 dripping sheets		- -	Well almost very	

Well almost very

2 Monday sweat	do	do		Well <u>very</u> (not a strong dash)	
3 Tuesday sweat	do	do		Well almost very in morning:	
4 Wednesday Shallow Bath	do			Well	a good deal of
5 Thursday sweat	do	do		Well	flatulence
6 Friday Shallow Bath	do			Well very	
7 <u>Saturday</u> sweat	do	do		Well <u>very</u> on slight fit of	

slight eruption on legs
fl at night not counted

flatulence at 5 P.M.

8 Sunday Shallow Bath   do   Well almost very, one bad, one slight fit of flatulence,
otherwise well

9 Monday sweat   do   do   Well – feeling vigorous all day,

10 Tuesday sweat   do   do   Well almost very (as on 8th)

11 Wednesday Shallow Bath   do   Well almost very. Then slight fit of flat.

12 Thursday sweat do   do   Well almost very. 2 baddish & 1 slight fit of flat:
<u>very much</u> flat in night

13 Friday Shallow Bath   do   Well not quite. 2 bad fits of & much continual flat.
eruption much diminished

14 <u>Sat.</u> sweat   do   do   Well almost very. 1 baddish 1 slight fit of fl: all night
very bad fl. with fright

15 Sund. Shallow Bath. 2 footbaths   do   Poorly – 2 very bad fits & much continued flat – do
in night. languid

16 Monday Sweat do 3 dripping sh.   Poorly, little; much continued flat: - do in night; languid
54° for 5'

17 Tuesd. Shallow Douche   Drip. Sh.   Poorly, much flat; excessive at night with slight trembling &
fright.

18 Wed   Sweat Douche   do   Well, but with much flatulence

19 Thrusd.   Shallow   Douche   do   Well feeling vigorous, but with several bad fits of fl & much
at night

20 Frid.	Shallow Douche	do	Poorly in morning, well afterward, not very much fl
21 Sat	Sweat Douch	do	Well in morning. poorly afterwards with very much fl.
22 Sund	Shallow Douche	do	Well but with good deal of fl.
	*		
23 Monday	Sweat * Douche	do	Well in morning, poorly in evening with very much fl.
24 Tuesd. **	Shallow Douche	do	Well, feeling vigorous all day, but in even[9] good deal of fl. excell night
25 Wed.	Sweat Douche	do.	Well very. At 5.30: long though slight fit of fl. & some afterward
26 Thurs	Shallow Douche	do	Poorly little with considerable fl
27 Friday	Shallow Douche	do	Well almost very with 3 slight fits of fl: at night considerable fl.
28 Sat	Sweat Douche	do (2 foot baths)	Well in morning. Poorly in afternoon, nausea, much discomfort & fl.
29 Sund	Shallow foot Shallow Drip: at 12' 30'		Poorly very with nausea slight sinking, several fits of excessive fl.
30 Mond	Sweat Shallow Douche	do	Well decidedly 4 slight fits of fl.
31 Tuesday	Sweat Douche	do	Well nearly, ["but" del] with very much fl. 6 or 7 baddish fits of

* St lb

11 0 0   Without Hat or Compress in grey trousers & shoes.

29th almost every trace of eruption gone

** Began working on Cirripedia.

August 1849

1 Wed	0 Sh: 0 Dr.	Well <u>very</u>, two very slight fits of fl.
2 Th	Sw: Sh: D: Dr.:	Well very 3 slight fits of fl.
3 Fri	Sw: Sh: D Dr.	Well <u>very</u> 2 very slight fits of fl
4 Sat	Sw. Sh. D Dr.	Well <u>very</u> no fit of fl. only few separate eruct.
5 Sund	Sh. O Sh. Foot B.	Poorly little, 6 or 7 fits of fl of which 2 or 3 bad ones: little nausea
6 Mon	Sw: Sh D Dr	Well in morning, after 7 about 6 fits of fl not very bad: night bad, wakeful, much fl
7 Tuesday	Sw Sh D Dr	Well, with 2 rather consid. Fits of fl
Wednesday	0 Sh: 0 Dr.	Well, barely, 5 or 6 fits of fl. of which one baddish
Thursday	Sw. Sh. D. Dr.	Well 4 or 5 slight fits of fl.
10 Friday	Sw. Sh. D. Dr.	Well in morning: <u>poorly</u> little afterwards, 4 or 5 fits of fl. of wh. One bad: night bad, oppressed, much fl
1 Sat	Sw. Sh. D Dr.	Well <u>very</u>, only one very slight fit of fl; night however with much. –
2 Sund	0 Sh 0. Dr.	Well barely 4 or 5 slight fits of fl.; night very good
3 Monday	Sw. Sh. D. Dr.	Well <u>very</u>, no fit of fl but some occas separate eruct: night with consid fl.
4 Tuesd	Sw Sh. D Dr.	Well <u>very</u> do do. <u>Night</u> or early morning, terrible fl headache, nausea, shivering, retching up with acid & clots blood
+ 5 Wed	Sh. Dr. (FB) Dr(FB)	much headache fl. nausea, one bad sickness, acid & slime: night excellent
6 Th[10]	Sw Sh D D	Well, but exhaust in morning. In evening little poorly. Night good but too heazy
7 Fri	Sw. Sh. D Dr.	Well 3 fits of fl night rather wakeful much fl.
8 Sat	Sw. Sh. D. Dr.	Well do night moderately good.
9 Sund	Sh. D. Dr.	Poorly little, much fl. – night fair
0 Mond.	Sw. Sh. D. Dr.	Well, 4 fits of fl. night fair but heazy.
Tuesd	Sw. Sh. D Dr.	Well <u>very</u> no fits of fl. but at <u>early</u> night much, good afterwards.
Wednesday	0 Sh. 0 D Dr.	Well almost very 3 fits of fl of wh. One longish night good, often wakeful
Th	Sw. Sh. D. Dr.	Well <u>very</u> no fits of fl & but very little occas. night good ["little" del] not much fl. often waking
Fri	Sw. Sh. D. Dr.	Well <u>very</u> do some reather uncomfortable feels- night good
Sat	Sw. Sh. D. Dr.	Well <u>very</u> do night so, so
Sund	0 Sh. 0 Dr.	Well: at 4 P.m. & after 4 fits of fl. night ["very" del] good,, rather heazy
Mond	Sw. Sh. D Dr.	Well <u>very</u> at l. one fit of fl. night uncomfort. often waking. yet stay heazy much fl
Tues	Sw. Sh. D Dr.	Well much fl. in afternoon to cleansing.[11] Night not very bad.

no eruption
4 to 6 fits of fl
every night, otherwise
good night

29 Wed	0 Sh. D Dr.	Well not quite, bowels uncomfort. 2 fits of fl. one long & <u>bad</u>: excellent
30 Th	Sw. Sh 0. 0	Poorly. Exhausted. Bowels wrong, Physic, <u>much fl</u>. from spice. night goodish.
31 Fri	0. 0. 0. 0.	Poorly. Bowels. not very much fl: night much fl

	3 P.M.	St	lb	oz	
* Tuesday 7th:	11"	2"	1		dressed as before

Go on till 10th of September[12]

7 double dashes[13]

eptember 1849

. Sat	Sw. Sh. D. Dr.		Well almost very. One fit of fl. not slight – Night uncomfort. much fl.
Sunday	Sw. Sh. D.		Well very . some occas. fl night bad very much fl wakeful discomfort
Monday	Sw. Sh. D. Dr.		Poorly a little, much fl night at first bad, then rather heazy
Tues	Sw ShO. 0 Dr	Travels	Poorly very, excessive fl; headache. night heazy, but otherwise pretty good
Wen	0. Sh. D. Dr.		Well but with many fit of fl not very bad. night pretty good
Th	Sw. Sh. D. Dr.		Well very . little occas. in evening. – night excellent, but long fit of fl in early morning
Fri	Sw. Sh. D. Dr.		Well very in morning: from long drive 3 consid. fits of fl night good
Sat	0. Sh D Sh		Well almost very, but 3 or 4 slight fits of fl night good
Sun	0 Sh. 0. Sh		Well almost very, one not very slight fit of fl night excellent
0 Mon	0 Sh. D. Sh.		Well almost very. one long but not bad fit of fl. night good.
1 Tu	0 Sh.		Well travelling. some fl. night bad
	Birmingham		
2 W.	Sh.		Well, not quit[e] 3 or 4 fits of rather bad fl. night excellent
3 Th.	Sh.		Well extremely but 1 fit of fl night uncomfortable
4 Fr.	Sh.		Well do do night no good
5 Sat.	Sh.		Bowels bad some fit of fl night good
6 Sund	0		Well do night excellent
7 Mon	Sh		Well very 1 fit of fl. night excellent
8 Tu	Sh		Well extremely 1 rather bad fit of fl night not bad
9 W.	Sh.		Well very 1 or two fits of fl night not good
0 Th.			Well do (travelling)[14] night ["bad" del] fair
1 Fri	Sw. Sh. D. Dr.		Well. 3 fits of fl, of which two bad – night much fl
2 Sat	Sw. Sh. D. Dr.		Well 5 fits of consid. fl. night bad, much fl. headach[e], fear
3 Sund	Packed.		Poorly in bed a good deal of fl. night good, too heazy
4 Mond	Sw. Sh. D. Dr.		Well, but 4 or 5 fits of fl. night fair
5 Tu	Sw Sh. D. Dr.		Well 4 fits of fl. of which two baddish night not very good
6 W.	0 Sh. D. Dr.		Well 3 fits of fl of which 1 bad night fair in morning 1 bad fl.
7 Th.	Sw. Sh. D. Dr.		Well do 1 rather bad night good
8 Fr.	Sw. Sh. D. Dr.		Well very , one slight fit of fl night fair
9 Sat	Sw. Sh. D. Dr.		Well very Little occas. night good
0 Sund.	0. Sh. 0. Sh.		Well very night wakeful

not very much fl.

Birmingham

3 double[15]

0th							
	St	lb			St	lb	oz
	11	3	0	21st	11	2	8

October   1849

1 Mon.	Sw. Sh. D. Dr.	Well _very_	night excellent, two slightest fits of fl
2 Tu.	Sw. Sh. D. Dr	Well _very_	night poor wakeful consid. fl
3 Wed	D. Sh. D Dr.	3 slight fits of fl	night good
4 Th	Sw. Sh. D Dr.	Well _very_, With fl before breakfast – from not working – night poor much fl rather wakeful
5 Fri	Sw. Sh. D. Dr	Well almost very. 2 fits of fl of wh[ich] one very slight. – night pretty good
6 Sat	Sw. Sh. D. Dr.	Well. 2 fits of fl of wh[ich] one bad night poor much fl
7 Sun	0 Sh. 0 Dr.	Well not perfectly 6 fits of fl night fair rather heazy
8 Mon	Sw. Sh. D Dr.	Well _very_ night poorish 8 consid. fits of fl.
9 Tu	Sw. Sh. D. Dr.	Well _very_ slightest erupt. on back night ogod
10 Wed	0 Sh. D. Dr.	Well _very_ do night very good
11 Th	Sw. Sh. D. Dr.	Well _very_ 1 perhaps slightest fit of fl night very good with fl except firs
12 Fri	Sw. Sh. D. Dr.	Well _very_ rash night very good, hardly got up for fl.
13 Sat	Sw. Sh. D. Dr.	Well _very_ (["little" del] bad boil) night very good – not much fl.
14 Sun	0 Sh. 0 0.	Well _very_ uncomf. from Boil night very good, very little fl
15 Mon [16]	Sw. Sh. 0 Dr.	Well _very_ do night good, in morning some fl
16 Tu	Sw. Sh. Dr. 0	Well _very_ do Some occas. fl night good, in morning some consid. fl.
17 Wed	0 Sh. 0 Dr.	Well _very_ Boil broke night good
18 Th	Sw. Sh. D. Dr.	Well very 2 not very slight fits of fl before breakfast. night fair
19 Fri	Sw. Sh. D. Sh.	Well _very_ night good with fl, oppressed.
20 Sat	Sw. Sh. D. Dr.	Well _very_ night poorish ["much" del] consid fl
21 Sun	0 Sh. 0 Dr.	Well _very_ (rash almost gone) night baddish much fl in early part
22 Mon	Sw. Sh. D. Dr.	Well. 3 fits of fl. of wh. [ich] one long night poorish
23 Tu	Sw. Sh. D. Dr.	Well almost very 2 fits of fl one very slight night poorish
24 W.	0 Sh. D Dr.	Well _very_ some occas. fl (rash gone) night good
25 Th	Sw. Sh. D. Dr.	Well _very_ ["(new boil coming)" del] night good
26 F.	Sw. Sh. D. Dr.	Well _very_ night first part baddish
27 Sat	Sw. Sh. D. D.	Well very, after tea one baddish long fit of fl, night poor, heaz very much fl
28 Sund	0 Sh. 0 0	Well 3 fits of fl of which one long. night fair
29 Mon	Sw. Sh. D. Dr.	Well 2 fits of fl of which one long night poor, wakeful yet Heazy
30 Tu.	Sw. Sh. D. Dr.	Well _very_ night poor
31 Wed.	0. Sh. 0. Dr.	Well not quite 7 fits of fl night pretty good

20 double dashes[17]

	St	lb	
18th	11	10	in summer cloths as before

& Ten days in November on same treatment[18]

849

November

Thurs 1st	Sw. Sh. D. Dr.		Well not perfectly. 4 or 5 fits of fl. night wakeful, heazy much fl.
Fri 2nd[19]	Sw. Sh. D Dr.		Well not perfectly. 4 or 5 fits of excessive fl. - night bad excessive fl.
3rd	Sw Sh D. Dr.		Well very. one fit of fl night fair
Sun 4th	Sh. Sh.		Well very one consid. fit of fl night poorish
M 5	Sh T[20]		Well, much fl. fatigue headache night good
6	Dr T		Well do do do
W 7	Dr T[21]		Well very night fair
Th 8	Dr T	London	Well much fl. night good
Fr 9	Dr T		Well do night good
Sat 10	Sw Sh. Sh.		Well very do
Sun 11	Sw Sh. Sh.		Well very do
M 12	Sh. D.		Well very night excellent. 1 slight fit fl.
13	Sw Sh. Sh. Dr		Well very night good
W 14	Sh. D.		Well almost very incipient cold uncomfort. night good.
Th 15	Packed Sh		Well very ["with" del] not well from cold night good.
16	Sh.		Well almost very 2 fits of fl London night good, wakeful
Sat 17	Dr.		Well do very 2 fits of slight fl do night poor
18	Sw. Sh. D.		Well not quite 3 fits of fl of which only one very bad night heazyish. consid. fl
M 19	Sw Sh. D.		Well not ["Boil" inserted] 5 or 6 fits of bad fl night with some consid. fits of fl.
20	Sw. Sh. Sh. Dr.		Well 5 fits of not bad fl. night with some consid. fits of fl
W 21	Sh. D.		Well 4 fits of fl night poor do
Th 22	Sh. 0 0 0		Poorly little. 4 or 5 fits of fl (Boil Broke) night pretty good
23	Sw. Sh. D.		Well very (one almost fit of fl) night good
Sat 24	Sh. D.		Well very rash night good
Sun 25	Sw. Sh. Sh.		Well very night not very good
M 26	Sh. D.		Well very (1 slight fit of fl after breakfast) night good
27	Sw. Sh. Dr Dr		Well very 1 fit of fl before breakfast night excellent
W 28	Sh. D.		Well very night good
Th 29	Sh. D.		Well very night excellent
Fr 30	Sw. Sh. Dr. Dr.		Well very night good

2 Weeks, to Nov. 10)   Sw. 5   D. 5   Dr. Twice[22]

11 Double dashes[23]

	St	lb	
7th	11	11	with flannel waistcoat

1849   December

Sat 1.	Sh. D.	Well <u>very</u> (rash continuous)	night poorish
Sund. 2nd	Sw. Sh. Sh.	Well not quite; in afternoon 6 or 7 fits of bad fl.	night poor much fl.
M. 3	Sh D	Well <u>very</u> night rather wakeful, poor	
Tu. 4	Sw. Sh. Dr. Dr.	Well <u>very</u> night rather wakeful but good	
Wed. 5	Sh. D.	Well <u>very</u> night little do do	
Th. 6	Sh. D.	Well <u>very</u> night often disturbed but goodish	
Fri 7	Sw. Sh. Dr. Dr.	Well <u>very</u> (little Boil broke / some rash) night good	
Sat 8	Sh. D.	Well <u>very</u> (little occas. fl. in evening no fl) night excellent	
Sun 9	Sw. Sh. Sh	Well <u>very</u> night not very good	
M 10	Sh. D.	Well <u>very</u> (some little occas. fl) night good	
Tu 11	Sw. Sh Dr. Dr.	Well <u>very</u> (consid. occas. fl) night poorish, much fl	
Wed 12	Sh. D.	Well <u>very</u> night good	
Th. 13	Sh. D.	Well <u>very</u> night not very good	
Fri. 14	Sw. Sh. Dr. Dr.	Well (two consid. fit & occas. fl) night bad, heazy, excessive fl	
Sat 15	Sw. Sh. Dr. Dr.	Well <u>very</u> (rash gone) night good	
Sun 16	Sw. Sh. Sh.	Well <u>very</u> (some occas fl) night pretty good	
Mon 17	Sh. D.	Well <u>very</u> (do) night do	
Tu 18	Sw. Sh. D.	Well <u>very</u> night do	
We 19²⁴	Sh. London	Well <u>very</u> night bad, wakeful, excessive fl night good	
Th 20	Dr. T²⁵ ["do inserted]	Well not quite; headache excessive fl night good	
26 ⌗			
Fi 21	Sh D.	Well <u>very</u> (no rash) night pretty good	
Sat 22	Sh. D.	Well <u>very</u> night excellent	
Sund 23	Sh. Sh.	Well <u>very</u> night pretty good ["wakeful" inserted]	
Mo 24	Sh. D.	Well <u>very</u> night very wakeful, one bad fit of fl in middle	
Tu 25	Sh. Dr. 0.	Well <u>very</u> (almost 1 fit of fl. night goodish, but good deal of fl early & ["late" del] morning	
Wed 26	Sh. D.	Well <u>very</u> (new boil) night wakeful very much fl	
Th 27	Sh. D.	Well <u>very</u> night wakeful excessive fl early in morning	
Fi 28	Sh. Dr. Dr.	Well <u>very</u> night rather wakeful, rather much fl, little in morning	
Sat 29	Sh. D.	Well <u>very</u> night good – With fl morning	
Sund. 30	Sh. Sh.	Well <u>very</u> (some occas. fl) night good – baddish fit of fl in M[orning]	
Mon 31	Sh. D.	Well <u>very</u> (not very comfortable) ["before Boil broke)" inserted] night go hardly any fl in m[orning]	

Nov 10th Dec 20 (six weeks) Sw. thrice, D. 4 times, Dr. twice[27]

28 double dashes[28]

1850 January

Tu 1st   Sh Dr. 0   Well not quite, in afternoon excessive fl. Little headach. Night wakeful very much fl.

Wed 2nd   Sh. D.   Well <u>very</u>   some occas fl   night wakeful rather much fl

Th 3   Sh. D.   Well <u>very</u>   do   night   much fl

Fr 4   Sh. Dr. Dr.   Well <u>very</u>   night wakeful   consid. fl

Sat 5   Sh. D.   Well <u>very</u>   night wakeful   do

Su 6   Sh. Dr. Dr.   Well <u>very</u>   night good, little wakeful, little fl

M 7   O D.   Well <u>very</u>   night excellent   do   very little fl.

Tu 8   Sh. Dr. Dr.   Well <u>very</u>   night good, little wakeful, consid fl m.[orning]

W. 9   Sh. D.   Well <u>very</u>   night do   do   Little fl

Th 10   Sh. D.   Well <u>very</u>   (2 slight fit of fl)   night good   do
                42°

F 11   Sh   Dr. Dr.   Well <u>very</u>   (some discomfort) night heazyish, rather much fl.

Sat 12   Sh. D.   Well <u>very</u>   night   poorish. wakeful. extreme fl

Su. 13   Sh. 0. 0.   Well <u>very</u>   night   do   do   do

M 14   Sh. D.   Well <u>very</u>   night good   E[29]   confinement

Tu. 15   Sh. Dr. Dr.   Well <u>very</u>   (some occas. fl) night good, heazyish, 2 or 3 baddish fits of Fl

W. 16   Sh. D.   Well <u>very</u>   night – consid. fl.

<u>Th. 17</u> <u>Sh.</u> D.[30]   Well <u>very</u> (some discomfort)   night heazyish, rather much fl

F. 18   Sw. Sh. Dr. 0   Well <u>very</u>   tired in evening   night often waking.   do

Sat 19   Sh. D.   Well.   3 fits of slight fl. G. unwell[31] night heazyish. 1 bad fit of fl

Su 20   Sh. 0. 0.   Well <u>very</u>   (some discomfort) night heazyish   consid. fl

M. 21   Sh. D.   Well <u>very</u>   night rather wakeful, rather much fl

Tu 22   Sw. Sh. Dr. Dr.   Well <u>very</u>   night good; little wakeful

W. 23   Sh. D.   Well <u>very</u>   night uncomfort Ge.y unwell[32]

Th. 24   Sh. D.   Well <u>very</u>   (tired in evening)   night good

Fi 25   Sw. Sh. Dr. Dr.   Well <u>very</u>   night very good

<u>Sat. 26</u>   Sh. D.   Well <u>very</u>   night good

Su. 27   Sh. 0. 0   Well <u>very</u>   (little oppressed in evening) night pretty good

M. 28   Sh. 0. 0   Well <u>very</u> (long continuous slight fl. in evening (Mitcham) night   do[33]

Tu 29   Sw. Sh. D.   Well, in afternoon not quite, several bad fits of fl   night not very good

W. 30   Sh. D.   Well not, increasing, very bad fl.   night excessive fl

Th. 31   Sh. D.   Well amost <u>very</u>, one not bad fit of fl   night poor oppressed, wakeful .

Dec. 21 to Jan 17 – four weeks, with D. 4 times per week & no lamp. Dripping twice per week

Jan 18th to Feb 12   three weeks with D. 4 times. Sw twice in six days. Dr. twice[34]
                            24 double dash[35]

1850 February

F. 1	Sw. Sh. Dr. Dr.	Well _very_ (some occasional fl) night wakeful, but very good
Sat 2	Sh. D.	Well _very_ do night very good
Sund 3	Sh. 0. 0.	Well 2 slightest fits of fl. discomfort. night wakeful, not very good
M 4	Sw. Sh. D.	Poorly, yet not much fl night languid yet rather wakeful
Tu 5	Sh. D.	Well _very_ (consid. occas. fl) night uncomfort, wakeful, exhausted.
Wed. 6	Sh.[36]	Poorly very much fl + night, bad sickness,[38] slight shivering
Th 7	Dr[37]	Poorly, better in evening night pretty good
Fi. 8	Dr	Well only about 2 or 3 slight fit night rather wakeful, good
Sat 9	Sw. Sh. Dr.	Well _very_ (2 barely fits of fl) night heazyish, much fl
Sun 10	Sh. D.	Well, in evening 1 bad fit fl. night heazy much fl
M. 11	Sh D.[39]	Well do do night pretty good

(brace grouping Wed. 6, Th 7, Fi. 8 labeled "London")

* ———————

Tu 12	Sw. Sh. Dr. D.	Well do 2 or 3 fits of fl night extreme fl.
W. 13	Sw. Sh. D.	Well _very_ 2 of the _slightest_ fits of fl night pretty good. consid fl.
Th 14	Sh. Dr. F.B.	Well _very_ do night very good
F 15	Sw. SH. D F.B.	Well _very_ some occas. fl night pretty good
Sd 16	Sh. Dr. Dr.	Well _very_ night good
Sun 17	Sw. Sh. D F.B.	Well _very_ Little occas fl night heazy, but goodish
M 18	Sh. Dr. DR.	Well _very_ night good
Tu 19	Sw. Sh. D FB	Well _very_ night good
W 20	Sw. Sh. Dr. Dr.	Well _very_ almost 1 fit of fl. night wakeful, poorish, much fl
Th 21	Sh. D. F. B.	Well _very_ do night not very good
F 22	Sw. Sh. Dr. F.B.	Well _very_ night poor much fl
Sat 23	Sh. D. F.B.	Well _very_ night heazish, rather much fl
Sun 24	Sw. Sh. Dr. F.B.	Well _very_ night poor, heazy much fl.
M. 25	Sh. D. F.B	Well _very_ night very poor. extreme fl
Tu 26	Sw. Sh. Dr. Dr.	Well _very_ (1 fit of fl night bad, ["exhausted" del] extreme fl
W 27	Sh. D. FB	Well. 2 fits of fl not bad, night poor wakeful. extreme fl
Th 28	Sw. Sh. D. FB	Well _very_ night bad, ["much" del] extreme fl.

15 Double[40]

	St	lb		
Feb. 26	11	13 ¾	(thick trousers Fl.[annel] W.[aistcoat])	15 double dashes

1850

March

F. 1	Sh. 0. F.B.	Poorly, light headache excessive fl. night bad excessive fl
Sat 2	Sw. Sh. D. Dr.	Poorly, little light headache several fits of fl ["Boil broke" inserted]
		night pretty good
Sun 3	Sw. Sh. D. F.B.	Well, very, one long fit of fl night poorish, wakeful much fl
M 4	Sh. D. F. B.	Well very night wakeful, not good
T. 5	Sw. Sh. Dr. Dr.	Well very night good, but consid fl.
Wed 6	Sh. D. F.B.	Well very almost fit of fl. night wakeful, goodish
Th 7	Sw. Sh. D.	Well very (some occas fl) night with consid fl
F. 8	Sw. Sh. Dr. Dr.	Well very (do) night pretty goodish
Sat 9	Sh. D.	Well very night goodish
Sun 10	Sw. Sh. Sh.	Well very night pretty good
M. 11	Sh. D.	Well not quite in evening 1 bad & 2 slight fits of fl night languid, pretty good
Tu 12	Sw. Sh. Dr Dr	Well very (some occas. fl) night good
W 13	Sw. Sh. D.	Well ["almost very" inserted] 1 longish & 1 slight fit of fl
		night, heazest, poorest, consid fl.
Th 14	Sh. D. F.B.	Well very night often waking consid fl.
F. 15	Sw. Sh Dr. Dr.	Well very (3 slight fits of fl. night poorish heaz yet wakeful. do
Sd 16	Sh. D. F.B.	Well very , yet poorly with occas fl night heazest, but pretty good
Sun. 17	Sw. Sh Sh	Well very 2 slight fits of fl. night poor wakeful
M 18	Sh. D.	Well very almost 1 fit of fl night pretty good
Tu. 19	Sw. Sh. D.	Well very night good
W. 20	Sw. Sh. Dr. 0.	Well not quite 5 or 6 slight fits of fl night poor, oppressed excessive fl
Th 21	Sh. D.	Well very (some occas fl) night pretty good
F. 22	Sw. Sh. Dr. F.B.	(2 & ½ ["slight" inserted] fits of fl.) night poorish extreme fl
Sat 23	Sh. D.	Well (4 slight fits of fl) night pretty good
Sun 24	Sw. Sh. Sh.	Well very night bad, heazy, 1 very bad fit of fl
M. 25th	Sh. D.	Well (in evening 2 or 3 bad fits of fl night much fl
Tu 26	Sw. Sh. Dr. Dr.	Well 3 or 4 slightest fit of fl night very much fl
W. 27	Sw Sh. D.	Well very some occas. fl & discomfort – night good
Th 28	Sh. D.	Well very night good. somewhat oppressed
F. 29	Sw. Sh. Dr Dr	Well very night very much fl
Sat. 30	Sw. D.	Well 4 fits of fl of which 1 bad night do heazy
Sun. 31	Sw. Sh. Sh.	Well 3 fits of fl night do do
		["11" del] 16 double dashes[41]

	St	lb	
March 27th	11	11 ¾ in thick trousers Fl. wt	/ all this must explain weariness in Evening

1850
April

M. 1	Sh. D.	Well very. 1 fit of not bad fl. Night consid fl heazish, pretty good
Tu 2.[d]	Sw. Sh. Dr. Dr.	Well very do night pretty good
W 3	Sw. Sh. D. FB	Well very 2 slight fits of fl night good but heazish
Th 4	Sh. D.	Well very 1 & almost 2 slight fits of fl night heazy
F. 5	Sw. Sh. Dr. Dr.	Well 2 slight fit & occas fl night heazish much fl
Sat 6	Sh. D.	Well 3 fits of fl night consid fl
Sun 7.	Sw. Sh. Sh.	Well 3 or 4 fits of fl night do
M. 8	Sw. Sh. D.	very much fl night poorish very much fl
Tu. 9	T[42]	do some headache night do do
W. 10[43]	T	do night better. do
Th. 11	T	do night pretty good. much fl
F. 12.	Sw. Sh. D.	Well very night very heazy. extreme fl
Sat 13	Sh. D.	Well very almost fits of fl night at first very much fl. then good
Su. 14	Sw. Sh. F.B.	Well very night very good
M. 15	Sh. D.	Well very (Boil) night at first very much fl; then good
Tu. 16	Sw. Sh. Dr. F.B.	Well very , almost 1 fit of fl. night good
W. 17	Sw. Sh. D.	Well very night good
Th. 18	Sh. D.	Well very almost 1 fit of fl night restless, but very good
F. 19	Sw. Sh. Dr.	Well very consid. occas. fl night very good
Sat 20	Sh. Dr. Dr.	Well very (Boil broke) night, later much fl.
Su 21	Sw. Sh. 0. 0.	Well very night heazish, do
M. 22	Sh. D.	Well very night poorish, much fl.
Tu 23	Sw. Sh. Dr. Dr.[44]	Well 2 slight fits of fl. (discomfort) night heazish
W. 24	Sw. Sh. D.	Well. 1 slight. 1 baddish fit of fl night ["do" inserted] pretty good
Th 25	Sh. D.	Well very night poorish. very much fl
F. 26	Sw. Sh.	Well very some occas fl night good
Sat 27	Sh. D.	Well very night very good
Sun. 28[45]	Sw. Sh. O	Well very some occas fl night good
M. 29	Sh. D.	Well very night very good, rather wakeful
Tu 30	Sw. Sh. D.	Well very almost 1 fit of fl. ["2 little boils" inserted]

(London — bracketed beside M. 8 – Th. 11)

night poorish, early extreme fl.

17 double dash[46]

		St	lb	oz
18th	at 2 oclock / with thin cloth trouser	St	lb	oz
	Left off Compress, & waistcoat flannel	11.	13 ["12" del] ¾

Some few evenings less tired

<u>1850</u>

May -- 1 --	Sh. D.	Well <u>very</u> . Some occas fl. night good	
Th 2	Sh. 0. 0.	Well 2 or 4 very slight fits, much discomfort night uncomfortable	
Fi. 3	Sh. 0 0.	Well 2. slight fits, evening do night do. but very much fl.	
<u>Sat 4</u>	Sw Sh. D	Well very. 1 slight fit & occas. fl. night pretty good	
S 5th	Sh D.	Well <u>very</u> night almost very good	
M 6	Sw. Sh. D.	Well <u>very</u> almost 1 fit of fl. night good	
Tu 7	Sw. Sh. D.	Well <u>very</u> night good ["but bad" del] 2 fits of fl in morning	
W. 8	Sh. D.	Well <u>very</u> night very good, heazish	
Th 9	Sw. Sh. D.	Well <u>very</u> night 3 bad fits of fl. acid from stomach	
F. 10	Sh. D.	Well. 3 bad fits of fl. night good	
<u>Sat. 11</u>	Sw. Sh.	Well. do night pretty good	
Sun 12	Sh. 0 0	Well not quite much l night considerable fl.	
M. 13	Sh. [London]	Well not quite excessive fl night pretty good	
Tu 14	Sw. Sh. D.	Well <u>very</u> almost 1 fit of fl. night consid. fl. heazish	
W 15	Sw. Sh. D.	Well <u>very</u> almost 1 fit of fl night much fl	
Th 16	Sh. D	Well <u>very</u> night consid. fl	
F. 17	Sw. Sh. D.	Well <u>very</u>. 1 fit of fl. from excitment[47] night rather much fl	
<u>Sat 18</u>	Sh. D.	Well. 2 rather bad fits of fl (Got Boil) night do	
<u>S. 19</u>	Sw. Sh. O. O.[48]	Work not at all extreme fl. night heazy 2 very bad fits of fl	
M. 20	Sh. D. Dr.	Well not quite 5 or 6 bad fits of fl night not very bad. consid fl	
Tu 21	D. Sw. Sh. Dr	Well not quite do do night much fl	
W. 22	Sh. D. Dr.	Well not quite 6 or 7 bad fits of fl (Boil ["first" inserted] broke) night heazish. much fl	
Th 23	Sw. Sh. D. Dr.	Well 2 fits of fl. one bad night much fl	
F 24	D. Sw. Sh. Dr	Well 3 fits of fl. one baddish night consid. fl	
<u>Sat 25</u>	Sh. D. F.B.	Poorly Little in excessive fl.: slight headache night at first much fl. after good	
S. 26	Sw. Sh. 0. 0.	Well not quite. much fl slight headach night pretty good	
M. 27	Sh. D. Dr.	Well <u>very</u> 1 long slight fit of fl night do heazish	
Tu 28	D. Sw. Sh. Dr.	Well <u>very</u> night very good	
W 29	Sh. D. Dr.	Well <u>very</u> almost 1 slight fit of fl night good. heazish	
Th 30	Sw. Sh. D. Dr.	Well very. 3 slight fits of fl night consid fl	Successiv Boils
F. 31st	Sh. D. Dr.	Well <u>very</u> night pretty good. rather wakeful	

12 double dashes

12 double d.[49]

	St.	lb	oz	
10	11	13	10	
28	11	12	8	(light plaid trousers.)

<u>1850</u>
June

Sat 1	D. Sw. Sh. Dr.	Well <u>very</u>	1 fit of fl.		night restless consid fl.
S. 2nd	Sw. Sh. O F.B.	Well very	2 slightest fits of fl.		night very good
M. 3	Sh. D.	Very much fl			
Tu 4	Dr.	do	(London)		
W 5	Dr.	do: in evening well			
Th 6	Dr	Well <u>very</u>			
F. 7	Sw. Sh. D. Dr.	Well <u>very</u> 1 long fit of fl		Boils	night pretty good
Sat 8	Sh. D. Dr.	Well <u>very</u>			night do
S. 9	Sw. Sh. 0. 0.	Well <u>very</u> 1 & almost 2 fits of fl			night pretty good
M. 19	Sh. D.	Well <u>very</u> do			night do
Tu 11	Sh. D. Travelling	Extreme fl			night good
W 12	O. D.	Well <u>very</u> 2 slight fits of fl			night very good
Th 13	D. Sw. Sh.	Well[50] <u>very</u> some occas. fl			night indifferent
F. 14	D. Sw. Sh	Well 3 or 4 fits of fl	(Malvern)		night good
Sat 15	D., S., Sh	Well <u>very</u> 2 longish fits of fl. yet very vigorous			night good
Su 16	D. O. O.	Well 2 or 3 do			night heazish good
M. 17	D. Sw. Sh	Well <u>very</u> do			night pretty good
Tu 18	Dr. Travelling	much fl			night good
W 19	Sh. D. Sitz[51]	Well <u>very</u> 2 slight fits of fl			night heaz much fl
Th 20	Sw. Sh. O Sitz	Well 3 fits of fl			night heazish do
F. 21	Sh D Sitz	Well <u>very</u> 1 or 2 slight fits of fl			night heazish, pretty good
Sat 22	Sw. Sh Dr Sitz	Well <u>very</u>			night uncomfort. very much fl
S. 23	Sh. O. O.	Well <u>very</u> 1 long fit of fl			night heazish with much fl
M 24	Sh D Sitz	Well 2 long fits of fl ["Evening" inserted] (Salad)			night pretty good
Tu 25	Sw. Sh. D.	Well <u>very</u> 1 long fit of fl			evening night good except mo
W 26	Sh. O. O.	Well 2 or 3 slight fits of fl			night wakeful good
Th 27	Sw. Sh. D. F.B.	Well <u>very</u> occas. fl. (new Boil)			night rather idle. good
F. 28	Sh. O. O.	Well <u>very</u> 1 do			night goodish, heazish
Sun 30	Sh. O O	Well 2 or 3 slight fits of fl.			night good.

5 double[52]

1850

July

M. 1	Sw. Sh. D.		Excessive fl	Boil broke	night baddish
Tu 2	Dr		do		night pretty good
W 3	Dr.	London	much fl		night good
Th. 4	Sw. Sh. D.		Well very	1 very slight fit of fl.	night very good
F 5	Sh. D.		Well very	some ocass fl.	night good
Sd 6	Sw. Sh. D.		Well very	2 fits of fl. of which one long	night good
Sun 7	Sh. 0. 0.		Well very	some occas fl	night good
M. 8	Sh. D.		Well very	1 long slight fit of fl	night moderate
T. 9	Sw. Sh. D.		Well very	1 do	night do morning bad fl
W 10	Sh. 0. 0.		Well not quite. Much fl		night good
Th. 11	Sw. Sh. D.		Well	2 or 3 long fits of fl	night do
F. 12	Sh. 0.	Boils	Poorly a little much fl		night good
Sd. 13	Sw. Sh. D.		Well very	some occas. fl	night pretty good
S. 14	Sh. O.		Well very	2 slight fits of fl	night indifferent
M. 15	Sh. D.		Well very	1 longish fit of fl	do
T. 16	Sw. Sh. D.		Well very	2 slight fits of fl	night good
W. 17	Sh.		Well very		night consid. fl
Th. 18	Sw. Sh. D.		Well very	some occas. fl	night do
F 19	Sh		Well very		night after first part good
Sat 20	Sw. Sh D.		Well very	1 slight fit of fl	night, pretty good
Sun 21	Sh.		Well not quite. several not bad fits of fl		night first part bad
M. 22	Sh. D.		Well	3 fits of fl. not bad	night fair
Tu. 23	Sw. Sh. D.		Well very some occas fl		night consid. fl. –
W. 24	Sh.		Well very	do	rather much fl
Th. 25	Sw. Sh. D.		Well very	1 long fit of fl	heazish
F. 26	Sh.		Well not quite	several slight fits of fl	not good
Sat 27	Sw. Sh. D.	Little Boil broke / new slight Boil	Well very		heazish do
S. 28	Sh.		Well not quite. heaz much slight fl continuous		heazish do
M. 29	Sh. D.		Well very	1 slight fit of fl	night good
T. 30	Sw. Sh. D.		Well very	do	considerable fl.
W. 31	Sh		Well very	1 long fit of fl	very much fl.

	St	lb		
9th	11	12	.	9 double dashes[53]

1850 August			Night
Th. 1	["Sw. Sh. D" inserted]	Well very	pretty good
F. 2	Sh	Well very	much fl
Sat 3	Sh	Well very	early part good. morning excessive fl. a◦
S. 4	Sh.	Well very 2 slight fits of fl	night moderate
M. 5	Sh. D.	Well 2 consid fits of fl.	night pretty good
Tu 6	Sw. Sh.	Well very 1 fit o fl	night at first uncomf then good
W. 7	Sh.	Well very do	moderate
Th. 8	Sw. Sh. D.	Well very do	good
F. 9	Sh	Well very 2 fits of fl	good
Sat 10	Sh	Well very consid occass fl	very good
Su 11	Dr. T.[54]	Well barely very much fl	good
M 12	Dr.	Well very 2 fits of fl	night indifferent heazish
T 13	Dr.	Well not quite much fl.	night heazish
W 14	Dr.	Well very 2 fitrs of fl	heazish
Th 15	Dr.	Well very	good
F 16	Dr.	Well very	good
Sd. 17	Dr	Well very	indifferent
S. 18	Dr	Well very almost fit of fl	poor, much fl
M. 19	Dr.	Well very	good. morning baddish fit
T. 20	Sw Sh. D.	Well very	pretty good. consid fl.
W 21	Sh.	Well. 2 baddish fits of fl	modest do
Th. 22	Sh. D.	Well very. 1 baddish fit of fl	consid fl
F 23	Sw. Sh.	Well very 2 mod. fits of fl.	do heazish
Sat 24	Sh. D.	Well very. 1 baddish 1 slight fit	do heazish
S. 25	Sh.	Well very Boil	good
M. 26	Sh. D.	Well very 2 fits of fl	indifferent consid fl.
T. 27	Sw. Sh.	Well very 1 slight fit of fl	pretty good
W. 28	Sw Sh	Well very broke	much fl
Th 29	Sh. D.	Well very 1 slight fit of fl.	baddish, oppressed much fl
F. 30	Sw. Sh.	Well very almost 1 fit of fl	pretty good
Sat 31	Sh. D.	Well very	good

Leith Hil [55]

11 double dashes[56]

1850 September   Night

Day			Night
Sun 1	Sh.	Well <u>very</u> <u>occas</u> fl (a little rash)	good
M. 2	Sh. D.	Well <u>very</u> do	consid fl
T. 3	Sw. Sh. D.	Well <u>very</u> much do	much fl.
W 4	Sh.	Well <u>very</u>	very much fl
Th 5	Sh. D.	Well <u>very</u> much fl.	much fl
F. 6	Dr. 0 London.	Well not quite. excessive fl. slight headache	excessive fl.
Sat 7	Sw. Sh D.	Well <u>very</u>	extreme fl (Willy ill)[57]
S. 8	Sh.	Well <u>very</u>, barely fit of fl & much occas	consider .fl
M. 9	Sh. D	Well <u>very</u>	rather much fl
Tu 10	Sw. Sh. D.	Well not quite. very much cont. fl	extreme fl. oppressed
W 11	Sh	Well do (Cold)	much fl. do
Th 12	Sh. D.	Well <u>very</u> 2 very slight fits of fl	pretty good
F. 13	Sw. Sh.D.	Well <u>very</u> 1 consid fit of fl	extreme lf
Sat 14	Sh. D.	Well very 2 slight fits of fl.	much fl
S. 15	Sh	Well <u>very</u>	do
M. 16	Sh. D.	Well <u>very</u> 1 fit of fl	rather much fl.
T. 17	Sw. Sh. D.	Well <u>very</u> 1 long fit of fl (rash continued)	very much fl.
W. 18	Sh.	Well several fits not bad of fl	do oppressed
Th. 19	Sh. D.	Well do do	do do
F. 20	Sw. Sh.	Well very 1 fit & almost second do	much fl.
Sat 21	Sh. D.	Well <u>very</u> 1 slight fit of fl occas. fl	pretty good
S 22	Sh	Well <u>very</u> some consid fl	1 do
M 23	Sh. D.	Well very 2 slight fits of fl much fl.	little oppressed
T. 24	Sw. Sh. D.	Well <u>very</u> 1 slight & occas fl	excessive fl. discomfort
W. 25	Sh.	Well <u>very</u> do do	rather much fl
Th. 26	Sh. D.	Well very 2 fits of fl	very much fl
F. 27	Sw. Sh. D.	Well <u>very</u> 1 fit of fl	rather much fl
Sat 28	Sh. D.	Well several sligh fits of fl	pretty good
S. 29	Sh.	Well barely do	do
M. 30	Sh.	Well <u>very</u> consid occas fl	excessive fl

8 double dashes[58]

1850	October			Night
Tu 1	Sw. Sh. D.	Well not quite, much fl		pretty good. oppressed
W. 2	Sh. D.	Well <u>very</u> almost 1 fit of fl		good
Th 3	Sh.	Well <u>very</u> some occas fl		consid fl
F 4	Sw. Sh. D.	Well <u>very</u> 1 small fit & ½ anoth		pretty good
Sat 5	Th. Sh. D.	Well <u>very</u>		do
Sun 6	S.	Well <u>very</u>		do
M. 7	Sh. D.	Well <u>very</u> 1 slight fit		do
T 8	Sw. Sh. D.	Well <u>very</u> 1 do almost two	persistent surface boil	indifferent, oppressed, much fl
W. 9	Sh.	Well very 2 fits of fl		night good
Th 10	Sh. D.	Well <u>very</u> 1 slight fit		wakeful. not much fl.
F 11	Sw. Sh. D.	Well barely 3 fits of fl		night little oppressed. much fl
Sat 12	Sh. D.	Well not quite. several fits of fl		shivering, vomit, very much fl + [59]
Sun 13	Sh.	Poorly a Little, excessive fl		later with consid. fl

**

M 14	Sh.	Poorly a Little excessive fl	Little Boil	extreme fl
T 15	Dr.	Well not quite extreme fl		rather much fl
W. 16	Dr.	Well many fits of fl		good
Th 17	Dr	Well almost very 3 or 4 fits of fl		good heazish
F. 18	Dr.	Well not quite, extreme fl		do do
Sat 19	Swim	Well almost very 3 fits of fl		do do
Sun 20	Swim	Well do		do
M 21	Swim	Poorly, excessive continued fl Little Boil		poorish
Tu 22	O	Well 3 or 4 not bad fit of fl 12 bad days![62]		good
W. 23	Sh	Well <u>very</u> 1 slightest fit of fl		good
Th. 24	Sh.	Well <u>very</u>		good
F. 25	Sh.	Well 3 fits of fl		good
Sat 26	Sh.	Well <u>very</u> 1 & nearly 2 fits of fl		modest. Little oppressed
Su 27	Sh.	Well <u>very</u> 1 fit of fl		moderately good
M 28	Sh	Well <u>very</u> rather uncomfortable		good heazish
Tu 29	Sw. Sh. D.	Well <u>very</u> 1 fit of fl		moderately good
W 30	Sh. D.	Well very 2 fits of fl		moderate
Th. 31	Sw. Sh.	Well 3 fits of fl		extreme fl.

(bracket grouping Oct 14–22: Ramsgate[61] Hartfield[60])

5 double dash[63]

Oct. 14 not tired in evening[64]

1850 November				Night
F. 1	Sh. D.	Well	3 fits of fl	much fl heazish
Sat 2	Sw. Sh. D.	Well very	2 or 3 slight fits of fl	consid fl
S 3	Sh	Will	3 baddish fits of fl	do pretty good
M. 4	Sw. Sh. D.	Well very	3 fits of fl slight	good
Tu 5	Sh. D.	Well very, but not quite in morning. 3 fits of fl		good
W. 6	Sw. Sh	Well several slight fits of fl		good
Th. 7	Sh. D	Well very 1 fit & some occas fl		moderate
F. 8	Sw. Sh.	Well. 1 baddish & 1 slight fit	poor ["very" inserted]	much fl
Sat.9	Sh. O	Poorly. bed feverish		bad
Sun 10	Packed	Poorly bed. much continued fl. (cold)	some bad fits of fl	
M. 11	Sw. Sh. D. F.B.	Well very	2 ½ fits of fl	much fl
Tu. 12	Sh. F.B. Well very	cold	2 or 3 fits of fl	good
W. 13	Sh. FB	Well very	1 consid. & 1 light fit of fl	pretty good
Th. 14	Sw. Sh. F.B.	Well very	1 fit of fl	poor excessive fl
F. 15	Sh. F.B.	Well very	2 consid fits of fl	pretty good
Sat 16	Sw. Sh. F.B.	Well. much continued fl (Mitcham)[65]		moderately good
Sun. 17	Sh. F.B.	Well very	1 fit of fl (Boils)	do
M. 18	Sw Sh F.B.	Well very	occas fl	do
Tu 19	Sh. F.B.	Well very	do	do
W. 20	Sw. Sh. D. F.B.	Well very	do	not very good
Th. 21	Sh. D.	Well very two fit in evening		do
F. 22	Sw. Sh.. F.B.	Well very	do	do
‡				
Sat 23	Sh. D. F.B.	Well very	occas. fl	do
Sun 24	Sh.	Well very	1 fit of fl evening	good
M 25	Sw. Sh. D. F.B	Well very	do	not very good
Tu 26	Sh. D. F.B.	Well very	do	do
W. 27	Sh. F.B.	Well several fits of fl.		indifferent
Th. 28	Sw. Sh. D. FB	Well very 1 fit in evening		poorish
F 29	Sh D. FB	Well very 1 fit		indifferent
Sat 30.	Sh. D.	Well very	do	pretty good

with rash

Little rash

4 dash[66]

1850 December		(Diary page 20)		Night
Sun. 1	Sw Sh	Well very	1 fit & almost another	indifferent
Mon 2	Sh. D.	Well very	2 fits one baddish	good
Tu 3	Sh. D.	Well very	1 fit	good
W 4	Sw. Sh.	Well	3 or 4 fits of fl	pretty good
Th 5	Sh. D.	Well very	2 fits of fl	good
Fr. 6	Sh	Well very	1 fit & occas	good
Sat 7	Sh. D.	Well very	occas fl bad, excessive fl.	slight shivers.
S. 8	Sw. Sh.	Well barely	3 or 4 fits of fl	goodish, but heasy
M. 9	Sh D	Well very	2 or 3 slight fits	good
Tu 10	Sh. D.	Well very	1 fit	good
W. 1	Sw. Sh.	Well very, but in eveng 1 bad fit		bad. vomit, excessive acid
Th 12	Sh F.B.	Poorly, extreme continued fl		good
F. 13	Sh.D.	Well very	1 fit & occas fl	wakeful but good
Sat 14	Sw. Sh. D.	Well very	do	indifferent
S. 15	Sh.	Well very	2 fits of fl	wakeful, poor much
M. 16	Sh. D.	Well	2 fits of fl	moderate
T. 17	Sh.	Well	much fl	moderate
W. 18	Dr.[67]	Well hardly, slight headache much fl		poor headache
Th. 19	Dr.	do	in evening very well	pretty good
F. 20	Dr	Well very though with fl		wakeful
Sat 21	Dr	do	do	good
Sun 22	Dr.	Well	3 or 4 fits of fl	indifferent
M. 23	Sw. Sh. D.	Well very	occas fl	heazish but good
Tu 24	Sh. D.	Well very	in evening 2 bad fit of fl	indifferent
W. 25	Sh.	Well very	occas fl.	Vomit, ["not acid" inserted], dazzle headache, excessive fl
Th. 26	Sh.	Poorly a little, much slight continued fl		heazish pretty good
F. 27	Sw. Sh D	Well very	occas fl.	good, little heazish
Sat 28	Sh. D.	Well very	1 slight fit	indifferent
Sun 29	Sh.	Well very	do & occas fl.	do
M. 30	Sh. D.	Well very	do do	do
T. 31	Sw. Sh.	Well	4 fits of fl	do

(The rows for W.18–Sat 21 are bracketed together with the note "London")

4 dashes[68]

24th began Tartar Emetic Ointment, & rubbed in for 12 days[69]

1851 January   <u>Night</u>

Day		Well	Fits		Night
Wed. 1	Sh. D.	Well <u>very</u>	1 fit of fl.		good
Th. 2	Sh. D.	Well <u>very</u>	occas fl.		pretty good
F. 3	Sw. Sh.	Well <u>very</u>	do		do
<u>Sat 4</u>	Sh. D.	Well <u>very</u>	do		wakeful do
Sun 5	Sh.	Well	4 fits of fl		good
M. 6	Sh. D.	Well <u>very</u>	1 fit of ["fl" omitted]		pretty good
T. 7	Sw. Sh. D.	Well <u>very</u>	do slight long continued		moderately good
W. 8	Sh. D.	Well <u>very</u>	do do		pretty good
Th. 9	Sh. D	Well very	do do		good
F 10	Sw. Sh.	Well very	3 fits of fl		indifferent
<u>Sat 11</u>	Sh. D.	Well <u>very</u>	2 fit		pretty good

———⚬ 70

Day		Well	Fits	Boils	Night
Su 12	Sh	Well	2 fits of fl. & occas		do
M. 13	Sh	Well	feeling poorly but not much flt		do heazish
T 14	Dr. T	Well; hardly	do 2 fits of do slight	Boils coming cause of unwelness	do do
W 15	Sh	Poorly a little	do do		
Th 16	Sh. D.	Well <u>very</u>	2 very slight fiits of fl	broke	indifferent
F. 17	Sh	Well very	2 fits of fl		do
<u>Sat 18</u>	Sh. D.	Well <u>very</u>	1 fit		do
Sun 19	Sh.	Well very	2 strong fits of fl another boil came		pretty good
M. 20	Sh. D.	Well <u>very</u>	1 fit		do
T. 21	Sh.	Poorly headache, excessive fl. from Boils			good
W. 22	Sh. D.	Well <u>very</u>	occas. fl		pretty good
Th. 23	Sh	Well <u>very</u>	1 very slight fit		do
F. 24	Sh. D.	Well <u>very</u>			mod. good
<u>Sat. 25</u>	Sh.	Well <u>very</u>			do heazish
Sun 26	Sh	Well <u>very</u>	1 fit. some discomfort ["very bad" insert]		indifferent
M. 27	Sh	Well	3 or 4 fits of fl do		do heazish
Tu 28	Sh.	Well <u>very</u>	1 slight fit		do good
W 29	Sh	Well <u>very</u>	occas fl		pretty good
Th 30	Sh	Well <u>very</u>	2 or 3 <u>very</u> slight fits	indiff.	heazish
F. 31	Sh. D.	Well <u>very</u>			moderately good

8 double dashes[71]

oz
Jan 4th (thick trousers & flannel w:)   12 7 4

["9th began Tartar"] , then crossed out.[72]

1851 February					Night
Sat. 1	Sh. D.	Well very,	1 slight fit	(new boils)	indifferent
Su. 2	Sh.	Well very	do		do
M. 3	Sh. D.	Well very	do & occas.		indifferent, heazish
Tu. 4	Sh.	Well in very not quite; much fl			indifferent
W. 5	Sh.	Poorly considerab[le] flat			half good
Th. 6	Sh.	Poorly a little	do		do
F. 7	Sh.	Well not quite. 2 or 3 bad fits		broken	indifferent
Sat. 8	Sh.	Well 2 consid fits of fl			pretty good
S. 9	Sh	Well 2 fits of fl			moderate heazish
M. 10	Sh. D.	Well very	almost 1 fit		do do
T 11 ♯	Sw. Sh. D.	Well very	1 slight fit		indifferent
W. 12	Sh. D.	Well very	do		pretty good
Th. 13	Sw. Sh. D.	Well very	1 sharpish fit		do heazish
F. 14	Sh. D.	Well very	1 slight fit, some discomf.		do
Sat 15	Sw. Sh. D.	Well very	do		indifferent
S. 16	Sh	Well 3 slight fits		pretty good	heazish
M 17	Sw. Sh. D.	Well very			moderately g.[ood] do
T. 18	Sh. D.	Well very	1 slight fit		heasy
W. 19	Sw. Sh. D.	Well 2 fits of fl			pretty good, heasz
Th 20	Sh	Well. 2 or 3 fits, not comfortable			heasy
F. 21	Sh.	Well 2 or 3 fits			heazish
Sat 22	Sh. D.	Well barely much fl		Lyell's visit	much fl. pretty good
S. 23	Sh	Well 2 or 3 fits of fl.			do heasz
M 24	Sh	Well bar[ely] do			do
T. 25	Sh. D.	Well. 2 or 3 fits of fl			heaszish
W. 26	Sh. Sw. Sh	Well very	1 fit of fl		heaszish
Th. 27	Sh. D.	Well 2 fits fl (Tartar Emetic O.[intment] in evening)[73]			do
F. 28	Sw. Sh. D.	Well almost very 2 slight fits			a little hea[s]y

2 double[74]

1851	March			Night
Sat. 1	Sh. D.	Poorly Little, heasz		heaszish. pretty good
S. 2	Sw. Sh.	Well 2 fits; in evening bad fl, to bed.		pretty good
M 3	Sh. D.	Well very. 1 fit of fl.		heaszish. do
T. 4	Sw. Sh. D.	3 sharpish fits of fl (Croton)[75]		good
W. 5	Sh. D	Well very. 1 fit of fl		good
Th 6	Sw. Sh. D.	Well 2 or 3 consid fl		good
F. 7	Sh. D.	Well very, heasy much fl		pretty good
Sat 8	Sw. Sh. D.	Well several fits of fl		do
Sun 9	Sh	Well do		do
M. 10	Sh. D.	Well almost very. 1 baddish fit (new Boil)		do
T 11	Sh	Well 3 fits of fl		do
W. 12	Sh. D.	Well. 3 fits of fl		moderately good
Th. 13	Sh.	Well very 1 sharp fit		do
F. 14	Sh. D.	Well 2 or 3 fits		not very good
Sat 15	Sh	Well 2 or 3 fits fatigued from shivering		poor. headache
Sun. 16	Sh	Poorly with Influenza	do	do
M. 17	Sh	Well very 1 fit do	["pretty" del]	barely good
T 18	Sw. Sh	Well much fl do	pretty good	
W. 19	Sh	Well barely do do		moderately good
Th. 20	Sw. Sh	Poorly influenza		do
F. 21	Dr.	do do		pretty good
Sat 22	Sh. D.	Well very		do
Sun 23	Sw. Sh	Well 2 or 3 fits of fl		good
M. 24	Sh	Several fits of fl		
T. 25				
W. 26				
Th. 27				
F. 8	Malvern & London no day without fits of fl. but got well[74]			
Sat. 29				
Sun 30			1 double[77]	
M. 31				

1851 April				Night	
T. 1	Sh	Well _very_	1 slight fit	pretty good	
W. 2		Well _very_	do	not very good, much fl	
Th. 3		Well _very_		pretty good	
F. 4		Well _very_	almost one fit	moderately good	
Sat 5		Well _very_	1 slight fit	do	
Su 6		Well _very_	1 consid fl	not very good	
M 7		Well _very_	almost fit	indifferent	
T. 8		Well very.	2 slight fits	pretty good	
W. 9		Well very	do	wakeful	indifferent
Th. 10		Well. Headache in after noon		Kew	Bad
F. 11	O	Poorly		Bad	
Sat 12	O	Poorly - vomit, not heavily		Bad	
Sun 13	Dr.	consid. fl	pretty well	moderate	
M 14	Sh	Well not very.	2 or 3 fits	pretty good	
T. 15					
W. 16					
Th. 17					
F. 18					
Sat 19					
S. 20					
M. 21					
T. 22		Malvern			
W. 23					
Th 24					
F. 25					
Sat 26		78			
S. 27	Sh.	2 or 3 fits, slight	oppressed	heaszish	
M 28	Sh.	do	do	do pretty good	
T. 29	Sh.	do	do	heaz	
W. 30	Sh	do	do	pretty good	

3 double dashes[79]

1851 May						Night
Th. 1	Sh.	Well barely	3 or 4 slight fits of fl. oppressed			oppressed
F. 2	Sh.	do	do	do		pretty good
Sat 3	Sh.	do	do	slightly		do
S. 4	Sh.	do	do	slightly do		do
M. 5	Sh	Well	3 fits of fl			moderately good
T. 6	Sh.	Well very	1 fit of fl			indifferent much fl
W. 7	Sh.	Well	2 fits of fl		slight eruption	moderately good
Th. 8	Sh	Well	do			pretty good
F. 9	Sh	Well	do			pretty good
Sat 10	Sh	Well	3 fits of fl			indifferent
Su 11	Sh	Well	3 fits of fl			pretty good. heasz
M. 12	Sh	Well very	1 fit of fl & occas.			indifferent. extreme. fl-
T. 13	Sh	Well very	occas.	Child Born 9° 30' [80]		very good
W. 14	Sh.	Well very	2 fits			moderately good
Sh. 2						
Th 15	Sh.	Well very	1 fit			pretty good
F. 16	Sh.	Well very	2 fits			moderately good
Sd 17	Sh.	Well almost very	2 sharpish fit			very good
Su. 18	Sh.	Well very	1 fit			moderately good
M. 19	Sh.	Well	2 or 3 slight fits uncomfortable		sl. Eruption	pretty good
T. 20	Sh.	Well very	2 fits of fl – oppressed			do
W. 21	Sh.	Well	2 or 3 fits do			do
Th. 22	Sh.	Well	do			indifferent
F. 23	Sh	Well	2 fits			pretty good
Sd 24	Sh	Well very				moderate
Sun 25	Sh	Well very 2 – slight fits				pretty good
M 26	Sh	Well very			Eruption almost gone	do
T. 27	Sh.	Well very	1 slight fit			very good
W. 28	Sh.	Well very	do			indifferent
Th. 29	Sh	Well very				very good
F 30	Sh	Well very	1 fit			pretty good
Sat 31	Sh	Well very	1 slight fit			good

3 double dashes[81]

1851 June   Night

Sun 1	Sh.	Well very	2 slight fits of fl	moderate
M 2		Well very	occas fl	wakeful good
Tu 3		Well almost very	2 or 3 slight fits	pretty good
W. 4		Well very		wakeful do
Th. 5		Well very		pretty good
F. 6		Well very	1 slight fit	do
Sat 7		Well very	1 longish fit	do
Su. 8		Well very	2 longish fits, squashy	Little oppressed
				pretty good
M. 9	82	Well very	do do	do do
T. 10		Well	2 or 3 fits	heasz do
W. 11		Well very	1 slight fit	good
Th. 12		Well not quite .	several fits, slight headache	pretty good
F. 13		Well very	2 fits of fl	wakeful indifferent
Sat 14		Well very	do	wakeful do
Sun 15		Well very		do do
M. 16		Well very	1 & ½ fit	pretty good
T. 17		Well very	occas fl	rather indifferent
W. 18		Well very	2 slight fits	do
Th. 19		Well very		wakeful indifferent
F. 20		Well very		do rather indifferent
Sat 21		Well very		do poor
Sun 22		Well very	2 slight fits	do rather indifferent
M. 23		Well	3 fits	do poor
T. 24		Well very	occas fl	very good
W. 25		Well very	1 fit	Little wakeful rather indifferen
Th. 26		Well very	1 & almost ½ other	pretty good
F. 27		Well not quite, consid fl.	slight headache	do
S. 28		Well very		do
Sun 29		Well very	1 & ½ fit	moderate
M. 30		Well very	occas fl	do

83

11 double dashes[84]

1851 July					Night		
Tu. 1	Well very	3 slight fits			pretty good		
W. 2	Well not quite, several fits, slight headache				pretty good		
Th. 3	Well very	2 fits			moderate		
F. 4	Well very	1 fit			wakeful	pretty good	after
Sat 5	Well very	1 fit		rather w.[akeful]	very good		
Sun 6	Well very	much occas fl		do	do		
Mon. 7	Well very	occas. fl			good		
T. 8	Well very	almost one fit		do		do	
W. 9	Well barely in evening		several slight fits		good		
Th. 10	Well very		sharply	do	very good		
F. 11	Well very	1 slight fit	wakeful		indifferent		
Sd 12	Well very	do			very good		
Sun 13	Well very	2 slight fits		rather w.[akeful]	do		
M. 14	Well very	occas. fl	(small Boil broke)		very good		
T. 15	Well very	1 fit			do		
W. 16	Well very	do			do		
Th. 17	Well very	2 slight fits			do		
F. 18	Well very				very good		
Sat. 19	Well very	1 fit & ½			moderate		
Sun 20	Well very	some occas fl	heazish		pretty good		
M. 21	Well very	1 slight fit			very good		
T. 22	Well	3 fits of fl (visitors)[85]			pretty good		
W. 23	Well very	1 fit			do		
Th. 24	Well very	occas fl			moderate		
F. 25	Well very	2 fits, slight discomfort			do (fear)		
Sat 26	Well not quite, several fits some bad (slight sinking)				poorish		
Sun 27	Well not quite, several slight fits, some discomfort				pretty good		
M. 28	Well	2 or 3 slight fits			do		
T. 29	Well	2 sharpish fits			moderate		
W. 30	Well very	1 fit			very good		
Th 31	Well very	1 & ½ fit			do		

London

			lb		
July 5ᵗʰ.	Light trousers & drawers, no fl. w	12	1	7

[8 double dashes][86]

1851 August						Night	
F. 1		Well very	2 fits			wakeful	moderate
Sat 2		Well very	2 or 3 baddish fit			do	pretty good
S. 3		Well very	2 or 3 fits			:	very good
M 4		Well very	2 fits			wakeful	pretty good
T 5		Well very					good
W 6		Well	slight headache	Kew			very good
Th 7		Well very					indifferent
F. 8		Well headache					moderate
Sat 9		Well barely					pretty good
Sun 10		Well very				:	indifferent
M. 11		Well very	almost 1 fit			wakeful	indifferent
T. 12		Well very					moderate
W 13		Poorly feverish, cold, much fl					very good
Th 14		Poorly Rheumaticks continued	slight fl			:	good
F 15		Well. 2 fits of fl	Little Rheumatism				pretty good
Sat 16		Well very	1 fit			indifferent, very much fl.	
Sun 17		Well very	2 fits, discomfort some,				pretty good
M 18		Well very	1 fit			heazish,	pretty good
T 19		Well	2 or 3 fits			do	do
W. 20		Well	2 or 3 fits			do	do
Th. 21		Well	do			:	pretty good
F. 22		Well very	1 fit				good
Sat 23		Well very	yet uncomfortable				pretty good
S. 24		Well very	occas. fl.				moderate
M. 25		Well	2 or 3 fits uncomfort				pretty good
T. 26		Well not quite	1 bad fit & much fl.				good
W. 27		Well not quite [88]	do			pretty good	
Th. 28	Sw. Sh. O F.B.	1 bad fit		heazish,		pretty god	
F. 29	Sh. D. F.B.	Well very				:	good
Sat 30	Sh. D. F.B.	Well very	1 consid. fit				moderate
S. 31	Sw. Sh. F.B.	Well very	do			heazish	do

London [87]

(5. double dashes)[89]

1851 September

						Night
M. 1	Sh. D. F.B.	Well	1 fit			Heayish, pretty good
T. 2	Sh. F.B.	Well very				good
W. 3	Sw. Sh. D. F.B.	Well very				moderate
Th. 4	Sh. F.B.	Well very				heazish. very good
F. 5	Sh. D. F.B.	Well very	almost 1 fit			do moderate
Sd 6	Sw. Sh. F.B.	Well very	evening uncomfort:			: poorish
Sun 7	Sh. F.B.	Well very	yet not very comfort:			: wakeful moderate
M. 8	Sh. D. F.B.	Well very	1 fit			moderate
T. 9	Sw. Sh. F.B.	Well very	almost fit			do
W. 10	Sh. D. F.B.	Well very	1 fit			pretty good
Th. 11	Sh	Well very	2 fits			moderate
F. 12	Sw. Sh. D.	Well very	1 fit			indifferent
Sat 13	Sh	Well very	2 fits			do
S. 14	Sh	Well	2 or 3 fits	Very tired in evening		moderate
M. 15	Sh. D.	Well	do	Speudo[90] - boils. --		good
Tu. 16	Sw. Sh.	Well very	1 fit			moderate
W. 17	Sh. D.	Well very	some occ.			wakeful. indifferent
Th. 18	Sh.	Well very	do			do good
F. 19	Sw. Sh. D.	Well very				very good
Sat 20	Sh.	Well very				first part bad moderate
Su 21	Sh	Well very	almost 1 fit	Small Boils	do	indifferent
M 22	Sw. Sh. D.	Well very			do	moderate
T. 23	Sh.	Well very	1 consid fit			pretty good
W. 24	Sh. D.	Well very				: wakeful. moderate
Th 25	Sw. Sh.	Well very	1 consid. fl:			pretty good
F. 26	Sh.	Well almost very	2 or 3 fits			moderate
Sat 27	Sh. D.	Well very	2 fits of fl.			pretty good
Sun 28	Sw. Sh	Well	3 or 4 slight fits			: do
M. 29	Sh. D.	Well very				do
T. 30	Sh	Well very	some occas fl.			good

(15 double dashes)

Best month since April 1850[91]

1851	October					Night		
W. 1	Sw. Sh. D.	Well very				good		
Th. 2	Sh.	Well very				indifferent		
F. 3	Sh. D.	Well very	1 slight fit		do	do		
Sat 4	Sw. Sh.	Well very	1 fit			early part. indifferent		
S. 5	Sh.	Well	2 or 3 slight fits			heazish	pretty good	
M. 6	Sh. D.	Well very	1 fit			good		
T. 7	Sw. Sh.	Well not quite	2 or 3 fits.			: languid good		

\# 92

W. 8	Sh	Well very		some occas fl.		indifferent restless		
Th. 9	Sh.	Well not quite	2 or 3 fits.	Heady		heaszish, pretty good		
F. 10	Sh	Well very	occas fl			wakeful pretty good		
Sat 11	Dr. T:	Well very				pretty good		
S. 12	Sh.	Well very				indifferent		
M 13	Sh	Well very	1 long fit			pretty good		
T. 14	Sh.	Well very	some occas			do		
W. 15	Sh	Well very. slight head. slight continued fl afternoon:				heasziest, indifferent		
Th. 16	Sh	Well very	occas fl. (Electric Chains[93] attc' waist)			Wakeful good		

(London — vertical label)

F 17	Sh	Well very				slightly so ["rather' inserted] indiff		
Sd 18	Sh.	Well very	1 cosid fit			very moderate		
S. 19	Sh.	Well very	(do neck)			heazish, good		
M. 20	Sh	Well very	almost fit			wakeful indifferent		
T. 21	Sh	Well 2 or 3 fits				: moderate		
W. 22	Sh	Well very	1 or 2 fits			pretty good		
Th. 23	Sh.	Well	3 or 4 fits		slight headache	moderate		
F. 24	Sh.	Well not quite	much fl			good		
Sd. 25	Sh	Well very	1 fit			good		
S. 26	Sh	Well very	some occas.			heazish. pretty good		
M. 27	Sh	Well very	do			: moderate		
T 28	Sh.	Well very	2 fits of fl not bad			do		
W. 29	Sh.	Well	3 or 4 fits			heazish pretty good		
Th. 30	Sh	Well	do			do good		
F. 31	Sh	Well very	occas fl			good		

(visitors' Lyells — bracketed vertical label)

	St	lb	oz		
Oct 1st	--	12	6	6	-- light trousers, drawers no flannel wt

[14 Double Dashes][94]

1851

<u>November</u>   <u>Night</u>

Day					Night
<u>Sat. 1</u>	Sh.	Well not quite. headache. much fl			very good
S. 2	Sh.	Well <u>very</u> some occas.			do
M. 3	Sh.	Well <u>very</u> slmost 1 fit			: very good
T. 4	Sh.	Well <u>very</u>			moderate, wakeful
W. 5	Sh.	Well <u>very</u> some occas.			pretty good
Th. 6	Sh.	Well <u>very</u> 1 slight fit			very good. not SU[95]
F. 7	Sh.	Well <u>very</u> do			: very good. do
<u>Sd 8</u>	Sh.	Well bar[el]y several fits			very good Seldom up
S 9	Sh.	Well do slight fits			good do
M. 10	Sh.	Well not quite several fits			good
T 11	Sh.	Well <u>very</u> 1 consid fit			moderate
W 12	Sh.	Well several fits			: ["very" del] good, not S.U.
Th 13	Sh.	Well <u>very</u>			indifferent
F. 14	Sh.	Well <u>very</u> (uncomfort. in evening)			good
<u>Sat 15</u>	Sh.	Well <u>very</u> 1 consid. fit (party)			poor
S. 16	Sh.	Well <u>very</u> some occas			good
M. 17	Sh.	Well <u>very</u>			moderate
T 18	Sh.	Well <u>very</u> 1 fit			good
W. 19	Sh	Well <u>very</u> 1 slight fit			: very good
Th. 20	Sh	Well <u>very</u> good: ["nearly" del]			morning bad
F. 21	O	Poorly a Little, headache, much fl			very good. not S.U.
<u>Sat 22</u>	Sh	Well <u>very</u>			very good. not S.U.
S. 23	Sh.	Well very 2 fits			very good hardly S U
M 24	Sh	Well <u>very</u>			: very good
T 25	Sh.	Well <u>very</u> almost fit			very good hardly S.U.
W. 26	Sh.	Well <u>very</u> 1 fit			goodish
Th 27	Sh.	Poorly a little consid fl			moderate
F. 28	Sh	Well barely do			moderate
<u>Sat 29</u>	Sh	Well bare[l]y			do
S. 30	Sh	Well <u>very</u> 1 or 2 fl			: very good

Capt. Sulivan [96]

12 double dashes[97]

1851 Dec.				Night
M. 1.	Sh.	Well _very_		very good. hardly U.
T. 2	Sh.	Well _very_	1 fit	good: do
W. 3	Sh.	Well _very_		very good
Th. 4	Sh.	Well _very_		do. hardly U
F. 5	Sh	Well _very_	(almost 1 fit)	Very good -- Not U
Sat 6	Sh.	Well _very_	1 fit	goodish
Sun 7	Sh.	Well _very_		good:
M. 8	Sh	Well _very_		_very good_ not U
T. 9	Sh	Well _very_		very good
W 10	Sh.	Well very	2 fits	good
Th 11	Sh	Well _very_	(some discomfort)	very good
F 12	Sh	Well _very_		good restless
Sat 13	Sh	Well.	2 or 3 baddish fit	good:
Sun 14	Sh	Well _very_		good
M. 15	Sh	Well _very_		do
T. 16	Sh	Well _very_	London 98	do
W. 17	Sh	Well _very_ [99]		do
Th 18	Sh.	Well _very_		goodish
Fr. 19	Sh.	Well _very_		_very good:_ not Up
Sat 20	Sh	Well _very_		good
Sun 21	Sh.	Well _very_	1 baddish fit	very good
M. 22	Sh.	Well _very_	almost 1 fit	goodish. consid fl. once U
T 23	Sh	Well _very_	consid fl. occas fl	well 1 consid fit
W. 24	Sh	Well _very_	1 fit	moderate. 3 or 4 baddish fits
Th. 25	Sh	Well _very_	1 consid fl	good 2 fits
F. 26	Sh.	Well _very_		good 2 fits
Sat 27	Sh	Well _very_	1 consid fl	good
Su 28	Sh	Well _very_	occas fl	wakeful much fl :
M. 29	Sh	Well _very_		several bad fits of fl
T. 30	Sh	Well _very_		good 2 fits
W. 31	Sh	Well _very_	1 fit	poorish. several fits

19 double – dashes

Best since Jan. 1850[100]

1852

January

						Night
Th 1	Sh.	Well very			moderate	3 or 4 fits
F. 2	Sh.	Well very	almost 1 fit		poorish	some bad fl
Sat --3		Sh.	Well very	2 or 3 fits		do do
Sun 4		Sh	Well very			good
M. 5		Sh	Well very		very good	not Up
T. 6		Sh	Well	2 or 3 fits		poorish. some bad fits
W. 7		Sh	Well not quite			very good
Th 8		Sh	Well	2 baddish fits		wakeful. poor:
F 9		Sh	Well very			very good
Sat 10		Sh	Well very			good:
Su 11		Sh.	Well not quite. several fits.			good heazish
M. 12		Sh	Well very			good:
T. 13		Sh	Well	2 or 3 bad fits		goodish
W. 14		Sh.	Well not quite, several fits[101]			poorish
Th 15		Sw. Sh. O F.B.	Well very	2 or 3 much fits		restless. uncomfortable:
F. 16		Sh. D. F. B.	Well very			good
Sat 17		Sh. D. F.B.	Well very	much occas fl		indifferent
Sun 18		Sw. Sh. O F.B.	Well very	do discomfort		1 bad fit:
M. 19		Sh. D. F.B.	Well very	some slight fl.		good
T. 20		S. O F.B.	Well	2 or 3 fits		do
W 21		Sw. Sh. D. F.B	Well very	1 fit		do
Th 22		O F.B.	Well very			indifferent. much fl.
F. 23		Sh. O. F.B.	Well very			goodish 2 or 3 fits
Sat 24		Sw. Sh. D. F.B.	Well very	1 fit		good: do
Sun 25		Sh	Well very	2 or 3 fits		goodish: do
M. 26		Sh. D.	Well very	do		good
T. 27		Sw Sh	Well very	do		good
W. 28		Sh. D.	Well very	do		good
Th. 29		Sw Sh	Well much fl.	London[102]		very good
Fr. 30		Sw. Sh.	Well barely	several fit		poorish
Sat 31		Sh. D.	Well	several fits		goodish

11 Double Dashes, but [103]
many poorish days.

<u>1852</u>

February

					<u>Night</u>
Sun 1.	Sh.	Well barely.	several fits		moderate
M. 2	Sw. Sh. D.	Well	do		good
T. 3	Sh.	Well barely	do		indifferent. much fl.
W. 4	Sh. D.	Well very	3 fits		moderate
Th. 5	Sw. Sh.	Well barely	do		good:
F. 6	Sh. D.	Well <u>very</u>	1 fit		good
<u>Sat 7</u>	Sw. Sh.	Well very	2 fits		very good
S. 8	Sh.	Well <u>very</u>			good
M 9	Sh. D.	Well <u>very</u>	(almost 1 fit)		good
T. 10	Sw. Sh.	Well <u>very</u>			good
W. 11	Sh D.	Well <u>very</u>			very good:
Th. 12	Dr	Well <u>very</u> .	almost 1 fit.	<u>Cold</u>	good
F. 13	Dr.	Well <u>very</u>	1 slight fit	do	moderate
<u>Sat 14</u>	Dr.	Well <u>very</u>	some occas fl.	do	pretty good
S. 15	Sh.	Well very	2 or 3 fits		do:
M. 16	Sw. Sh. D.	Well <u>very</u>	1 fit		heazish good
T 17	Sh.	Well <u>very</u>	occas fl.		good :
W. 18	Sw. Sh D.	Well <u>very</u>			moderate
Th. 19	Sh. O	Well <u>very</u>	occas fl		indifferent
F. 20	Sw. Sh. D.	Well <u>very</u>			good
<u>Sat 21</u>	Sh.	Well <u>very</u>			good
S. 22	Sw. Sh.	Well <u>very</u>	occas fl		good
M. 23	Sh D.	Well <u>very</u>			very good
T. 24	Sw Sh.	Well <u>very</u>	1 slight fit		moderate
W. 25	Sh D.	Well <u>very</u>			good
Th. 26	Sw. Sh.	Well <u>very</u>			goodish
F. 27	Sh.	Well <u>very</u>	some occas. & discomfort		indifferent
<u>Sat 28</u>	Sw. Sh. D.	Well <u>very</u>	do		moderate:
S. 29	Sh.	Well <u>very</u>			good

[104]

18 Double Dashes[105]

six & ½ weeks of Treatment.[106]

1852 March: --					Night
M. 1	Sh.	Well very			very good
T. 2	Sh.	Well very			pretty good
W. 3	Sh.	Well very	1 bad fit, slight headache		good
Th. 4	Sh.	Well barely	2 or 3 fits	do	heaszish. good
F. 5	Sh.	Well very			good
Sat 6	Sh.	Well very	almost 1 fit		very good
S. 7	Sh	Well very	2 fits		very good hardly U.
M 8	Sh	Well very			indifferent Wakeful
T. 9	Sh	Well very			good
W. 10	Dr.	Poorly in afternoon. Headache	Vomit	London	bad
Th. 11	Dr.	do	do		pretty good:
F. 12	Sh.	Well very	1 slight fit		good
Sat 13	Sh.	Well very			very good
S. 14	Sh	Well very	1 in evening. Boil under arm.		heazish good
M. 15	Sh	Well very	poorly from boil wh. didn't break		good
T. 16	Sh	Well very			very good
W. 17	Sh	Well very			indifferent:
Th. 18	Sh	Well very	almost 1 fit		good
F. 19	Sh	Well barely	several fits in afternoon		heaszish. good
Sat 20	Sh	Well barely	do do		do good
S. 21	Sh	Well very	1 fit		very good
M. 22	Sh.	Well very	1 or 2 fits		good
T. 23	Sh	Well very			very good
W. 24	Sh	Well very		Rugby [107]	wakeful do:
Th. 25	Sh.	Well very			good
F. 26	Sh. Dr.	Well very			wakeful moderate
Sat 27	Dr.	Well very	1 fit		do
S. 28	Dr.	Well very	2 or 3 fits heasy		good
M 29	Dr.	Poorly	several slight fits	Shrewsbury [108]	very heasy
T. 30	Dr.	Well not quite	2 slight fits		good
W. 31	Dr.	do			good

15 Double Dashes[109]

1852 April						Nights
Th. 1	Dr.	Well <u>very</u> , occas fl				very good
F. 2	Sh.	Well <u>very</u> almost fit				very good
<u>Sat 3</u>	Sh.	Well <u>very</u> occas fl				do
Sun 4	Sh.	Well <u>very</u> 1 fit				good
M 5	Sh	Well <u>very</u>				very good
T. 6	Sh.	Well <u>very</u>				very good. Hardly Up. –
W. 7	Sh.	Well <u>very</u>				moderate
Th. 8	Sh.	Well not quite evening. continued fl. slight headache				good
F. 9	Sh.	Well <u>very</u> evening not comfortable				very good
<u>Sat 10</u>	Sh.	Well <u>very</u> a cold				indifferent ;
S. 11	Sh.	Poorly . Cold, Sundays stomach not bad				moderate ;
M. 12	Dr. ["Well <u>very</u>" del] but Poorly. cold.					indifferent.
T. 13	Sh	Poorly. heasy Languid ["do" del]				moderate:
W. 14	Sh.	Poorly - little heaz				pretty good
Th. 15	Sh.	Well <u>very</u> 1 consid fit				moderate
F. 16	SH.	Well <u>very</u> do				good
<u>Sat 17</u>	Dr.	Poorly little several fits slight headache. Cold				good :
Sun 18	Dr.	Poorly Cold				goodish
M. 19	Dr.	Poorly little do				very good
T. 20	Dr.	Well <u>very</u>				do
W. 21	Sh.	Well <u>very</u> 1 baddish fit (slight cold)				do
Th. 22	Sh.	Well <u>very</u> occas fl				do
F. 23	Sh	Poorly little much fl. slight headach		visitors 110		heazish do
<u>Sat 24</u>	Sh	Well <u>very</u> occas fl			good	
Sun 25	Sh	Well <u>very</u> do				very good:
M. 26	SH.	Well <u>very</u> 1 consid fit				do
Tu 27	Sh.	Well <u>very</u> slight Cold				do
W. 28	Sh.	Well <u>very</u>				Moderate
Th. 29	Sh.	Well <u>very</u> almost fit				pretty good
F. 30	Sh.	Well <u>very</u>				good

(14 Double dashes) Continued cold[111]

April 20 20 12. 10 Cloth J[acket] & Trousers & flannel wastc[t].

<u>1852 May</u>   <u>Night</u>

<u>Sat. 1</u>	Sh.	Well <u>very</u> , almost fit		very good:
Su 2	Sh.	Well very	2 fits	good
M 3	Sh.	Well <u>very</u>	1 fit	indifferent:
T. 4	Sh.	Well <u>very</u>	do	good
W. 5	Sh.	Well <u>very</u>	almost 1 fit	indifferent wakeful
Th 6	Dr.	Well barely. cold & headache		very good
F. 7	Sh.	Well <u>very</u>		good
<u>Sat 8</u>	Sh.	Well	2 or 3 fits	Moderate
S. 9	Sh.	Well barely		pretty good;
M. 10	Sh.	Well <u>very</u>		do. 1 bad fit
T 11	Sh.	Well <u>very</u>	1 consid fit	good
W. 12	Sh.	Well	2 or 3 fits	heazish good
Th. 13	Sh.	Well barely	3 a fit, slight headach	do. do.
F. 14	Sh.	Well <u>very</u>		moderate
<u>Sat 15</u>	Sh.	Well <u>very</u>	1 fit	good
S. 16	Sh	Well	2 bad fits	heazish good
M 17	Sh.	Well <u>very</u>	1 fit	do do
T 18	Sh.	Well <u>very</u>	occas fl.	good
W. 19	Sh.	Well <u>very</u>		very good
Th. 20	Sh.	Well <u>very</u>		wakeful. goodish
F 21	Sh	Well very	2 or 3 fits	good:
<u>Sat 22</u>	Sh.	Well <u>very</u>		very good.
Sun 23[112]	["Sh" lightly del]	Well <u>very</u>		very good
M. 24	Sh	Well <u>very</u> (some occas)		very good
T 25	Sh.	Well <u>very</u>		good
W. 26	Sh.	Well <u>very</u>	nearly a fit	very good
Th. 27	Sh.	Well <u>very</u>		very good
F. 28	Sh.	Well <u>very</u>		good:
<u>Sat 29</u>	Sh.	Well <u>very</u>	almost 1 fit	goodish
S. 30	Sh.	Well <u>very</u>	1 baddish fit	very good:
M. 31	Sh.	Well	some occas. fl	goodish

17 double dashes[113]

1852 June						Night
T. 1	Sh.	Well very				good
W 2	Sh.	Poorly		vomit at night		very bad
Th . 3	Dr.	Well	London	114		good
F. 4	Dr.	Well very				bad
Sat 5	Dr.	Poorly	Cold		Wakeful	good :
Su 6	Sh.	Well very	Cold		do	good
M 7	Sh	Well very	Cough		very poor	
T. 8	Sh	Well very			very good	
W 9	Sh	Well very	almost 1 fit			do
Th. 10	Sh.	Well very	do		not up..	do:

115

F. 11	Sw. Sh. D. F.B.	Well very	1 fit	["very" del]		good
Sat 12	Sh F.B.	Well very			moderate	
Su 13	Sh. D. F.B.	Well very			very good	
M. 14	Sw. Sh F.B.	Well very	1 fit discomfort		moderate	
T. 15	Sh. D. O	Well barely	2 or 3 fits	tooth ach	very good	
W. 16	Sh O. O.	Well very	1 consid fit		good	
Th 17	Sw. Sh. D. F.B.	Well ["very" del]	2 or 3 fits			very good
Fr. 18	Sh. D. F.B.	Well very	2 fits		indifferent	
Sat 19	Sh. F.B.	Well very	do		good	
116 S 20	Sw. Sh. D. ["F.B." del]	Well barely face-ache poorly			heazish good	
M. 21	Dr	Well barely	do not much flatulence		good	
T 22	Dr.	Well	toothach		very good	
W. 23	Sh	Well	toothache ["out & chloroform" del]		good	
Th 24	Dr.	Well	tooth out & chloroform		good	
F 25	Dr.	Well very			indifferent	
Sat 26	Sh.	Well very			very good	
S. 27	Sh.	Well ["very" del]	2 or 3 fits		heazish moderate	
M. 28	Sh.	Well ["very" del]	do		do do	
T. 29	Sh.	Well ["very" del]	do		do do	
W. 30	Sh	Well	do		do do	

Nine ["Eight" del] Double Dashes[117]

    (Ten Days Treatment)[118]

1852 July					Night
Th. 1	Sh.	Well	2 or 3 fits.	heazish as during usual days	good:
F. 2	Sh.	Well very			good
Sat -3	Sh	Well very	1 fit		pretty good
S. 4	Sh	Well	2 or 3 fits (heazy)		good
M. 5	Sh	Well very	1 fit		very good
Tu 6	Sh.	Well very	1 slight fit		very good :
W. 7	Sh	Well very	1 fit		very good.
Th. 8	Sh.	Well very			very good:
F. 9	Sh	Well very	2 fits		very good
Sat 10	Sh.	Well very	occas fl		good:
S. 11	Sh.	Well barely	much fl		good
⚞ 119					
M. 12	Sw. Sh. D.	Well very			moderate
T. 13	Sh	Well	2 baddish fits		goodish:
W. 14	Sh. D.	Well very			very good
Th 15	Sw. Sh.	Well	2 fits		very good
F. 16	Sh. D.	Well very			very good
Sat 17	Sh	Well very	2 fits		good
Sun 18	Sw. Sh. D.	Well very	1 fit		good
M 19	Sh	Well	2 fits		heazyish pretty good:
T 20	Sh D.	Well very			baddish
W. 21	Sw. Sh.	Well very	1 fit		do
Th 22	Sh D.	Well very		wakeful	moderate
F 23	Sh.	Well	2 or 3 fits		very good
Sat 24	Sh. D.	Well very	do		heasy moderate
S. 25	Sw. Sh	Well barely		heaz. flat	very heaz
M 25	Sh. D.	Well very	1 fit		goodish
T 27	Sh.	Well barely much fl			good heazish
W. 28	Sw. Sh. D.	Well very			good
Th 29	Sh	Well very			very good
F. 30	Sh. D.	Well very			good
Sat 31	Sw. Sh.	Well very	2 fits		moderate:

12 Double Dashes[120]

1852 August					Night
Sun 1	Sh.	Well	2 or 3 fits		wakeful good
M. 2	Sh. D.	Well <u>very</u>			<u>very</u> good
T. 3	Sw. Sh. D.	Well <u>very</u>			very good
W. 4	Sh	Well <u>very</u>	1 fit		very good:
Th. 5[121]	Sh. D.	Well <u>very</u>	do		moderate
F. 6	Sw. Sh.	Well <u>very</u>	do		good
<u>Sat 7</u>	Sh.	Well <u>very</u>			good
S. 8	Sh	Well <u>very</u>			good
M 9	Sw. Sh. D.	Well <u>very</u>			very good
T. 10	Sh. D.	Well <u>very</u>			good
W. 11	Sh	Well	2 slight fits		good
Th. 12	Sw Sh.	Well very	2 fits		good
F. 13	Sh D.	Well <u>very</u>			good [written in small letters] "is
<u>Sat 14</u>	Sh. D.	Well <u>very</u>	2 slight fits		indifferent
S. 15	Sw. S	Well <u>very</u>			goodish
M 16	Sh D.	Well <u>very</u>			indifferent
T. 17	Sh D.	Well <u>very</u>			moderate
W. 18	Sw. Sh	Well <u>very</u>	1 bad fit		very heasy . poor
F 20	Sh. D.	Well <u>very</u>	1 fit		good
<u>Sat 21</u>	Sw. Sh. D.	Well <u>very</u>			wakeful good
S. 22	Sh	Well barely			good
M. 23	Sh	Well			goodish:
T 24	Sh.	Well <u>very</u>			very good
W. 25	Sh.	Well <u>very</u>	almost 1 fit		goodish
Th. 26	Sh.	Well <u>very</u>	do (tired in evenings)		wakeful indifferent
F. 27	Sh.	Well <u>very</u>		heaz	very good
<u>Sat 28</u>	Sh.	Well	3 or 4 fit	heasz	very good
S. 29	Sh	Well <u>very</u>	1 fit		very good
M. 30	Sh.	Well	3 or 4 fits		good
T. 31	Sh.	Well <u>very</u>	1 fit		good

122

Six weeks treatment: not much good effect extremely tired in Evening.

I do not think last treatment did me much good.[123]

17 Double Dashes[124]

1852 September				Night
W. 1	Sh.	Well very.		good
Th. 2.	Sh.	Well very	1 fit	good:
F. 3	Sh.	Well	2 consid. fit	wakeful moderate
Sat 4	Sh.	Well very	1 fit	Sh. 2 good
S. 5	Th	Poorly. excessive fl. headache vomit. Trs[125]		poor
M 6	Sh.	Well very		good
T. 7	Sh.	Well very	1 fit	very good
W. 8	Sh.	Well	2 fits	Wakeful poorish
Th. 9	Sh.	Well very.	1 fit	heasy. moderate
F. 10	Sh.	Well very		goodish
Sat 11	Sh	Poorly. headache		goodish
S. 12	Dr.	Well very		good
M. 13	Dr.	Well very		very good
T 14	Dr.	Well very	Leith Hill [126]	goodish
W. 15	Dr.	Well very		very good ["ish" del]
Th. 16	Dr.	Well very		good
F. 17	Sh	Well.	2 or 3 fits heasz	goodish
Sat 18	Sh.	Well very		good
S. 19	Sh.	Well very	1 fit	good
M. 20	Sh.	Well very	almost fit	goodish
T. 21	Sh	Well very	1 fit	good
W. 22	Sh.	Well very	do	very good
Th. 23	Sh.	Well very	2 fits	heaszish good
F. 24	Sh	Well very	1 fit	good
Sat 25	Sh.	Well very		very good
S. 26	Sh.	Well very	2 consid fits	very good
M. 27	Sh.	Well very	almost 1 fit	indifferent
T. 28	Sh.	Well. evening extreme fl. headache.		good
W. 29	Sh.	Well very		good
Th 30	Sh.	Well very	1 consid fit	indifferent

Eleven double dashes[127]

1852 October				Night
F. 1	Sh.	Well very		moderate
Sat 2	Sh.	Well very		good :
S. 3	Sh.	Well very	almost 1 fit	indifferent
M 4	Sh.	Well very		good
T. 5	Sh.	Well very	almost 1 fit	good
W. 6	Sh.	Well very	1 fit	goodish
Th. 7	Sh.	Well very		indifferent
F. 8	Sh.	Well	2 fits fl	goodish
Sat 9	Sh	Well very	almost fit	wakeful. goodish:
S. 10	Sh.	Well very	1 fit	good
M 11	Sh.	Well very		very good
T. 12	Sh.	Well very		wakeful, good
W. 13	Sh.	Well very		very good
Th. 14	Sh.	Well very		goodish
F. 15	Sh.	Well very	Dinner Party[128]	goodish
Sat 16	Sh.	Well very		moderate
Su 17	Sh.	Well very	two fits	good
M 18	Sh.	Well very		restless good
T 19	Sh	Well very		indifferent
W 20	Sh.	Well very	1 fit	do
Th 21	Sh.	Well very		good
F 22	Sh.	Well very		poorish
Sat 23	Sh.	Well very	Dinner Party [129]	good
S 24	Sh.	Well very	almost fits[130]	poorish
M. 25 [131]	Sh.	Well very		good
T. 26	Sh.	Well very		very good
W. 27	Sh.	Well very		goodish
Th 28	Sh.	Well very		goodish
F. 29	Sh.	Poorly	excessive fl. headache	very good
Sat 30	Sh.	Well very		goodish
S. 31	Sh.	Well very	2 fits	goodish

22 Double dashes

(Best month since Jan. 1850) [132]

1852 November						Night
1. M	Sh.	Well	very			Heazish. goodish
2. T	Sh.	Well	very			moderate
3. W.	Sh.	Well	very			good :
4. Th	Sh.	Well	very			good :
5. F	Sh.	Well	very			good
Sat 6	Sh.	Well	very	almost fit		good
S. 7	Sh.	Well	very			good
M 8	Sh.	Well	very			good
T. 9	Sh.	Well	very			good
W 10	Dr.	Well	very			poor
Th. 11	Dr.	Well	very	1 fit		very good
F. 12	Dr	Well	very			very good
Sat 13	Sh.	Well	very	2 fits slight headache in evening		wakeful
S. 14	Sh.	Well	very			good
M. 15	Sh.	Well	very	1 fit		very good
T. 16	Sh.	Well	very	1 fit		good
W. 17	Sh.	Well	very	2 fits	London[133]	poor
Th. 18	Dr.	Well	very			very good
F. 19	Sh.	Well	very			very good
Sat 20	Sh	Well	very	1 fit		goodish
S 21	Sh.	Well	very	almost fit		good
M 22	Sh	Well	very			wakeful indifferent
T. 23	Sh.	Well	very	almost fit		one fit. very good
W. 24	Sh.	Well	very			very good.
Th. 25	Sh	Well	very			goodish
F. 26	Sh.	Well	very			good
Sat 27	Sh	Well	very	almost fit		moderate
S. 28	Sh.	Well	very			good
M. 29	Sh.	Well	very			good
T. 30	Sh.	Well	very			(i.e. often waking & restless, considerable fl but ["not" del] hardly sitting up. indifferent

(23 double dashes)

1849   Dec.   28 double dashes
1850   Jan.   24 double dashes[134]

1852. -- December						Night: --
W. 1	S	Well	<u>very</u>			restless indifferent
Th. 2		Well	<u>very</u>			goodish, 3 fits
F 3		Well	<u>very</u>			<u>very</u> good
<u>Sat 4</u>		Well	<u>very</u>			good
S 5		Well	<u>very</u>			very good : --
M. 6		Well	<u>very</u> (slight occas fl.)			wakeful moderate
T. 7		Well	<u>very</u>			indifferent
W. 8		Well	<u>very</u>			goodish
Th. 9		Well	very	two fits		good
F. 10		Well	<u>very</u>			good
<u>Sat 11</u>		Well	very	two fits		moderate
S. 12		Well	<u>very</u>	some occas. fl		wakeful indifferent
M. 13		Well	<u>very</u>	do		very good
T. 14		Well	<u>very</u>	do		good
W. 15		Well	<u>very</u>			good
Th. 16		Well	<u>very</u>			wakeful indifferent
F. 17		Well	<u>very</u>			moderate
<u>Sat 18</u>		Well	very	2 fits		good.
S. 19		Well	<u>very</u>			poorish
M. 20		Well	<u>very</u>			wakeful. moderate
T. 21		Well	very	almost fit	no Tea	pretty good
W. 22		Well	<u>very</u>			wakeful indifferent
Th. 23		Well	<u>very</u>	1 fit		wakeful, restless, consid. fl
F. 24		Well	<u>very</u>			pretty good
<u>S. 25</u>		Well	<u>very</u>	1 fit		Little wakeful good:
S. 26		Well	very	2 fits		wakeful goodish:
M. 27		Well	very	do		slept well good.
T. 28		Well	<u>very</u>			goodish
W. 29		Well	<u>very</u>			good
Th. 30		Well	<u>very</u>			good
F. 31		Well	<u>very</u>	consid occas fl		goodish:

24 double dashes [135]

1853 January[136]   Night

Sat 1	Well	very .	some fl. yet poorly	good
S. 2	Well	very	2 fit. uncomfortable	goodish
M. 3	Well	very		poorish
T. 4	Poorly a little not much fl: Boil. --			good
W. 5	Poorly			wakeful. poor
Th. 6	Well very yet rather poorly			goodish
F. 7 [137]	Well barely	consid fl	acid sickness.	do
Sat 8 Dr.	Poorly	in	even[in]g shivering	bad at first. then good
S. 9	Poorly		Boil broke	do do
M. 10	Well not quite			wakeful moderate
T. 11	Well not quite		1 fit	goodish:
W. 12	Well			good
Th. 13	Well very	get Boil not well painful in night		much fl:
F. 14	Well very	2 fits		good
Sat 15	Well very	core extracted Party		moderate
S. 16	Poorly very. excessive fl. ["Bad" del] Vomiting			good
M. 17	Well very	occas. fl		good
T. 18 [138]	Well very	do		goodish
W. 19	Well very			wakeful. goodish
Th 20	Well very	occas fl		goodish
F. 21	Well very	1 fit		goodish
Sat 22	Well very	2 or 3 fits		moderate
S. 23	Well very	almost fit	heasyish good	
M. 24	Well barely	Much fl activities		good
T 25	Well very	almost fit	heasyish good	
W. 26	Well very	1 fit	heasz :	
Th 27	Poorly very	acid vomiting Excessive fl headach		good
F 28	Well very Two fits			goodish
Sat 29	Well very		poor	
S. 30	Well consid fl		good	
M 31	Well very	1 fit	good	

11 Double Dashes

<u>1853 February</u> [139]   <u>Night</u>

Date		Well			Night
T. 1		Well <u>very</u>	London [140]		goodish.
W. 2		Well <u>very</u>			goodish
Th. 3		Well <u>very</u>	(sty in rg eye)		Wakeful
F. 4		Well <u>very</u>			do indifferent
<u>Sat. 5</u>		Well <u>very</u>			good:
S. 6		Well <u>very</u>			goodish
M. 7		Well <u>very</u>	almost fit		good
T. 8		Well <u>very</u>	do		good
W. 9		Well <u>very</u>	1 fit		good
Th. 10		Well <u>very</u>	Do		good
F. 11		Well <u>very</u>	2 fits (slight boil begun) failed		heaszish good
<u>Sat 12</u>		Well <u>very</u>	1 slight fit		good
S. 13		Well <u>very</u>			good
M. 14		Well <u>very</u>	1 fit		good
T. 15		Well <u>very</u>	do		very good
W. 16	Dr.	Well <u>very</u>	Cold		heaszish very good
Th 17	Dr.	Well <u>very</u>	do		good
F. 18	Dr.	Well <u>very</u>	Cough		indifferent
<u>Sat 19</u>	Dr.	Well very	consid fl. in evening		good:
S. 20	Dr.	Well very	do		good
M. 21	Sh	Well very	do		indifferent
T. 22		Well <u>very</u>	1 fit		goodish
W. 23		Well <u>very</u>			good
Th 24		Well very			heaszish indifferent:
F. 25		Well very, in evening poorly			do goodish
<u>Sat 26</u>		Well <u>very</u>			moderate
S. 27		Well <u>very</u>			poor
M. 28		Well <u>very</u>			goodish

Nine Double Dashes

1853 March [141]				Night	
T. 1	Well very			goodish	
W. 2	Well very			do	
Th. 3	Well very			good	
F. 4	Well very	2 or 3 fits		poorish	
Sat 5	Well very	do		heazish	good:
S. 6	Well very	almost fit		indifferent	
M. 7	Well very	["do" del]		very good	
T. 8	Well very	almost fit		good	
W. 9	Well very			good, morning bad	
Th. 10	Poorly	headache ["slight" inserted] sickness		goodish	
F. 11	Well very	2 or 3 fits	baddish in evening	good	
Sat 12	Well very	almost fit		goodish	
S. 13	Well very	1 fit		heazish good	
M 14	Well very			good	
T 15	Well very			good	
W 16	Well very	some fl from London [142]		good	
Th 17	Well very	1 fit		goodish	
F. 18	Well very in morning; Poorly in evening: dazzling & headache.			heazish	
Sat 19	Well very			good:	
S. 20	Well very			good	
M. 21	Well very			good	
T. 22	Well very	almost fit		good	
W. 23	Well very	1 fit		goodish	
Th. 24	Well very			poorly	
F. 25	Well very	1 fit		wakeful goodish	
Sat. 26	Well very			heasyish good	
S. 27	Well very			wakeful	
M. 28	Well very			do	good
T. 29	Well very			good	
W. 30	Well very	2 or 3 fits		heaszish	very good:
Th. 31	Well very			do	do

18 Double dashes

<u>1853 April</u> [143]   <u>Night</u>

F. 1	Well <u>very</u>			very good
<u>Sat 2</u>	Well <u>very</u>			moderate
S. 3	Well <u>very</u>			heazish very good
M. 4	Well <u>very</u>			good
T. 5	Well <u>very</u>			do
W. 6	Well <u>very</u>	1 fit		do
Th. 7	Well <u>very</u>			do
F. 8	Well <u>very</u>			wakeful do:
<u>Sat 9</u>	Well <u>very</u>	almost fit		moderate
S. 10	Well very	2 or 3 slight fits	heazish ["very" inserted]	good.
M. 11	Well <u>very</u>	almost fit		heasy goodish
T. 12	Well <u>very</u>	do		goodish
W. 13	Well <u>very</u>			good
Th. 14	Well <u>very</u>	1 fit		goodish
F. 15	Well <u>very</u>			very good
<u>Sat 16</u>	Well <u>very</u>			very good
S. 17	Well <u>very</u>			very good
M. 18	Well <u>very</u>	Little swimming[145]		goodish

London [144] (bracketed beside April 3–8)

T. 19 Well very. ["much" del] continued slight flatulence; yet heazish good
            well in evening: but cold with a pain & oppression of Breathing.

W. 20	Well <u>very</u>	some continued. some 2nd fever chest pain		do – goodish
Th 21	Well <u>very</u>	almost fit		good
F. 22	Well <u>very</u>			Little wakeful goodish
<u>Sat 23</u>	Well <u>very</u>	1 fit		good
S. 24	Well <u>very</u>			rather wakeful goodish
M. 25	Well <u>very</u>			Little heazish very good
T. 26	Well <u>very</u>	almost fit		moderate
W. 27	Poorly sickness frm indigestion			goodish
Th. 28	Well <u>very</u>	1 consid fit	Tea[146]	very good
F. 29	Well <u>very</u>		do	very good
<u>Sat 30</u>	Well <u>very</u>			good

20 double dashes

1853 May			Night
S. 1	Well	consid fl	good
M 2	Well very		moderate
T. 3	Well very	1 fit	poorish
W. 4	Well very	considerable continued fl	moderate
F. 5	Well very	do	do
Sat 7 [147]	Well very		goodish
S. 8	Well		do
M 9	Well		Wakeful Poor:
T. 10	Well very	almost one fit	very good
W 11	Well very	do	good
Th 12	Well several fit		heasy;
Sat. 14	Well very		do poorish
S. 15	Well very	yet poorly with small Boil	do goodish
M. 16	Poorly. yet not much fl		shiverzy poorish
T. 17	Poorly	do	good
W. 18	Well very	some fl	very good
Th. 19	Well very		moderate
Sat 20	Well very		goodish
Sat 21	Well very		moderate
S. 22	Well barely		poorish
M 23	Well very		good :
T 24	Well very	some fl	good
W. 25	Well very		good
Th. 26	Well very	1 baddish fit	good
F. 27	Well very	do	moderate
Sat 28	Well very		moderate
Sun 29	Well very	almost fit	good
M. 30	Well very		good
T. 31	Well very		good

13 Double dashes

1853 June				Night
W. 1[148]	Well very	London	1[149]	goodish
Th 2	Well very			good
F 3	Well very	i fit		good
Sat 4	Well very yet much fl.	Crystal Palace[150]		good
S. 5	Well very			very good
M. 6	Well very	almost fit		rather wakeful goodish
T. 7	Well very			very good
W. 8	Well very	2 consid fit		goodish
Th 9	Well very	1 fit		good
F 10	Well very	almost fit		restless wakeful poorish:
Sat 11	Well	3 or 4 fit		moderate
S. 12	Well very	i fit		good
M 13	Well very			good
T. 14	Well very			good
W. 15	Well very			moderate
Th. 16	Well not much fl	very slight sickness		goodish
F. 17	Well very			very good
Sat 18	Well very			good
S. 19	Well very	i fit		good
M. 20	Well very			indifferent
T. 21	Well very : I fit baddish			good
W. 22	Well very			good
Th 23	Well very			good
F. 24	Well very	2 or 3 fits		wakeful moderate
Sat 25	Well very			do moderate
S. 26	Well very			goodish
M 27	Well very			wakeful goodish
T. 28	Well very tired			rather w-- goodish
W. 29	Well very	very tired. consid fit		goodish
Th 30	Well very	do		good

15 Double Dashes. –

1853: -- July: --			Night: --
F. 1	Well very		goodish
Sat 2	Well very	1 or 3 fits	moderate
Sun 3	Well very		good
M. 4	Well very		goodish
T. 5	Well very		indifferent
W 6	Well very		goodish
Th. 7	Well very		indifferent
F. 8	Well very	2 or 3 fits	good
Sat 9	Well barely.	much continued fl. vomited. a litt[le]	moderate
Sun 10	do	do	goodish
M. 11	Poorly	in evening bad vomtiting	Bad
T. 12	Well very		good
W. 13	Well very		good
Th 14	Well very	[Eastbourne][151]	good
F. 15	Well very	2 or 3 fit	Dreadful vomiting from Crab
Sat 16	well very	weakish	good
S. 17	Well very	1 longish fit	wakeful goodish
M 18	Well very	languid	heaszish, good
T. 19	Well very	do	goodish
W 20	Well very		very good
Th 21	Well very		very good
F. 22	Well very	languid	good
Sat 23	Well barely.	headache	good. very:
S. 24	Well do	slight do	heazish. goodish
M. 25	Poorly	very heasy	do do
T. 26	Well barely	weak & languid	goodish
W. 27	Well very,	2 or 3 fits, but better.	good
Th. 28	Well very		goodish
F. 29	Well very		goodish
Sat 30	Well very (2 fits)		good
S. 31	Well very		heazish good

11 Double – Dashes

August 1853					Night
M. 1	Well	very			good
T. 2	Well	very			good
W. 3	Well	very			goodish
Th. 4	Well	very			good:
F. 5	Well	very			good
Sat 6	Well	very	i fit		goodish
S. 7	Well	very	do		moderate
M. 8	Well	very			good
T. 9	Well	very	i fit		moderate
W. 10	Well	very			goodish
Th. 11	Well	very	2 fits		goodish
F. 12	Well	very			good
Sat 13	Well	very			goodish:
S. 14	Well	very			goodish
M. 15	Well	very	Hermitage[152]		indifferent
T. 16	Well	very			do
W. 17	Well	very			very good
Th 18	Well	very			good
F. 19	Well	very	I fit		poorish:
Sat 20	Well	very			goodish
S. 21	Well	very.	heasy consid fl	heayish	good
M 22	Well	very			good
T. 23	Well	very			good
W. 24	Well	very		cold	goodish:
Th. 25	Poorly with a cold				
F. 26	do		do		
Sat 27	Well	very		wakeful	goodish
S 28	Well	very			do
M. 29	Well	very			good
T. 30	Well	very			good
W. 31	Well	very			good

17 Double Dashes, but I think I am not so strict

as I used to be. –

September 1853				Night	
Th. 1	Well very	some occas fl		good.	
F. 2	Well very	i fit [153]		good	
Sat 3	Well very			good	
S. 4	Well very	consid fl.	slight headache	good	
M 5	Well very	i fit		good	
T. 6	Well very	2 fits		goodish	
W. 7	Well very			good	
Th 8	Well very			moderate	
F. 9	Well very			indifferent	
Sat 10	Well very			goodish	
S 11	Well barely,	several fits		goodish	
M 12	Well very	i fit		moderate	
T 13	Well very	very tired		heazish	good
W. 14	Well very			do	good
Th 15	Well very	tired		good	
F. 16	Well very			good	
Sat 17	Well very			goodish	
S 18	Well very	2 fits		moderate	
M 19	Well very			good	
T 20	Well very	i fit		moderate	
W. 21	Well very	do		very good	
Th 22	Well very	several fits & headache from Crystal Palace [154]		good	
F 23	Well very			goodish	
Sat 24	Well very	i fit		good	
S 25	Well very			good	
M 26	Well very			moderate	
T. 27	Well very			poor	
W. 28	Well very	2 or 3 fit		goodish	
Th. 29	Well very			good	
F. 30	Well very [155]	2 or 3 fits		goodish	

13 double dashes

1853	October: --				Night
Sat 1:	Well very				good
S. 2	Well	several fits of fl			goodish
M 3	Well very				good
T 4	Well very	2 or 3 fits			good:
W 5	Well very				good.
Th 6	Well very	headach & much fl	London 156		moderate
F 7	Well very	do			do
Sat 8	Well very				very good
Sun 9	Well very			wakeful	very good
M 10	Well very			do	do
T 11	Well very	i baddish fit		do	good:
W 12	Well barely	headach & cold			good
Th. 13	Well barely	i fit			good
F. 14	Well very	almost fit			good
Sat 15	Well very				poorish
S. 16	Well very				good
M 17	Well very	i baddish fit			good
T 18	Well very	do			goodish
W 19	Well very				poorish
Th 20	Well ["very" del] 3 fits barely				good
F. 21	Well ["barely much fl" del] very				good
Sat 22	Well very	2 or 3 fits			good
S. 23	Well very	----			goodish:
M 24	Well very	do		heazish	good
T. 25	Well very	do		do	good
W. 26	Well very	d		["do" del]	goodish
Th. 27	Well very	d		do	good
F 28	Well very				goodish:
Sat 29	Well very				good
S. 30	Well very				good
M 31	Well very				good

8 double - Dashes

1853	November							Night
1. T	Well <u>very</u>	I fit						moderate
2. W	Well <u>very</u>							good
3. Th.	Well <u>very</u>	do						good
4. F	Well <u>very</u>	do						goodish
<u>Sat 5</u>	Well <u>very</u>							moderate
S. 6	Poorly	sickness, headache						good
M. 7	Well ["very" del]	<u>sick</u> at night, slight sinking						Poor
T. 8	Well barely	much fl						goodish
W. 9	Well very[157]							good
Th 10	Well <u>very</u>	almost fit						slight sinking at night
F 11	Well <u>very</u>	1 slight fit						moderate
<u>Sat 12</u>	Well very	1 slight fit [158]						goodish

Sun 13.	S.W.	F.B	Well very	2 fits				moderate
M. 14	D.		Well <u>very</u>	some ocas fl				good
T. 15		F.B.	Well <u>very</u>	i fit considerable				goodish
W. 16	S.W. D.	F.B.	Well <u>very</u>		wakeful			good
Th. 17		F.B.	Well <u>very</u>	some occas				good
F. 18		F.B.	Well <u>very</u>					good
<u>Sat 19</u>	S.W.		Poorly from		Sorry Back			Poor then good
S. 20	D. ,	F.B.	Well <u>very</u>					wakeful good
M. 21	D.	F.B.	Well <u>very</u>	1 or 2 fits				do goodish
T. 22	SW.	F.B.	Well <u>very</u>					good
W. 23	D.	F.B.	Well <u>very</u>					do good
Th. 24		F.B.	Well <u>very</u>					no tea. sleepy.good.[159]
F. 25	S.W.	F.B.	Well <u>very</u>	do		do		goodish
<u>Sat 26</u>	D.	F.B.	Well <u>very</u>	do	half	do		good
S. 27		F.B.	Well <u>very</u>	some occas fl		do	do	good
M. 28	S.W.[160]	D. F.B.	Well very	do				good
T 29	} London	Sick & Heasish						
W. 30		<u>Poorly</u>[161]						

12 Double Dashes

1853	December				Night: --
Th. 1	(London)	Well very			
F 2	SW. D. F.B.	Well <u>very</u>	almost a fit		goodish
<u>Sat 3</u>	F.B.	Well <u>very</u>	do	tea <u>wakeful</u>, indifferent, much fl	
Sun 4	D. F.B.	Well very	2 slight fits	coffee	good
M 5	SW F.B.	Well <u>very</u>		coffee	good
T. 6	D. F.B.	Well <u>very</u>		coffee rather wakeful	good
W. 7	F.B.	Well very	two fits	coffee	good
Th 8	SW. D. F.B.	Well <u>very</u>	coffee	rather w.[162] indifferent palpitations	
F. 9	F.B.	Well very	tea	not more wakeful	good
<u>Sat 10</u>		Well <u>very</u>	(London)[163]	tea. <u>rather</u> wakeful	good
S. 11	Sw. D. F.B.	Well <u>very</u>			good
M 12		Well very (Barely)	in ev[enin]g much fl		good
T. 13	D. F.B.	Well <u>very</u>	almost fit	coffee not wakeful[164]	good
W. 14	SW. F.B.	Well very	2 fits		moderate
Th. 15	Sh D. F.B.	Well <u>very</u>	slight, acid sickness		good
F. 16	Sh. F.B.	Well <u>very</u>	i fit	tea	good
<u>Sat 17</u>	SW. <u>Sh</u>. F.B.	Well <u>very</u>		do	good
S. 18	Sh. F.B.	Well very	2 slight fits	do	goodish
M 19	Sh. Sh. F.B.	Well very – ["do" del]	2 fits	do consid fl	good
T. 20	Sw. F.B.	Well very	3 or 4 fits	d	goodish
W. 21	Sw. O O	Well barely	several fits		good
Th. 22	Sh. F.B.	Well <u>very</u>	1 fit		consid fl.
F. 23	SW. [165] Dr. D. F.B.	Well very	slight acid sickness at Lunch		good
<u>Sat 24</u>	Sh. F.B.	Well very	2 consid fit		good
S. 25	Sh. D. F.B.	Well <u>very</u>	166		goodish
M. 26		Well <u>very</u>	i fit		goodish
T. 27		Well <u>very</u>	almost fit		do
W 28		Well <u>very</u>	i fit	wakeful ["goodish" del]	much fl
Th. 29		Well <u>very</u>			very good
F. 30		Well <u>very</u>			very good
<u>Sat 31</u>		Well <u>very</u>	i fit		do

12 double Dashes

	St	oz
Dec. 23	13	5 ½

1854. January   <u>Night</u>: --

Sun 1	Well <u>very</u>			very good
M 2	Well <u>very</u>			very good
T. 3	Well <u>very</u>			very good
W. 4	Well <u>very</u>			good
Th 5	Well <u>very</u>			moderate
F 6	Well	several fits from party [167]		goodish
<u>Sat 7</u>	Well <u>very</u>			goodish
S. 8	Well <u>very</u>	1 fit		goodish
M. 9	Well <u>very</u>			good
T 10	Well <u>very</u>	almost fit		moderate
W 11	Well <u>very</u>		Wakeful	moderate
Th 12	Well very	2 fits		moderate
F. 13	Well <u>very</u>	1 fit		goodish:
<u>Sat 14</u>	Well <u>very</u>	do		do
Sun 15	Well <u>very</u>	do		moderate
M 16	Well very	2 or 3 fits		goodish
T 17	Well <u>very</u>	almost fit		good
W 18	Well <u>very</u>			goodish:
Th 19	Well <u>very</u>			good
F 20	Well <u>very</u>	London[168]		good
<u>Sat 21</u>	Well <u>very</u>			good
S. 22	Well <u>very</u>	|———————————————| [169]	good
M 23	Well very	2 or 3 fits	½ Lemon ["thrice" "twice" del] thrice	good
T 24	Well <u>very</u>	(some occas. fl)	(Whole Lemon Twice a day)	moderate[170]
W. 25	Well <u>very</u>	some occasional		good
Th 26	Well <u>very</u>	do		good:
F. 27	Well <u>very</u>			goodish
<u>Sat 28</u>	Well <u>very</u>			good
S. 29	Well <u>very</u>			good
M. 30	Well <u>very</u>		no fit of fl	good
T. 31	Well <u>very</u>	i fit		goodish

16 Double Dashes

1853 February					Night
W. 1	Poorly. Bad headache.	Sickness	(London)[171]		Bad
Th 2.	Well _very_	1 slight fit			indifferent
F 3	Well _very_	occas fl			moderate
Sat 4	Well _very_	do			good:
Sun 5	Well _very_				goodish
M. 6	Well _very_	i fit	(slight cold)		goodish
T 7	Well _very_			wakeful	poorish
W 8	Well _very_			one baddish fit	moderate
Th. 9	Well _very_				good
F 10	Well _very_			one consid fit	good
Sat 11	Well _very_				good
Sun 12	Well _very_				goodish
M 13	Well _very_	one consid fit			good
T 14	Well _very_		(Dinner party)[172]	goodish	
W 15	Well _very_				indifferent
Th 16	Well very	2 fits			good
F 17	Well _very_			hardly any fit	very good
Sat 18	Well _very_	almost a fit			good
S. 19	Well _very_	i fit			very good
M. 20	Well _very_	do			very good
T 21	Well _very_	do			good
W 22	Well _very_	do			very good
Th 23	Headach		⎫		moderate
F 24	do		⎬ London[173]		goodish
S. 25	Well _very_		⎭		good
S. 26	Well _very_				good
M 27	Well _very_				good
T. 28	Well _very_				good

⎡ 15 Double Dashes   17 in long month ⎤
⎣   & include two visits to London. --   ⎦

1854 March						Night
W. 1	Well very	almost fit				good
Th. 2	Well very	2 consid. fits				moderate good:
F. 3	Well very	some occas fl				good:
Sat 4	Well very	i fit				heasy, good.
S. 5	Well very					goodish.
M. 6	Well very	i bad fit & Discomfort				good
T. 7	Well very	1 slight fit	do			good
W 8	Well very	2 fits	(Left off Lemon) [174]			goodish
Th 9	Well very	i fit				good
F. 10	Well very	i fit				goodish
Sat 11	Well very					good
Sun 12	Well very					good
M. 13		at night sickness				
T. 14		Rather Poorly				
W. 15	Hartfield for Franky [175]					
		Well				
Th. 16		Well very				good
F. 17		Well very				goodish
Sat 18	Well very					goodish
Sun 19	Well very	i fit				good
M. 20	Well very	do				good:
T. 21	Well very	2 fits				very good
W. 23	Well very					very good
Th. 23	Well very					good
F. 24	Well very				heazish	good
Sat 25	Well very	heasy				good
S. 26	Well very					good
M. 27	Well very	some occas fl				good
T. 28	Well very	2 consid fits	wakeful			goodish
W. 29		Poorly in even[in]g				bad
Th 30	Very Poorly	much vomiting	Bad Boil			bad
F. 31	do	Boil broke in noon				bad

10 Double Dashes

1854	April			Night:
Sat. 1	Well but ill from Boil, which broke in early morning			very restless.
S. 2	Poorly	with do		goodish
M. 3	Sick in early morning			heasyish, goodish
T. 4	Poorly sick – Boil better			do good
W. 5	Well very	i fit	(Half Lemon)[176]	do do
Th. 6	Well very			very good
F. 7	Well very	2 or 3 fits		good
Sat 8	Well very	i fit		good
S. 9	Well very	2 fits		heasyish, good
M 10	Well very	1 fit		good
T. 11	Well very	2 fits		heasyish, good
W. 12	Well very	2 fits		good
Th. 13	Well very	i fit		good
F. 14	Well very			good
Sat 15	Well very	2 fits		good
S. 16	Well very			good
M. 17	Well very	2 bad fits		goodish
T. 18	Well very	2 bad fits		good;
W. 19	Well very	some occas fl	restless	goodish:
Th 20	Well very	2 fits		good
F. 21	Well very	i fit		very heasy --------
Sat 22	Well very			heasy good
S 23	Well very	several slight fits	very heasy	heayish good
M 24	Well very	occas fl	heasyish slight sinking.	bad fl
T. 25	Well very	2 or 3 fits	do much fl.	almost sick
W. 26	Well very	1 long fit	heay	considerable fl.
Th. 27	Well	2 or 3 slight fits	heazish	better
F. 28	Well very	2 slight fits	do	good
Sat 29	Well	much fl	Dinner Par[t]y[177] good	
S. 30	Well very	2 or 3 fits		goodish

Only 3 Double Dashes & two of these not good!

1854 May				Night
M. 1	Well very			good:
T. 2[178]	Well very	very well yet consid fl.		good:
W. 3	Well very			good, --
Th. 4	Well very			good.
F. 5	Well very			good.
Sat 6	Well very			good.: --
S. 7	Well very	2 consid. fit		good
M. 8	Well very			restless, goodish
T. 9	Well very	2 fits		heasyish good.
W. 10	Well very	1 fit		good.
Th 11	Well very	do		good
F. 12	Well ["very" del] very			goodish,
Sat 13	Well very			good
S. 14	Well very			good
M. 15	Well very	2 fits		goodish
T. 16	Well very		(Slightly heasy.)	good
W. 17	Well very			good
Th. 18	Well very		rather wakeful	goodish
F. 19	Well very			goodish
Sat 20	Well very			good.
S. 21	Well very			good.
M 22	Well very			restless goodish,
T 23	Well very	heazy		goodish.
W. 24[179]	very well London			good
Th. 25[180]				
F. 26				
Sat 27				goodish. --
S 28	Well very			good
M. 29	Well very			very good
T. 30	Well very			very good
W. 31	Well very			do

Eight Double, but night much better.

1854	June. –		Nights: --
Th. 1	Well very		goodish.
F. 2	Well very		good
Sat 3-	Well very		good.
S. 4	Well, but in afternoon one very bad fit of fl		good.
M. 5	Well very		goodish.
T. 6	Well barely several bad fits		good.
W. 7	Well very		good:
Th. 8	Well very	restless	goodish.
F. 9	Well very 2 baddish	restless,	poorish
Sat 10	Poorly & sickness & bad headache from Crystal Palace [181]		good
S. 11	Well very some occas.		good
M 12	Well very		good: --
T. 13	Well very (some occas fl.)		goodish
W. 14	Well very i fit		poorish
Th 15	Well 2 or 3 fits		goodish:
F 16	["Well very" del] Poorly sickness, headache		good
Sat 17	Well very		goodish
S. 18	Well very	wakeful	good
M 19	Well very i fit	restless	goodish.
T 20	Well very		good :
W. 21	Well very ⎤		goodish.
Th. 22	Well very ⎬ London[182]		good.
F. 23	Well very ⎦	restless	good:
Sat 24	Well very		very good.
S 25	Well very 1 slight		very good
M 26	Well very		good
T. 27	Well very		good.
W 28	Well very 2 fits		goodish
Th 29	Well very		good
F. 30	Well very		good

15 Double Dashes.

1854 July			Night
Sat 1	Well very		moderate
S. 2	Well not quite,	2 Boils	good. –
M. 3	Poorly, sickness		poorish
T. 4	Rather poorly		goodish
W. 5	Cold	Bad Boil	do
Th. 6	Cold	rather poorly	do
F 7	Cold		do
Sat 8	Well	2 or 3 fits	goodish:
S. 9	Well	do	good.
M. 10	Well very	(some occas fl)	goodish.
T. 11	Well very	2 or 3 fits	goodish
W. 12	Well very	do	good.
Th. 13	Well	Hartfield[183]	
F. 14	Well		goodish
Sat 15	Well very		good
S. 16	Well very		goodish.
M. 17	Well very		goodish
T. 18	Well very [184]		good :
W. 19	Well very		good
Th. 20	Well very		good
F. 21	Well very		goodish:
Sat 22	Well very		goodish
S. 23	Well very		moderate
M 24	Well	2 fits	moderate:
T. 25	Well very		do
W. 26	Well very		good
Th. 27	Well very		goodish
F. 28	Well very		good
Sat 29	Well very		good
S. 30	Well very		good.
M. 31	Well very		good:

12 Double Dashes

1854 August			Night: --
T. 1	Well but sick in Evening (London.)[185]		moderate
W. 2	Well		good:
Th 3	Well very		good
F. 4	Poorly, feverish, Boil		feverish
Sat 5			bad
S. 6			do
M 7	Bad Boil, Lumbago : very poorly. --		do
T. 8			do
W. 9			goodish
Th. 10	Better		good
F. 11	Well very		good.
Sat 12	Well very		good.
S. 13	Well very		good:
M. 14	Well very [186]	i fit	goodish.
T 15	Well very 1 fit		good.
W. 16	Well very do		good
Th 17	Well very		good
F 18	Well very some fl.	restless	good
Sat 19	Well very		good
S. 20	Well very		good
M 21	Well not quite – several fit	heazish	good
T. 22	Well very	do	good
W. 23	Well very	do	good
Th. 24	Well very	do	good
F. 25	Well very	do	good
Sat 26	Well very	do	good
S 27	Well very	do	good
M. 28	Well very		good.
T. 29	Well very		good.
W 30	Well very		good.
Th. 31	Well very as far as stomach. but very p from S.E.[187]		wretched[188]

10 Double Dashes

1854 September					Night—
F. 1	Well very				good: --
Sat 2	Well very				good
S. 3	Well very				good
M. 4	Well	much fl	(work)[189]	heazish	good.
T. 5	Well very		(work)		good.
W 6	Well very	30 drops of Cordial Aloes	no work		good
Th. 7	Well very	20 drops of do	no work		good:
F. 8	Well very	10 drops purged	5 work	10 drops twice a day w^d be enough [190]	good:
Sat 9	Well	consid fl			good:
S. 10	Well	do			good:
M. 11	Well	do			goodish
T. 12	Well very	i fit			good.
W. 13	Well very	, do			good
Th 14	Well very	almost fit			moderate
F. 15	Well very				do
Sat 16	Well very barely, oppressed				good:
S 17	Well very				good.
M 18	Well				good
T. 19	Well very				good.
W. 20	Well very				good.
Th. 21	Well very				good.
F. 22[191]	Well very				good
Sat 23	Well very				good
S. 24	Well very				moderate
M. 25	Well very	(little Boil)			poorish:
T. 26	Well very				goodish
W. 27	Well very				moderate
Th 28	Well very	some fl			good.
F. 29	Well very				good:
Sat 30	Well very				good.
					good.

15 Double Dashes

1854 October				Night.
Sunday 1	Well very	2 baddish fits		good.
M. 2	Well very			good. : --
T. 3	Well very			poorish.
W. 4	Well very		heasy	goodish
Th. 5	Well very	very heasy	do	poorish
F. 6	Well very		very do	good
Sat 7	Well very [192]		do	poorly, almost sinking
S. 8	Well very		do	moderate
M. 9	Well very		wakeful	poorish
T. 10	Well		do	goodish.
W. 11	Well very	Leith Hill[193]	do	do
Th. 12	Well very		do	good: -
F. 13	Well very		do	good
Sat 14	Well very		["do" del]	good
S 15	Well very		very good	
M. 16	Well very			good
T. 17	Well very			good
Th. 19	Well very			poorish:
F. 20	Well very			goodish.
Sat. 21	Well very			goodish.
S 22	Well very			poorish.
M. 23[194]	Well very			good:
T. 24	Well very			moderate.
W. 25	Well very			goodish.
Th. 26[195]	Well very			goodish:
F> 27	Well very		wakeful	good
Sat 28[196]	Well very		do	moderate
S 29	Well very		do	do
M. 20	Well very			goodish
T. 31	Well very	2 fits		do

(Nine Double Dashes)

	St.		
Oct. 31	13	; 8	lb

<u>1854 November</u>

					night: --
W. 1	Well <u>very</u>				goodish. –
Th. 2[197]	Well <u>very</u>	London[198]			good: --
F. 3	Well <u>very</u>				good: --
<u>Sat. 4</u>	Well <u>very</u>				good. –
Su 5	Well <u>very</u>				goodish –
M. 6	Well <u>very</u>		some occas		do.
T. 7	Well <u>very</u>				good
W. 8	Well <u>very</u>		one fit	face tickling	poorish
Th 9	Well <u>very</u>		oppressed occ	restless	goodish
F. 10	Well <u>very</u>			do. acid sickness,	poor
<u>Sat 11</u>	Well		afternoon poorly, much fl	wakeful	goodish –
S. 12	Well barely				moderate
M. 13	Well <u>very</u>				good
T. 14	Well <u>very</u>				moderate
W 15	Well <u>very</u>				good: --
Th. 16	Well very				goodish
F 17	Well <u>very</u>		20 drops of li Tinct. Aloes[199]		good
Sat 18	Well <u>very</u>				goodish
S. 19	Well <u>very</u>		1 w.[200]	very wakeful	moderate
M. 20	Well barely	(boil)	(4 w?)[201]	do do	do
T 21	Well <u>very</u>			do do	do acid sick
W. 22	Well <u>very</u>	i f		rather wakeful	goodish
Th 23	Well <u>very</u>			much ft.	do
F. 24	Well <u>very</u>				goodish
<u>Sat 25</u>	Well <u>very</u>				good
S. 26	Well <u>very</u>		some occas fl		very good.
M. 27	Well <u>very</u>	do			very good.
T. 28	Well <u>very</u>				good:
W. 29	Well <u>very</u> [202]				good
Th. 30	Well <u>very</u>				good

15 Double Dashes

1854 December			Night
F 1 [203]	Well very		good: --
Sat. 2	Well very		good:
S. 3	Well very		goodish.
M. 4	Well very		good
T. 5	Well very		good.
W. 6	Well very		poor
Th. 7	Well very		moderate
F. 8	Well very	Sty in Eye	good.
Sat 9	Well	several fits	goodish
S. 10	Well very		restless not good
M. 11	Well very		rather wakeful. goodish
T 12	Well very	i badd[ish] fit	good
W. 13	Well very		good
Th. 14	Well very		moderate
F. 15	Well very		goodish_
Sat 16	Well very		good.
S 17	Well very		good
M 18	Well very		good.
T 19	Well very		good:
W. 20	Well very	Children Ill.-- [204]	goodish.
Th 21	Well very		moderate:
F 22	Well very		good.
Sat 23	Well very		good.
S. 24	Well very	Sickness	goodish
M. 25	Well moderate		moderate
T. 26	Well very		do do
W. 27	Poorly rather		goodish
Th 28	do		good.
F 29	Well barely		good
Sat 30	Well very		good.
S. 31	Well very		very restless

13 Double Dashes.

			Night: --
1855			
Jan:			
M. 1[205]	Well very		bad.
T. 2	Well very		moderate
W. 3	Well very		good
Th 4	Well very		goodish
F. 5	Well very		poor. acid sick: --
Sat. 6	Well barely		moderate
S. 7	Poorly	sick in evening	baddish
M. 8	Well very		very restless extreme fl.
T. 9	Much flatulence		do do
W. 10[206]	Consid fl		good but fl.
Th. 1	Well very		goodish
F. 12	Well very		good:
Sat 13	Well very		good.
S. 14[207]	Well very		goodish
M 15[208]	Well very		do.
T. 16	Well very		good
W. 17			
Th. 18			
F. 19			
Sat 20			
S. 21			
M. 22			
T. 23			
W. 24			
Th. 25 [209]			
F. 26			
Sat 27			
S. 28			
M. 29			
T. 30			

W. 31

Notes

Abbreviations Used

Autobiography: 1958. *Autobiography of Charles Darwin, 1809–1882. With the Original Omissions Restored.* Edited by Nora Barlow. London: Collins.

Beagle diary: 1988. *Charles Darwin's* Beagle *Diary*. Edited by Richard Darwin Keynes. Cambridge: Cambridge University Press.

Collected Papers: 1977. *Collected Papers of Charles Darwin*. Edited by Paul Barrett. 2 vols. Chicago: University of Chicago Press.

Correspondence: 1985. *Correspondence of Charles Darwin*. Edited by Frederick Burkhardt et al. 15 vols. Cambridge: Cambridge University Press.

DAR: Darwin Archive, Cambridge University Library.

Emma Darwin (1904): 1904. *Emma Darwin, Wife of Charles Darwin: A Century of Family Letters*. Edited by Henrietta Litchfield. 2 vols. Cambridge: Cambridge University Press.

Emma Darwin (1915): 1915. *Emma Darwin: A Century of Family Letters, 1792–1896*. Edited by Henrietta Litchfield. 2 vols. London: John Murray.

Emma's diary: 1824–82. Diary owned by Professor Richard Darwin Keynes, on loan to the Cambridge University Library, in DAR 242.

G. Darwin, "Recollections": Darwin, George. 1882. "Recollections of My Father," DAR 112, B4–B23.

Herbert, "Recollections": Herbert, J. M. 1882. "Recollections," DAR 112, B57–B76.

Life and Letters: 1888. *The Life and Letters of Charles Darwin, Including an Autobiographical Chapter*. Edited by Francis Darwin. 2 vols. New York: D. Appleton.

More Letters: 1903. *More Letters of Charles Darwin*. Edited by Francis Darwin and A. C. Seward. 2 vols. New York: D. Appleton.

Notebooks: 1987. *Charles Darwin's Notebooks, 1836–1844*. Edited by Paul H. Barrett, Peter J. Gautrey, Sandra Herbert, David Kohn, and Sydney Smith. Ithaca, N.Y.: British Museum (Natural History) and Cornell University Press.

"Reminiscences," *L&L*: Darwin, Francis. 1882–87. "Reminiscences of My Father's Everyday Life." In *Life and Letters*, 1: 88–136.

"Reminiscences," ms: Darwin, Francis. 1882–87. "Reminiscences of My Father's Everyday Life." Manuscript. DAR 140.3.

Preface

    1. Darwin to Fox, 1863, *Correspondence*, 11: 438.

Chapter 1

    1. *Correspondence,* 1: 94, 230; 2: 353. *The New English Dictionary* defines "knock up" as "to overcome or make ill with fatigue; to exhaust, tire out."

    2. *Correspondence,* 1: 16, 25; *Autobiography,* 47.

    3. *Autobiography,* 48; Desmond and Moore 1991, 27; G. Darwin, "Recollections."

    4. *Correspondence,* 1: 16; Herbert, "Recollections."

    5. *Autobiography,* 44, 61.

    6. *Autobiography,* 61–62; Herbert, "Recollections."

    7. The account of the events of the Birmingham Music Festival on 8 October 1829 is based on the printed program of the festival and a detailed report, "Birmingham Musical Festival," published in the *Birmingham Journal.* The report emphasized the richness and variety of the operatic events and praised Malibran's "talismanic witchery of . . . voice and look," which held the large audience "spell-bound." *Correspondence,* 1: 93–94.

    8. Herbert, "Recollections"; *Correspondence,* 1: 73–74, 76, 101. Darwin would later tell his son Francis that, as a result of the accident, Owen suffered from a permanent impairment of the eye that had been injured. "Reminiscences," ms, 107.

    9. *Correspondence,* 1: 81, 82, 88, 106, 325. This explanation of mental stress being a cause of Darwin's lip disorder is similar to that given in Bowlby 1990, 100–101.

    10. Herbert, "Recollections." The medical books that Darwin possessed—Paris's *Pharmacologia,* Duncan's *Edinburgh New Dispensatory,* and *Zoonomia,* vol. 2, by his grandfather, Dr. Erasmus Darwin—recommended that arsenic be used externally in cancer and skin diseases and internally (usually in the form of Fowler's solution) as the treatment for fevers, headaches, periodical diseases, and "many anomalous diseases of the skin." It was also recognized that arsenic was "one of the most virulent poisons" and that when taken medicinally its toxic effects should be carefully watched for and its use should be stopped if these effects appeared. While it was stated in Colp (1977, 7) that Darwin met with Dr. Henry Holland in February 1829, and that this physician may have prescribed arsenic for him, it now appears that he met not with Dr. Holland but with Edward Holland, his nonmedical second cousin. *Correspondence,* 1: 76, note 2.

    11. *Correspondence,* 1: 143.

    12. *Autobiography,* 68.

Chapter 2

    1. In April 1831, after reading Humboldt's *Narrative,* Darwin wrote in a letter that his head was "running about the Tropics" and that he could "hardly sit still." Many years later, a friend remembered how, when Darwin spoke of Humboldt's descriptions, he showed his excitement by vehemently rubbing his chin. *Correspondence,* 1: 122; *Life and Letters,* 1: 144–45; *Beagle* diary, 3.

2. *Beagle* diary, 3; *Correspondence,* 1: 131–36.

3. *Correspondence,* 1: 382; *Beagle* diary, 3.

4. *Correspondence,* 1: 143, 148, 156.

5. *Beagle* diary, 10–12, 15; *Autobiography,* 79–80.

6. *Autobiography,* 80; *Beagle* diary, 8, 12, 13; *Correspondence,* 1: 163, 176, 180.

7. He was apprehensive not only that he might die from heart disease but that if it became known that he had this disease it would prevent him from going on the *Beagle.* Therefore, he made no mention of palpitations in letters to family and friends or in his conversations with the captain of the *Beagle,* Robert FitzRoy. On 19 November 1831, FitzRoy wrote to Captain Francis Beaufort, the Admiralty hydrographer in charge of the *Beagle* voyage, "Darwin has not yet shone one trait which has made me feel other than glad when I reflect how much we shall be together." F. Darwin 1912. Darwin would continue to conceal his palpitations and feelings of anxiety and depression from FitzRoy during the next six weeks that the two were together at Plymouth.

8. On 19 November, Captain Alexander Vidal of the Royal Navy told Darwin that during his eight years of surveying the African coast he had "buried 30 young officers," and "a boat never was sent up a river, without its causing the death of some of the party." *Beagle* diary, 7. At this time, among the many naturalists who explored the Tropics, "some of the best succumbed to tropical diseases." Mayr 1992, 136.

9. On 17 September, he grimly wrote to Susan: "I have been in capital spirits ever since all was fixed [his resolution to go on the *Beagle*], & if I go to the bottom, I shall go on this one point like a rational creature." *Correspondence,* 1: 156. He may have been fearful of drowning for several reasons: "he could . . . never learn to swim especially well" ("Reminiscences," ms); he had only been on a sailing ship in May 1827, when he crossed the English channel for a visit to Paris, and he had two fearful childhood memories of water: a "fear & astonishment of white foaming water" when the carriage he was riding in crossed a broad ford, and hearing a story about people accidentally being pushed into a canal because they were on the wrong side of the horse that was towing a ferry. "I had," he remembered, "the greatest horror of this story." *Correspondence,* 2: 438. He may have felt a combination of old and new horrors when, on 21 November, he recorded that a *Beagle* sailor "slipped overboard & was not seen again." *Beagle* diary, 8.

10. On 13 September, Darwin's Cambridge friend Charles Whitley wrote him: "I desire greatly to see you again. You may be drowned, shot or feversmitten, or I may die from pure vexation & disappointment before you return, & I should certainly like to shake hands once more before we separate." Ten days after receiving this letter, Darwin replied that a meeting was not possible and that "I have nothing particular to say excepting that all is finally settled, & I have sealed away about half a chance of life.—If one lived merely to see how long one could spin out life.—I should repent of my choice.—As it is I do not." *Correspondence,* 1: 154, 168.

11. *Beagle* diary, 19–20, 34, 35; *Correspondence,* 1: 201–34; *Life and Letters,* 1: 193.

12. *Beagle* diary, 18.

13. Moorehead 1969, 252. Sago was a starch preparation made from the stems of sago palms, and it was used medically as a nutrient and a demulcent.

14. *Life and Letters*, 1: 197–98; *Beagle* diary, 18.

15. *Beagle* diary, 23, 42–43; *Correspondence*, 1: 247.

16. *Beagle* diary, 41.

17. *Beagle* diary, 44–45, 65.

18. *Beagle* diary, 56; Moorehead 1969, 160.

19. Colp 1977. The receipts and memoranda book was the Darwin family medical scrapbook, containing medical information and prescriptions by Dr. Robert Darwin, Charles Darwin, and Emma Darwin.

20. *Beagle* diary, 67–68.

21. *Correspondence*, 1: 231; *Beagle* diary, 64. Charles Musters, volunteer first class on the *Beagle*, had been a friend and companion to Darwin since the start of the voyage.

22. *Correspondence*, 1: 256.

23. Forty-three years later, Darwin would refer to this sentence in *Autobiography*, 126.

24. *Correspondence*, 1: 311–12. The servant was Syms Covington (1816–61), who remained in Darwin's employ as secretary-servant from 1833 until 1839, at which point he emigrated to Australia.

25. Moorehead 1969, 208; *Beagle* diary, 193.

26. According to Francis Darwin: "Like most delicate people he [Darwin] suffered from heat as well as from chilliness; it was as if he could not hit the balance between too hot and too cold. "Reminiscences," ms, 90. This sensitivity to changes in temperature may have made Darwin especially prone to suffer heat stroke.

27. Moorehead 1969, 208; Darwin, *Journal of Researches*, 1839, 148.

28. Darwin, *Journal of Researches*, 1845, 128.

29. *Beagle* diary, 194; *Correspondence*, 1: 342.

30. *Beagle* diary, 199; Moorehead 1969, 213.

31. *Beagle* diary, 214–15; FitzRoy 1839, 319–20.

32. *Correspondence*, 1: 410–11, 418; *Beagle* diary, 262–63; *Life and Letters*, 1: 198.

33. Colp 1977, receipts and memoranda book, Dr. Robert Darwin's prescriptions. In 1833 Darwin had made a note to purchase calomel. Moorehead 1969, 184.

34. While Arthur Keith thought that the illness was typhoid fever (Keith 1955, 212), it has been postulated that it may have been typhus fever (Kohn 1963, 253). However, typhus fever is more likely to occur in epidemics and to run a course of two weeks, whereas Darwin's illness does not appear to have been part of an epidemic, and its course of five to six weeks fits the course of typhoid fever. Although Darwin believed that the illness resulted from drinking "sour new made" wine, and this belief has been supported by a recent biographer (Browne 1995, 280), the onset of typhoid is insidious and could have occurred before the incident with the sour wine, and the long duration of the fever distinguishes it from a form of food poisoning. I thank Professor Leonard Wilson for

writing me a letter discussing his reasons for believing that Darwin's 1834 illness was typhoid fever. See Wilson 1978.

35. *Correspondence*, 1: 418, 435; Darwin, *Journal of Researches*, 1839, 394, 395; *Life and Letters*, 2: 238.

36. Darwin, *Journal of Researches*, 1839, 403–4; *Beagle* diary, 315, note 1; Goldstein 1989, 597. In one of his pocket notebooks, Darwin first recorded the *Triatoma* attack: "The giant bugs of the Pampas; horribly disgusting to feel numerous creatures nearly an inch long and black and soft crawling in all parts of your person—gorged with your blood." Moorehead 1969, 236.

37. In June 1835, Darwin "caught" a triatome in the bed in which he had been sleeping, in Copiapo, Chile. In July, he caught and kept a "very thin" triatome at Iquique, Peru. He then had it suck blood for ten minutes from the finger of a *Beagle* officer, observing that it "caused very little pain; became bloated and globular & 5 or 6 times the original size; 18 days afterwards was again ready to suck; being kept 4½ months became of proper proportions, as thin as at first; I then killed it. A most bold and fearless insect." Since the triatome's sucking inflicted little pain, there may have been occasions when Darwin had been bitten by one or more bugs and not been aware of their biting. Darwin, *Journal of Researches*, 1839, 404; Porter 1983, 316; K.G.V. Smith 1987, 89, note 2913, 96, note 3423.

38. *Beagle* diary, 323; Goldstein 1989, 597.

39. Catherine wrote him from Shrewsbury on 28 January 1835, but there was a delay of about seven months before he received her letter.

40. *Correspondence*, 1: 424.

41. In March 1835, Darwin had written Caroline that "our voyage has at last a definite & certain end fixed to it" and that the *Beagle* was expected "to arrive in England in September 1836." *Correspondence*, 1: 433.

42. *Correspondence*, 1: 459.

43. In December 1835, Darwin's Cambridge mentor, J. S. Henslow, sent Robert Darwin a pamphlet of published "extracts" from Darwin's *Beagle* letters to Henslow. After reading this, Robert Darwin wrote Henslow a note expressing some of the feelings he felt for his son: "I thought the voyage hazardous for his happiness, but it seems to prove otherwise and it is highly gratifying to me to think he gains credit by his observation and exertion. There is a natural good humored energy in his letters just like himself." *Correspondence*, 1: 473.

44. *Correspondence*, 1: 471, 490, 497.

45. FitzRoy to Beaufort, 26 January 1836, in F. Darwin 1912, 548.

46. *Beagle* diary, 433–34; *Correspondence*, 1: 495.

47. *Correspondence*, 1: 495; Desmond and Moore 1991, 186; Browne 1995, 339.

48. *Life and Letters*, 1: 193.

49. *Correspondence*, 1: 503.

Chapter 3

1. *Autobiography*, 82–84, 100–101; *Correspondence*, 1: 512, 517; 2: 2, 4–5.

2. *Autobiography*, 83; *Correspondence*, 2: 11.

3. *Correspondence*, 2: 10, 52, note 6, 69. He served as one of two secretaries of the Geological Society from 16 February 1838 until 19 February 1841.

4. *Correspondence*, 2: 47, 49, 50–52, 431. According to the *Oxford Dictionary of National Biography*, Henry Holland (1788–1873) was a distant cousin of the Darwins and Wedgwoods, physician in ordinary to Queen Victoria 1852, and physician to Darwin's brother Erasmus. James Clark (1788–1870) was naval surgeon, 1809–15, and physician in ordinary to Queen Victoria 1837; he was created baronet in 1837. Holland and Clark knew each other and were leading London physicians and socially prominent.

5. Porter and Porter 1989, 74–75.

6. *Correspondence*, 2: 59. *Journal of Researches* was first published in 1839, as the third volume of *The Narrative of the Voyages of HMS Ships* Adventure *and* Beagle, edited by Captain Robert FitzRoy.

7. *Correspondence*, 2: 69–70, 80.

8. *Correspondence*, 2: 85. Darwin's plan of bringing out a work entitled "Geological Observations on Volcanic Islands and Coral Formations" was announced in an 1838 advertisement by the publisher Smith Elder, but was then abandoned. The first part, *Coral Reefs*, appeared in May 1842. The second part, *Volcanic Islands*, was published in November 1844.

9. *Notebooks*, 263.

10. *Notebooks*, 276. Prior to writing this passage, Darwin had become familiar with examples of men being persecuted and resisting persecution. When he was growing up, he may have observed how the conservative community in Shrewsbury regarded his father as a holder of "heretical views." And Robert Darwin may have told him how his grandfather, Dr. Erasmus Darwin, had been publicly ridiculed for holding liberal and evolutionary ideas during the period when England was opposing the French Revolution. As a youth he came to "revere" his uncle Josiah Wedgwood II as "the very type of an upright man" who would not "swerve an inch from what he considered the right course."

When he was at Edinburgh University, he witnessed how a paper read by a member of the Edinburgh Plinian Society was censored from the society's minutes because it stated a materialist position on the nature of organisms and mind. When he was at Cambridge University, he may have first heard from William Whewell about the condemnation of Bruno and Galileo by the Inquisition and about Copernicus's hesitation in publishing his heliocentric theory, and he may have been impressed by Whewell's belief that both Bruno and Galileo had brought punishment upon themselves by needlessly provoking the authorities. In his last year at Cambridge, when he read John Herschel's *Preliminary Discourse on the Study of Natural Philosophy*, and then thought of making "even the most humble contribution" to science, he may have been impressed by Herschel's observation that those who had previously advanced in science had done so by overcoming existing prejudices.

During the first year of the *Beagle* voyage, Darwin read in the first volume of Lyell's

Principles of Geology how the French naturalist Buffon had been forced by the faculty of theology at the Sorbonne to recant some of his ideas that contradicted the Bible. Colp 1986, 9–10.

11. *Correspondence*, 2: 84–85, 86–87, 431.

12. *Correspondence*, 2: 91–92, 96, 431; Colp 1980.

13. *Notebooks*, 527, 532; *Correspondence*, 2: 431.

14. *Correspondence*, 2: 444–45, note 1; *Emma Darwin* (1904), 1: 418, 420.

15. *Notebooks*, 539. This account of the influence of Comte's ideas on Darwin's evolutionary thinking is based on Schweber 1977, 241–64.

16. *Notebooks*, 329–30, 395–96.

17. Darwin kept his journal from August 1838 until December 1881. All references to it are based on the original manuscript (DAR 158, 1–76) or on citations from this manuscript in the chronology sections of *Correspondence*. For an account of how Darwin came to write the journal, see Colp 1980, 20–21, and *Correspondence*, 2: 430.

18. *Correspondence*, 2: 117–18, 125, 432.

19. *Correspondence*, 2: 432; Desmond and Moore 1991, 274–76.

20. *Correspondence*, 2: 144. Lady Catherine de Bourgh was a character in Jane Austen's *Pride and Prejudice* who possessed the following characteristics: "though this great lady was not in the commission of the peace for the county, she was a most active magistrate in her own parish . . . [so that] whenever any of the cottagers were disposed to be quarrelsome, discontented, or too poor, she sallied forth into the village to settle their differences, silence their complaints, and scold them into harmony and plenty." *Pride and Prejudice*, chap. 30.

21. *Correspondence*, 2: 149–50.

22. *Correspondence*, 2: 150–51, 161–62; Desmond and Moore 1991, 277.

23. *Correspondence*, 2: 166, 169. For a discussion of the religious differences between Charles and Emma at this time, see Keynes 2001, 49–51.

24. *Correspondence*, 2: 150, 169, 171. While Darwin never explained what he feared about participating in his wedding, it may have involved the fear of being in the center of a grave and formal public event and having to speak formally in front of a group of individuals who would evaluate his appearance and behavior. It may have been a form of stage fright that he would experience whenever he had to be present at formal scientific meetings.

25. *Correspondence*, 2: 170–71.

26. *Emma Darwin* (1904), 1: 441–43; *Correspondence*, 2: 433.

Chapter 4

1. *Emma Darwin* (1904), 1: 458, 461; Emma Darwin's diary, 12 March 1839; *Correspondence*, 2: 305.

2. *Emma Darwin* (1904), 1: 464; *Correspondence*, 2: 433.

3. In his Recollections, Thomas Butler writes that "Southey" (presumably the au-

thor Robert Southey [1774–1843]) was on the coach with him and Darwin and that the coach was going from Birmingham to Shrewsbury. Butler, "Recollections," 13 September 1882, DAR 112, A10–A12. Darwin traveled on this coach on 12 September 1839. *Correspondence*, 2: 433. Southey traveled frequently in England in the 1830s, but because of illness he did not travel after 1839. Southey 1855, 560–62. Thus it seems likely that Butler met Darwin on 12 September 1839. Thomas Butler was the son of the Reverend Samuel Butler, headmaster of Shrewsbury School while Darwin was there. He and Darwin were together at Shrewsbury School and then at Cambridge University.

4. *Correspondence*, 2: 227, 234.

5. *Correspondence*, 2: 270, 434. At this time flatulency was defined as "an undue formation and accumulation of air in the stomach or intestines, with frequent rejection of it." Copeland 1858, 1: 1043. Individuals suffering from this accumulated air would try to reject it by belching. Darwin's earliest recorded reference to flatulency and belching was in a notebook he kept on the mental development of his eldest child, William Erasmus Darwin. Here he recollected that in May 1840, when William was four and a half months old: "I one day made a loud snoring noise which I had never done before; he [William] instantly looked grave and then burst out crying. Two or three days afterwards, I made through forgetfulness the same noise with the same result." It seems likely that the "loud snoring" noises that Darwin made were belchings. Five months later, on 30 October 1840, Emma and her husband each noted—she in her diary, he in his notebook on his son—that when Darwin belched, William would respond to the belching by "patting" his father's "mouth, during [the] emission of sound." Darwin's notebook observations on William are published in *Correspondence*, 4: appendix 3, 415, 418.

6. *Emma Darwin* (1904), 2: 9, 10.

7. *Correspondence,* 2: 260, 261; 6: 344. In 1855, after Henslow had sent him a program of public lectures that he had given, Darwin replied: "You little know how difficult, not to say impossible & how awful it would be to many, & to myself for one; to lecture or lecturette to a crowd of people. I would sooner pay 50£ for a good lecturer to come here; but in the same proportion as I sh^d. dread such an undertaking, so do I honour you for all you do." *Correspondence*, 5: 481.

8. *Correspondence*, 2: 253–56; *Emma Darwin* (1904), 2: 9.

9. *Correspondence*, 2: 261–63, 270.

10. *Autobiography*, 98.

11. *Correspondence*, 5: 14, 15, 17; *Emma Darwin* (1904), 2, 142; Keynes 2001, 171.

12. *Correspondence*, 2: 434.

13. For more information on this prescription, see Dr. Robert Darwin's prescriptions in the receipts and memoranda book, in Colp 1977. Emma's diary mentions "calomel" on 22 and 23 September, "bismuth" on 25 September, and "no more bismuth" on 1 October. Emma's diary also contains references to the use of new kinds of foods such as oysters and artichokes, partridge and pudding, hare and oysters, which may have been intended as a treatment for her husband's illness.

14. *Correspondence*, 2: 278.

15. Colvin 1971, 571–72. In this same letter, Maria Edgeworth comments: "You know that he [Darwin] says he was ill in consequence of the [*Beagle*] sea voyage—that he was never a single day free from sea-suffering. But Dr. Holland tells us that the voyage was not the cause, only the continuance of his suffering—for that before he went to sea he was subject to the same." While Darwin appears to have told Dr. Holland that he had pre-*Beagle* vomiting, none of his early letters indicate that he had stomach symptoms that were as severe as his vomiting and flatulence of 1840. That his pre-*Beagle* stomach upsets were not serious is suggested by his 1849 recollection to Henslow of their 1830–31 associations: "Ah those were delightful days when one had no such organ as a stomach, only a mouth and masticating appurtenances." *Correspondence*, 4: 236.

16. *Correspondence*, 2: 279.

17. In his 1865 medical notes to Dr. John Chapman, Darwin wrote that "for 25 years" he had been having "extreme spasmodic daily & nightly flatulence." *Correspondence*, 13: 482. In 1869, he wrote William Preyer that his health had been "poor since 1840." Letter to William Preyer, 29 March 1869. DAR 147, 254–56. In 1873, he wrote Francis Galton that his health had been "bad for last 33 years." *Life and Letters*, 2: 356.

18. *Autobiography*, 98.

19. Bowlby 1990, 238; *Correspondence*, 2: 270, 279.

20. *Autobiography*, 98.

21. Goldstein 1989, 594–97.

22. Goldstein 1989, 597–98. While Goldstein believes that Chagas' disease became arrested in the 1850s, I believe that, judging from the course of Darwin's symptoms, it could have become arrested in the early 1840s.

23. For an account of the different opinions on Chagas' disease, see chapter 20.

24. In the 1830s, because of faulty ventilation and lighting (caused by the use of open-gas flare-burners), Athenaeum Club members complained of the "stupefying effects of gas" and of needing "copper lungs," and the bindings of many of the books in the Athenaeum's Library were injured. It was not until 1841 that some of these faults were temporarily (and then not very effectively) corrected. Ward 1926, 50–52. Darwin had become a member of the Athenaeum in June 1838, and although for most of the rest of the year he, in the words of his brother Erasmus, could "hardly live out of the Athenaeum," he did not (as far as can be determined) complain of respiratory distress. There is no record of how often he frequented the Athenaeum during his 1839 malaise and first exacerbation of illness in 1839–40. His second exacerbation occurred when he was in Maer. *Correspondence*, 2: 94, note 2; Browne 1995, 384, note 31.

25. *Correspondence*, 2: 298.

26. *Autobiography*, 35–36; *Correspondence*, 2: 305.

27. *Correspondence*, 2: 303, 318–19, 434–35.

28. *Autobiography*, 120, 131–32; *Correspondence*, 2: 279–80, 434; 4: appendix 2, 410–23.

29. *Autobiography*, 99; *Correspondence*, 2: 435; Charles Darwin, "Notes on the Effects Produced by the Ancient Glaciers of Caernarvonshire, and on the Boulders Transported by Floating Ice," *Collected Papers*, 1: 163–71.

Chapter 5

1. *Correspondence*, 2: 305.
2. Winslow 1971, 1–2.
3. Clark 1846, 2, 3–4.
4. Pike 1974, 297–98; Sheppard 1971, 16.
5. *Emma Darwin* (1904), 2: 32, 36.
6. E. Darwin 1796, 2: 674; 1798, 98.
7. *Autobiography*, 114; Topham 1997, 50–54.
8. *Correspondence*, 2: 324; Topham 1997, 50–54; Browne 1995, 442.
9. *Correspondence*, 2: 345.
10. *Correspondence*, 2: 435; Desmond and Moore 1991, 303.
11. *Emma Darwin* (1904), 2: 50.
12. *Correspondence*, 2: 435; Browne 1995, 443.
13. *Correspondence*, 2: 345.
14. *Correspondence*, 335.
15. *Correspondence*, 2: 360; Desmond and Moore 1991, 306–7; Browne 1995, 445.
16. Browne 1995, 445; Calvin 1998, 6; *Correspondence*, 3: 311.
17. *Correspondence*, 3: 2.
18. In 1858, he wrote this one line entry in his journal for June: "June 14th Pigeons: (interrupted)." His parenthetical "(interrupted)" communicated that, as he was working on the pigeon section of his big book on natural selection, he learned that Alfred Wallace had independently discovered his theory. *Correspondence*, 7: 503.
19. *Correspondence*, 3: 7, 25.
20. *Correspondence*, 3: 43, 395; Desmond and Moore 1991, 317. Darwin's paternal uncle, Charles Darwin, grandfather Erasmus Darwin, mother, and daughter Mary Elea-nor had all died suddenly, and his physician father had frequently observed instances of sudden death. Between 1829 and 1832, he learned about the sudden deaths of the sister of his friend Fox, his Cambridge friend Marmaduke Ramsay (who had been planning to go with him to Teneriffe), his young *Beagle* friend Charles Musters, and his cousin Fanny Wedgwood. Emma had been Fanny's sister and intimate companion and believed she would be reunited with Fanny in a future life. Emma may have spoken about Fanny with her husband. *Correspondence*, 1: 83–84, 128–30, 231, 268–69; Bowlby 1990, 39–40, 56–57; *Emma Darwin* (1904), 1: 346–47.
21. Hensleigh Wedgwood (1803–91) was a barrister and philologist who had some-times been Darwin's intellectual confidant.
22. Colp 1986, 17–19; *Correspondence*, 3: 44.
23. Browne 1995, 447; *Correspondence*, 3: xv.

24. *Correspondence*, 3: 47–57; Desmond and Moore 1991, 325.

25. *Correspondence*, 3: 254; Colp 1986, 20–22, 30–31.

26. Huxley 1918, 1: 29–30, 194–95. In May 1845, when Hooker was giving several public lectures, Darwin wrote him the following: "I shall be glad to hear how the lectures go on that you do not find them very terrific: the very thought of such a deed as lecturer to a whole class, makes me feel awe-struck." *Correspondence*, 3: 186.

27. *Correspondence*, 3: 166. That many of Darwin's friends considered him to be a hypochondriac may refer to a prevalent view that hypochondria (although understood to have a physical inheritable basis) reflected a weakness of moral fiber. "There was, after all, something self-pitying and at times self-serving about the hypochondriac's continual troubles." Baur 1988, 27–28.

28. *Correspondence*, 3: 211.

29. *Life and Letters*, 1: 387.

30. Hooker 1899. During his Down visits, Hooker also observed Darwin's retchings. In February 1849, when he was climbing the Himalayan Mountains in India, he wrote to Darwin: "I never thought more of you than amongst the Snowy passes, where the rarified air affects me at rather low elevations; sometimes I go on retching for hours & what with headache & its concomitant sensations I doubt if I ever could reach 18000 ft. perhaps not 16000." *Correspondence*, 4: 205.

31. *Correspondence*, 4: 49–50.

32. *Correspondence*, 3: 253.

33. Browne 1995, 470–71; Stott 2003, 83–86.

34. *Correspondence*, 4: 74–86.

35. Rudwick 1974, 97–185; Herbert 2005, 283–92.

36. Darwin persisted in believing in his marine theory until 1861. In that year, Thomas Francis Jamieson went to Glen Roy and wrote a paper presenting new evidence that the parallel roads had been formed by Ice Age lakes. He sent his paper to Darwin, who wrote him: "Your arguments seem to me conclusive. I give up the ghost. My paper is one long gigantic blunder. . . . How rash it is in science to argue because any case is not one thing, it must be some second thing which happens to be known to the writer." Darwin then sent Jamieson's letter to Lyell, along with the following note: "I think the enclosed is worth your reading. I am smashed to atoms about Glen Roy. My paper was one long gigantic blunder from beginning to end." *Correspondence*, 9: 255–57.

37. *Life and Letters*, 1: 288; *Correspondence*, 3: xiii, 84, 141, 287; 5: 198. A record of Darwin's 1844–48 attendance at meetings of the councils of the Geological Society is published in the chronology sections of *Correspondence*, vols. 3 and 4.

38. *Correspondence*, 4: 50–51, 53, 55; Desmond and Moore 1991, 347–49; Hooker 1899.

39. *Correspondence*, 3: 272–73, 274–75.

40. *Correspondence*, 4: 108–9, 111, 384; Geikie 1895, 130; Desmond and Moore 1991, 352. Darwin's illness and recovery is recorded in Emma's 1848 diary for 18–24 February.

41. *Correspondence,* 4: 53–54, 55–56, 58–60, 61, 74, 384.

42. "Reminiscences," ms, 94; *Autobiography,* 138; "Reminiscences," *L&L,* 1: 100, 102; *Emma Darwin* (1904), 2: 117–18.

43. "Reminiscences," ms, 23; "Reminiscences," *L&L,* 1: 100; Keith 1955, 23; *Correspondence,* 11: 167.

44. "Reminiscences," *L&L,* 1: 90–91, 93–94, 100; Atkins 1974, 25–26; Keynes 2004, 15–21.

45. Darwin to Asa Gray, 29 January 1876, Gray Herbarium, Harvard University; "Reminiscences," ms, 32.

46. *Emma Darwin* (1904), 2: 275; G. Darwin, "Recollections"; "Reminiscences," ms, 32.

47. "Reminiscences," *L&L,* 1: 103–4, 115.

48. *Autobiography,* 138.

49. Darwin 1929, 120.

50. "Reminiscences," *L&L,* 1: 101.

51. "Reminiscences," ms, 30, 37.

52. Brace 1894, 320; "Reminiscences," *L&L,* 1: 89.

53. Brace 1894, 320; Higginson 1900, 284; Mrs. Jane Loring Gray, 1868. Darwin began sitting in a "Highchair . . . supported on a high stool" in the 1840s and kept this up for the rest of his life. *Life and Letters,* 1: 388.

54. *Correspondence,* 2: 409; 3: 338, 141. For an account of Darwin's treatments, see chapter 6.

55. *Correspondence,* 4: 29–30, 383.

56. *Correspondence,* 4: 15, 55, 56, 91–92.

Chapter 6

1. Edgar Cockell was surgeon and apothecary at Down, circa 1840–55, and a member of the Royal College of Physicians. He was in attendance when Emma gave birth to Mary Eleanor on 23 September 1842. *Correspondence,* 2: 332–33.

2. *Correspondence,* 3: 86.

3. Royle and Headland 1865, 602. "Bitters were substances which were bitter to the taste—this was held to be due to an inherent "bitter principle"—and which were thought to act as "tonics" by giving a "salutary" stimulation to stomach and system in general. There was a variance of medical opinion about the use of bitters in dyspepsia. Dr. Holland held that their use had been "too large and indiscriminate" and that "there are various states of stomach in which the ordinary dose and strength of bitter infusions are injurious; while obvious good is got from a more moderate employment of the same means . . . the best mode of using bitters is in direct combinations with the aperient which may be necessary. Thereby a smaller quantity of the latter is usually rendered effectual; and the noxious effects of repetition materially abated." Holland 1840, 378–79. Dr. Brinton would write: "The various vegetable bitters claim peculiar notice . . . because

their effects [in dyspepsia] are more uniform and beneficial than those of most other medicines . . . most of them increase the appetite . . . their prolonged use produces such invigorating effects on the constitution, as to almost suggest some definite chemical purpose being subserved by their addition to the constituents of the organism, beyond any merely alternative effect." Brinton 1859, 385–86.

4. Moorehead 1969, 252.

5. Headland 1852, 107.

6. "Reminiscences," *L&L,* 1: 96.

7. *Correspondence,* 3: 247.

8. Royle and Headland 1865, 186. "Bismuth, some of the effects of which may perhaps be regarded as tonic, is still more useful as a remedy against that form of dyspepsia which constitutes the 'morbid sensibility of the stomach' specified by older writers. Here its effects in allaying flatulence and nausea, and in preventing vomiting, and (still more) in checking the pain produced by food, are so marked, that we may fairly accept the term of sedative often applied to it." Brinton 1859, 388.

9. Colp 1986, 22–23; *Emma Darwin* (1904), 2: 81.

10. *Correspondence,* 3: 264, 265, note 6, 287; *Emma Darwin* (1904), 2: 85. For the history of galvanism, see Licht 1967, 18–19, 24–30, and Rowbottom and Susskind 1984, chapters 3 and 4. Dr. Darwin's views on galvanism are not known.

11. *Correspondence,* 3: 325. Opium had been used by Darwin's grandfather (who had caused his grandmother, and then his uncle Tom Wedgwood, to become addicted to the drug), and by his father (see Dr. Darwin's prescriptions in Colp 1977, receipts and memoranda book). His brother Erasmus may have been addicted to opium. *Correspondence,* 2: 236.

12. *Correspondence,* 3: 326. The use of mercuric chloride was controversial. Some considered it a poison and were against its use. Royle and Headland 1865, 212. Henry Holland, however, wrote that mercuric chloride was "one of the most valuable remedies we possesse" and "on the whole as safe a medicine as Calomel in the hands of the practitioner." Holland 1855, 539–40.

13. *Correspondence,* 3: 327. Darwin would again use a form of galvanism in 1851.

14. *Correspondence,* 2: 399. Darwin would also report psychosomatic sensory changes in a letter to Dr. Henry Bence Jones on 2 August 1870.

15. *Correspondence,* 3: 68.

16. *Correspondence,* 3: 327; 4: 10, 24; 13: 245.

17. *Correspondence,* 4: 142–43, 144, 145, 146, 147, 384.

18. *Correspondence,* 4: 209.

19. *Correspondence* 4: 182–83, 385.

20. *Correspondence,* 4: 239, 269, 384–85.

21. Stott 2003, 85, 98, 145, 176, 259; *Correspondence,* 4: 136, 154; Browne 1995, 448.

22. *Correspondence,* 4: 227.

23. *Correspondence,* 7: 462.

24. "At night . . . anything which had vexed or troubled him [Darwin] in the day would haunt him, and I think it was then that he suffered if he had not answered some troublesome person's letter." "Reminiscences," *L&L,* 1: 102.

25. Darwin's account book for 1848 contains a payment to Dr. Holland of 1/1/0 [one pound, one shilling] on 17 December. There are no entries of payments to Dr. Holland in January and February 1849. *Correspondence,* 4: 209. For a discussion of the concept of "suppressed gout," see chapter 16.

26. Emma's diary for 1849 lists the following medicines for successive days in January: 8, "½ gr cal[omel]"; 10, "29 ½ cal[omel]"; 21, "1 ½ g. calomel"; 26, "began bizmuth." Although it is not specified who these medicines were for (and they are not mentioned in Darwin's health diary), since they were medicines favored by Dr. Darwin and previously used by Darwin, it seems likely that they were for Darwin's use. The medicines may have been suggested by Dr. Holland, who greatly favored the use of mercury medicines.

27. Sulivan urged Darwin to try hydropathy during a visit to Down in the fall of 1848, when Dr. Darwin was still alive. Darwin then wrote to Shrewsbury asking for his father's opinion. His father replied that he should try hydropathy, but not until spring. Bartholomew Sulivan to Joseph Hooker, not dated (but probably written soon after Darwin's death), DAR 107: ff 43–47. Fox wrote Darwin soon after his father's death, mentioning several cases that had benefited from Dr. Gully's hydropathy. *Correspondence,* 4: 209.

28. Browne 1995, 493.

29. Gully 1846, 192, 193. Italics in original.

30. Darwin's account book for 1849 has a payment to Dr. Gully on 14 February. Letters between Darwin and Dr. Gully have not been found. *Correspondence,* 4: 219.

31. *Correspondence,* 4: 209, 219, 226, 227, 385; Browne 1995, 493–94.

32. *Correspondence,* 4: 224–25.

33. Gully 1846, 127–28, 161; *Correspondence,* 4: 225, note 1; Browne 1995, 494–95.

34. The aim of hydropathy treatment was "to produce a counteraction, resembling as nearly as possible in its character that which it is intended to remove—namely, a nervous irritation . . . that amount of cutaneous irritation which is exhibited in a rash or itchy eruption. A good deal of friction is therefore desirable." Gully 1846, 158.

35. "A very nice part of treatment to adjust is the amount of *exercise.* In the majority of cases, it should be very sparingly used, because in exercise there is an exertion of the seat of the will, the brain and the spinal cord, which are already kept in an irritated state by the digestive disorder. . . . These cases require all the acumen of the practitioner; for on the question of exercise hinges that of the amount of water treatment, much of the latter demanding more of the former, and vice versa. . . . The rule to determine the amount and kind of exercise in nervous dyspepsia is to watch the effect of walking on the viscera." Gully 1846, 159–60.

36. As regards the diet in nervous dyspepsia, "the remedies should be chiefly *negative*—the withdrawal of irritating food and beverage . . . of all the forms of indigestion the *nervous* requires the most accurate adaptation of diet to the Protean changes of the

functions—changes which no writing could convey to the reader . . . professional experience alone can detect the causes for its daily or weekly alteration." Gully 1846, 154–55.

37. "The foot baths . . . afford by the combined cold and friction, an amount of nervous stimulation to the centre of nutrition, which tends to dissipate the congestion of its nerves; and thus it is that this simple remedy so often brings instant relief to malaise, or pain of stomach or head." Gully 1846, 158.

38. Since some patients needed to take hot water with food, "drinking cold water requires in many instances . . . to be very gradually applied. . . . In proportion as the positive remedies produce a sedative effect on the stomach, the quantity of water may be increased and its temperature decreased." Gully 1846, 156.

39. *Correspondence*, 4: 224–26.

40. *Correspondence*, 7: 462.

41. Dr. Gully had introduced the "lamp bath" into the process of hydropathy. "Up to that time the system had but one sudorfic process, the blanket sweat—by means of which several blankets with an eiderdown on the top. This was a powerful though slow process of inducing perspiration, taking from one to two hours. The lamp bath, by greatly curtailing the time of the sudorfic process, had its merits and to a certain extent superseded the blanket pack." Metcalfe 1912, 73. An eiderdown was a quilt or pillow that was stuffed with the feathers of the eider duck.

42. *Correspondence*, 4: 227, 242.

43. *Correspondence*, 4: 225, 226, 227, 234.

44. *Correspondence*, 4: 225.

45. *Correspondence*, 4: 225, 226, 234, 235, 246.

46. *Correspondence*, 4: 224. "It has been said of Dr. Gully by one who knew him: 'As a doctor no one ever consulted Dr. Gully without feeling himself in the grasp of a master mind. His profoundness, penetration, and resources were remarkable, and such as none could forget who ever consulted him. His was a deeply philosophical as well as a medical mind, and it was the intimate feeling of his profoundness and might that gave Dr. Gully such power of fascination over patients. At the sick bed his presence always gave relief and assurance. No one could ever look into his ruddy face, mostly lighted up with a smile, and not debit the consciousness that he was equal to the emergency, however great it might be.'" Metcalfe 1912, 73–74.

47. *Correspondence*, 4: 225, 226, 239.

48. *Correspondence*, 4: 234–35.

49. *Correspondence*, 4: 246.

50. *Correspondence*, 4: 385.

Chapter 7

1. *Correspondence*, 4: 240, 249, 269. The date when Darwin resumed work on barnacles is specified in his health diary.

2. Lewis 1909.

3. Henrietta Litchfield, autobiography, DAR, 246.

4. G. Darwin, "Recollections."

5. Notes to health diary for December 1849 and January 1850.

6. *Correspondence*, 4: 335, 353.

7. *Correspondence*, 4: 354.

8. G. Darwin, "Recollections."

9. Keynes 2001, 148–53, 154, 156–60, 165–68.

10. *Correspondence*, 5: 14. "My Maer illness" refers to Darwin's prolonged illness at Maer in the summer and fall of 1840, when Emma was pregnant with Annie. For an account of this illness, see chapter 4.

11. *Emma Darwin* (1904), II, 142; Keynes 2001, 171; *Correspondence*, 5: 15, 17.

12. *Correspondence*, 5: 18–19, 20.

13. *Correspondence*, 5: 23, note 7.

14. Fanny Wedgwood to her husband, Hensleigh Wedgwood, 23 April 1851, quoted in Bowlby 1990, 296.

15. *Correspondence*, 5: 23, note 7.

16. For a discussion of the meaning of this diagnosis and the possibility that Annie may have died from tuberculosis, see Keynes 2001, 199–208.

17. *Correspondence*, 5: 24.

18. Since Darwin stopped keeping his health diary when he was at Malvern (see health diary for 15–26 April 1851), the nature and intensity of his stomach illness can only be inferred from his letters to Emma and the correspondence of Fanny Wedgwood and Emma.

19. Letters quoted in Bowlby 1990, 296.

20. Colp 1987, 25–26; Keynes 2001, 195–98.

21. Colp 1987, 24. (Whereas I formerly stated that Darwin wept with his sisters Marianne and Caroline at the time of his mother's death, I now believe that the extent of his weeping is undetermined.) Bowlby 1990, 297.

22. It is not known what Darwin and Dr. Gully said to each other about their future contacts when Annie died. There appears to have been no contact between them for the next twelve years. Darwin sometimes commented that he could not visit Dr. Gully in Malvern because he feared that such a visit would stimulate painful memories of Annie.

23. *Correspondence*, 5: 83.

24. Tartar emetic ointment, when applied to the skin, was an irritant that produced vesicles and pustules. It was used as a counterirritant in coughs and chronic lung disease. See Haller 1975, 238–41.

25. Royle and Headland 1865, 586–87.

26. *Medical Times and Gazette*, 10 May 1856, 464.

27. *Association Medical Journal*, 15 March 1856, 214. The electric chain was used in England in the 1850s and 1860s. In 1866 it was recommended by a group of distinguished

London medical authorities, including Sir Henry Holland. In 1867, however, Dr. Julius Althaus stated that the current generated by the chains was "liable to great and sudden variations within a short time," that the chains caused sloughs and cicatrices, and that they "may aggravate the disorder for the relief of which they were brought into play." Colwell 1922, 104–5.

28. Tea and coffee were both held to be cerebral stimulants and antisoporifics. It was also held that they were "sedatives" that sometimes relieved the "stupor" caused by stimulants or the "drowsiness of fatigue," by counteracting the plethoric state of the brain and thus restoring the brain to its normal state. Royle and Headland 1865, 321, 460.

29. Lemon juice was used as a refrigerant, antalkaline, and antiscorbutic, and it was used to treat rheumatism. Royle and Headland 1865, 326.

30. Aloes was the inspissated juice from the leaves of different species of the aloe plant. This juice in small doses was a tonic, in larger doses a cathartic. Royle and Headland, 1865, 630–34. "Cordial aloes" was aloes in an alcoholic beverage. "Liquor infusion aloes" was the dilution of the juice of aloes by another liquid.

31. *Correspondence*, 5: 83. *The English Dialect Dictionary* (London, 1902) has the following definitions of *heaze:* To breathe thickly and with difficulty, to wheeze: to cough or "hawk"; As cattle when they clear the windpipe, or force up phlegm; *Heazy.* Adj. hoarse breathing with difficulty, wheezing: *fig.* creaking.

32. "Reminiscences," *L&L,* 1: 102. These nocturnal obsessions had become severe during Darwin's 1848–49 illness.

33. *Life and Letters,* 2: 236–38.

34. *Correspondence,* 4: 252. Darwin's 16 August visit to Chevening is dated by his 9 August (1849) letter to Lady Mahon, published in *Correspondence* 13, *Supplement, 1822–1864,* 373. Darwin would later recollect that Lord Stanhope once asked him, "Why don't you give up your fiddle-faddle of geology and zoology, and turn to the occult sciences?" *Autobiography,* 112.

35. *Correspondence,* 4: 256; *Diary,* 23 September 1849.

36. *Correspondence,* 4: 363, note 7.

37. *Correspondence,* 4: 354–55, notes 5 and 6; 4: 363, note 2 at top of page.

38. Woodham-Smith 1972, 317.

39. *Emma Darwin* (1904), 2: 153; *Correspondence,* 5: 55.

40. In a May 1854 letter to Hooker, Darwin wrote: "The last grand thing we were at together answered, I am sure, very well & that was the Duke's Funeral." *Correspondence,* 5: 194. "Everyone from the Queen to the costermonger, went to Chelsea. They assembled in vast crowds before the Hospital was open. On the privileged day thousands failed to gain admission; on the first public day there was a stampede in which two people were killed and dozens injured. The rain fell in torrents, and the crowds went dripping through the glittering darkness to the catafalque they had waited so long to see." Fletcher 1951, 92.

41. The diary has the following entries for 1853: 4 June: "well very got much ft. Crystal Palace"; 22 September: "well very several fits & headache from Crystal Palace."

42. Fortescue 1930, 13, 30.

43. *Emma Darwin* (1904), 2: 168; *Emma Darwin* (1915), 2: 154; G. Darwin, "Recollections."

44. On 29 May, Darwin wrote Hooker that he and Emma "in a very profligate manner have just taken a pair of Season-tickets to see the Queen open the Crystal Palace." *Correspondence*, 5: 194. Sydenham was about ten miles north of Down and had a special railway station. It is not known how—whether by train or coach—the Darwins traveled to Sydenham.

45. *Correspondence*, 5: 321.

46. There were two houses at Hartfield, Sussex, which were about a quarter of a mile apart and which the Darwins visited: Hartfield Cove, home of Charles Langton and his wife, Charlotte Wedgwood, who was Darwin's sister-in-law; and the Ridge, home of Sarah Elizabeth Wedgwood, Darwin's maternal cousin. *Emma Darwin* (1904), 2: 98–99.

47. G. Darwin, "Recollections."

48. The diary shows that when Darwin had visited Hartfield four years earlier, in October 1850, he had "excessive" flatulence.

49. *Correspondence*, 5: 83, 100.

50. Diary entry for 2 November 1849 and note on this entry; *Correspondence*, 4: 303; 5: 9.

51. Wilson 1977, 440–41.

52. *Correspondence*, 4: 368–69.

53. *Correspondence*, 5: 83.

54. *Correspondence*, 4: 257–60, note 3 on 259; 5: 100.

55. *Correspondence*, 5: 194–95. For Hooker's heart condition, see chapter 5. For Darwin's views on hereditary illness, see chapter 16.

56. Emma's 1854 diary records that Francis and Leonard came home unwell from Sarah Wedgwood's home on 13 and 15 December, respectively. On 22 December, she recorded "Franky's fit." *Correspondence*, 5: 253, note 2, upper page.

57. Although Dr. Darwin had previously stated that London air was bad and country air good, at one time he did state that in "old cases" of whooping cough a "change of air" was "often *very* useful." Colp 1977, receipts and memoranda book, Dr. Robert Darwin's entries on "Hooping Cough."

58. However, in March 1855, all of the Darwin children (except for William) had whooping cough. *Correspondence*, 5: 289.

59. See chapters 13 and 14.

Chapter 8

1. *Correspondence*, 5: 537. Although Darwin wrote in his 1876 autobiography that he

doubted that barnacles were "worth the consumption of so much time," in 1873 he had commented that the "rigorous and long continued work" on barnacles was an example of his mental energy. *Autobiography*, 118; *Life and Letters*, 2: 357.

2. *Correspondence*, 5: xv, 166.

3. Health diary entries for 29, 30 November 1854.

4. *Correspondence*, 4: 344; 5: xvii; Browne 1995, 513–16.

5. *Correspondence*, 5: chronology, 537.

6. *Correspondence*, 5: xviii–xix, 326, 331.

7. *Correspondence*, 5: 248.

8. Secord 2000, 212–13, 423–24, 429–33, 476–77, 505–6.

9. *Correspondence*, 6: 56, 58.

10. Wilson 1970, xliii–xlvi; *Correspondence*, 6: 78, 89, 522.

11. Darwin, *Natural Selection*, 1975, ed. Stauffer, 8–10.

12. *Correspondence*, 6: 174.

13. *Correspondence*, 6: 135–36.

14. Darwin to Hooker, 13 July [1856], *DAR*, 114.3, 169. In referring to himself as a "Devil's Chaplain," Darwin was also influenced by recollections of Cambridge in the 1830s, when he had witnessed the activities of the apostate priest Robert Taylor, who published *The Devil's Pulpit* and had been called "the Devil's Chaplain." Desmond and Moore 1991, 84–85.

15. *Correspondence*, 6: 236, 432.

16. *Correspondence*, 6: 238–39, 248, 304–5.

17. *Correspondence*, 6: 274, 305, 324, 385; Desmond and Moore 1991, 443–44.

18. *Correspondence*, 5: 84, 147. "Bugbear" was a sort of hobgoblin in the shape of a bear that was supposed to devour naughty children. It was also "an object of (needless) dread; an imaginary terror," according to the *Shorter Oxford English Dictionary*.

19. *Correspondence*, 6: 460, 476.

20. *Correspondence*, 6: 238, 335, 346.

21. *Correspondence*, 6: 335.

22. The receipts and memoranda book in Colp 1977 contains an undated prescription, in Darwin's handwriting, for a mixture of muriatic acid and nitric acid, to be taken in ten drops, twice a day, one hour before meals. Darwin would again take a course of "nitro-hydrochloric acid" in early 1860; see chapter 10.

23. "As this acid [hydrochloric acid] has been discovered in the natural gastric juice, it is often proposed for use in morbid conditions of that secretion, especially when there is a deficiency of acid in it. Hydrochloric acid may be used in Phosphaturia; it has been employed by some in Putrid Fevers; and it may be given as an Alternative in the same cases as Nitric acid, doing most good when combined with the latter, so as to form Nitro-muriatic acid." Royle and Headland 1865, 51.

24. *Correspondence*, 6: 377.

25. Metcalfe 1912, 57.

26. *Correspondence*, 6: 384, 385, 524.

27. *Emma Darwin* (1904), 2: 271.

28. *Correspondence*, 6: 386, note 5.

29. *Correspondence*, 6: 476.

30. *Correspondence*, 6: 385.

31. *Correspondence*, 7: 81.

32. Dr. Lane would be at Moor Park from 1854 to 1859, then at the hydropathy establishment at Sudbrook Park from 1860 into the 1870s. In the 1880s his address was in Harley Street, London. The *Times*, 13 July 1889, and the 1890 *Medical Directory* state that Dr. Lane died on 11 July 1889 at age sixty-seven. There are no obituaries of Dr. Lane in *Lancet*, *British Medical Journal*, or in medical biographical dictionaries, and little is known about the details of his life. The references to him are contained in the *Medical Directory*, 1865 and 1890; *Times*, 15 June 1858, p. 11, and 13 July 1889, p. 1; and Metcalfe 1912, 57.

33. *Correspondence*, 6: 385. Darwin was referring to Dr. Gully's beliefs in homeopathy and clairvoyance. Dr. Henry Holland's collection of medical essays, *Medical Notes and Reflections,* had an essay, "On Medical Evidence," that contained the following passage:

> And here I must advert to another circumstance which renders strict attention to laws of evidence a matter of peculiar obligation at the present time. This is the tendency, so marked in modern physiology, to carry its researches in to the more abstruse questions connected with vitality, the nervous power, and the relations of mental and material phenomena—inquiries justifiable in themselves, but needing to be fenced round by more than common caution as to testimony, and the conclusions thence derived. Yet here especially it is that such precautions have been disregarded;—partly it may be, from the real difficulty and obscurity of those who have taken it into their hands. Holland 1855, 10–11.

Opposite this passage, in the copy of this volume in Darwin's library, there is written in Darwin's handwriting "gully."

34. *Correspondence*, 6: 416.

35. *Correspondence*, 6: 476. Darwin possessed a copy of this book, because he would write Fox: "I send you by this Post D^r. Lane's Book, which you can keep as long as you like." *Correspondence*, 7: 90. Darwin's extant library (at Cambridge University Library and Down House) does not contain a copy of Dr. Lane's *Hydropathy*.

36. Lane 1857, 85–86.

37. Lane 1882, 2–3. Similar episodes of acute flatulence were observed by Darwin's geologist friend David Forbes, who recollected that "on one or more occasions, while Darwin was in his house, pains of such a violent character had seized him that he had been compelled to lie down for a time and had occasioned his host the greatest alarm." Judd 1910, 119.

38. Lane 1882, 5–6.

39. "Reminiscences," ms, 86; *Correspondence*, 7: 249.

40. Lane 1882, 5–6.

41. *Correspondence,* 6: 476.

42. *Correspondence,* 6: 404.

43. *Correspondence,* 7: 9.

44. *Correspondence,* 7: 70, 95, 504.

45. *Correspondence,* 7: 80. The military review at Aldershot occurred on 23 and 24 April 1858. The review had been scheduled to have been a "sham battle," but this had been cancelled, presumably because of inclement weather. *Times,* 26 April 1858, 8. Darwin had "intensely" enjoyed the "sham battles" at Cobham in 1854.

46. *Correspondence,* 7: 80, 81.

47. Darwin, *Natural Selection,* 1975, ed. Stauffer, 368–69, 370–71; Darwin, *Origin of Species,* 1859, 242.

48. *Correspondence,* 7: 84.

49. *Correspondence,* 7: 84–85, note 4.

50. *Correspondence,* 7: 78–79, 82–84, 85–86, 90, note 3.

51. *Correspondence,* 7: 80, 81, 87, 248. The anonymous author of *Three Chances* had also written *The Fair Carew; or, Husbands and Wives* (published in 1851, reprinted in 1869). Darwin enjoyed it for the "beauty of the heroine," although the details of her beauty were scarcely depicted. "Reminiscences," ms, 58.

52. *Correspondence,* 7: 81, 87, 89, 90.

53. *Correspondence,* 7: 92, 95.

Chapter 9

1. *Correspondence,* 7: 138.

2. *Correspondence,* 7: 107.

3. *Correspondence,* 7: 119.

4. Moody 1971; Desmond and Moore 1991, 470.

5. *Correspondence,* 7: 115–16.

6. *Correspondence,* 7: 118, 120, 121.

7. *Correspondence,* 7: 121. It has been suggested that Charles Waring suffered from Down Syndrome. Keynes 2001, 225–26.

8. *Correspondence,* 7: 125.

9. *Correspondence,* 7: 124.

10. *Correspondence,* 7: 127, chronology, 504.

11. *Correspondence,* 7: 138, 140.

12. *Correspondence,* 7: 137.

13. Colp 1981, 205–11.

14. *Correspondence,* 7: 116–18.

15. *Correspondence,* 7: 119–20.

16. Colp 1981, 212–13.

17. *Correspondence,* 7: 138.

18. *Correspondence*, 7: 503.

19. Darwin later recollected that the published Linnean Society papers "excited very little attention.... This shows how necessary it is that any new view should be explained at considerable length in order to arouse public attention." *Autobiography*, 122.

20. *Correspondence*, 7: 196. In the middle of October, before going to Moor Park, Darwin had written a paper on the importance of bee pollination in *Leguminosae* for the *Gardener's Chronicle*. After returning from Moor Park, he came to believe that working on this paper had been deleterious to his health. In a 23 November letter to Hooker he wrote: "I can do nothing after 12. [Up until 12 he worked on the "abstract."] That confounded Leguminous paper in G. Chronicle was done in afternoon & the consequence was I had to go to Moor Park for a week, & I am resolved I will not attempt mental work in the afternoon: my head, I do assure you, will not stand it." *Correspondence*, 7: 206, 207, note 5.

21. *Correspondence*, 7: 247.

22. Pepsine had been discovered in 1839 by the German physiologist Theodor Schwann and was then given—either in liquid or solid form—in cases of dyspepsia. Royle and Headland 1865, 713. Dr. William Brinton wrote:

> Pepsine has, I must confess, disappointed me in most of the cases of dyspepsia in which I have tried it; even after a careful selection of those which seemed best adapted for its use. Perhaps it is not often . . . that dyspepsia is caused by a mere deficiency of gastric juice; and certainly our existing means of diagnosis do not enable us to detect such cases with the accuracy that could be wished. While in many of those varieties of indigestion in which we are entitled to suspect graver and more constitutional causes, it is difficult to see how the scanty solution of a single alimentary constituent . . . can effect much benefit. Occasionally, indeed, I have found pepsine produces considerable disturbance, even in cases where no great irritability of stomach appeared to be present. Brinton 1859, 385.

23. *Correspondence*, 7: 504.

24. "Reminiscences," ms, 75; G. Darwin, "Recollections."

25. *Correspondence*, 7: 269. At this time playing billiards had become a passionate avocation for George Darwin, and Darwin had bought a book with accounts of famous billiard games. *Correspondence*, 7: 263.

26. During his later years, Darwin would sometimes play billiards with his sons. In 1876, he built a billiard room in Down House, which was perhaps mainly intended for the use of his sons. After about a dozen billiard games, this room was converted into Darwin's study. G. Darwin, "Recollections."

27. *Correspondence*, 7: 280.

28. *Correspondence*, 7: 284.

29. *Correspondence*, 7: 299–300. Darwin recorded *Adam Bede* in his reading notebook for July 1859 as being "excellent." *Correspondence*, 4: appendix 4: 128: 25. The novel did him "a world of good" because of its engrossing portrayal of the goodness in

the character of Dinah Morris, a young Methodist lay preacher who "makes everything seem right she says and does," whose looks and voice are vividly remembered by those who have met her, and who becomes happily married to the novel's protagonist, Adam Bede.

30. *Correspondence*, 7: 308.

31. *Correspondence*, 7: 317.

32. *Emma Darwin* (1904), 2: 187.

33. *Correspondence*, 7: 187.

34. *Correspondence*, 7: 320.

35. *Correspondence*, 7: 328.

36. Judd 1910, 117.

37. *Correspondence*, 7: 332.

38. In "Things for a Week," notes that were written in May and October 1859, under the heading "Physic," he first wrote "Magnesia," "Soda & Potash" (for his stomach), "Sal-volatile" [carbonate of ammonia], "Smelling-salts," "Spice-Bottle," and "Brandy" (as stimulants). To these, at some unknown time, he later added: "muriatic [hydrochloric acid] (for stomach), "Tincture of Senna" (a laxative), and "Lotion for Head."

39. *Correspondence*, 7: 336.

40. *Correspondence*, 7: 331–32, notes 1 and 3 at top of 332. Ilkley House had opened three years previously and would become a center of English hydropathy, rivaling Malvern. Metcalfe 1912, 105–9.

41. *Correspondence*, 7: 331.

42. *Correspondence*, 7: 342–43.

43. *Correspondence*, 7: 348–49, notes 1 and 2.

44. *Correspondence*, 7: 332.

45. *Correspondence*, 7: 365–66.

46. *Correspondence*, 7: 368.

47. *Correspondence*, 7: 351, 370, 371, 374.

48. *Correspondence*, 7: 351, 388.

49. *Correspondence*, 7: 383–84, 387–88.

50. *Correspondence*, 7: 362–64, 384–85, 388–89.

51. *Correspondence*, 7: 375, 398.

52. *Correspondence*, 7: 377.

53. *Correspondence*, 7: 348–49.

54. *Correspondence*, 7: 356.

55. *Correspondence*, 7: 362. This appears to be the only time that Darwin had a swollen leg.

56. *Correspondence*, 7: 377. Dr. Smith was fifty-five years old. He has been described as "able and conscientious," yet not in good health and not vigorous in his hydropathic work. Metcalfe 1912, 107.

57. *Correspondence*, 7: 393.

58. *Correspondence*, 7: 382, 396–98, 403–4.

59. *Correspondence*, 7: 383–84, 387–88, 391–92.

60. *Correspondence*, 7: 390–91.

61. *Correspondence*, 7: 434.

62. *Correspondence*, 7: 398, 400.

63. *Correspondence*, 7: 409.

64. *Correspondence*, 7: 418. Huxley later observed that Darwin had "an acute sensitiveness to praise and blame." *Life and Letters*, 1, 533.

65. *Correspondence*, 7: 444, 449.

Chapter 10

1. *Correspondence*, 7: 504.

2. *Correspondence*, 7: 441, 444, 449. Darwin would never return to Ilkley for hydropathy.

3. *Correspondence*, 8: 45.

4. In his *Essay on the Action of Medicines in the System*, Dr. Headland explained that oxaluria was a condition caused by "some fault in the complicated processes of assimilation and nutrition" and that treatment was intended to interrupt and neutralize the formation of oxalic acid and urea during the digestive process. *Correspondence*, 8: 133–34, note 2.

5. *Correspondence*, 8: 133, 215.

6. *Correspondence*, 8: 115.

7. *Correspondence*, 8: 154.

8. *Correspondence*, 8: 160.

9. *Correspondence*, 8: 157.

10. The visit is recorded in Emma's diary for 1860. In 1859, Darwin had given Miss Butler a presentation copy of *Origin*. *Correspondence*, 8: 556.

11. *Correspondence*, 8: 232, 252, 264.

12. *Correspondence*, 8: 268.

13. *Correspondence*, 8: 260.

14. *Correspondence*, 8: 551. Sudbrook Park was used as a hydropathy establishment by a succession of individuals; Dr. Ellis from the 1840s to 1860; Dr. Lane from 1860 to 1877; by a man named Borstal; then by a man named Hammond, after which its hydropathy use ceased. Metcalfe 1912, 56–57.

15. *Correspondence*, 8: 270–72.

16. *Correspondence*, 8: 272. Almost two years to the day after he received Hooker's letter, Darwin remembered how he had been warmly encouraged by its contents, and he wrote Hooker: "It is not your approbation of my scientific work (though I care for that more than any one's); it is something deeper. To this day I remember keenly a letter you wrote me from Oxford, when I was at the water-cure, & how it cheered me, when I was utterly weary of life." *Correspondence*, 10: 283.

17. *Correspondence*, 8: 274.

18. In 1873 Dr. Lane sent Darwin his book *Old Medicine and New.* In this letter of acknowledgment, addressed to "My dear D^r. Lane," Darwin wrote:

I am very much obliged for the present of your little book, which I will read as soon as I have finished another in hand. I never forget how much I owe to Hydropathy, although the last time I tried it, it seemed to do me harm. The days which I spent at Moor Park have left a most pleasant recollection on my mind. I hope you & all your family are well, & I beg you to give my kind & grateful remembrances to Lady Drysdale & M*rs* Lane." Darwin to E. W. Lane, 23 June 1873, Library of the American Philosophical Society.

In 1882, Dr. Lane was on "Personal Friends Invited" list for Darwin's funeral. Freeman 1978, 185.

19. *Correspondence*, 8: 435.

20. *Correspondence*, 8: 458.

21. *Correspondence*, 8: 510, 511.

22. *Correspondence*, 9: 20, 32.

23. *Correspondence*, 9: 69.

24. *Correspondence*, 9: 390–91.

25. *Emma Darwin* (1904), 2: 193.

26. *Correspondence*, 9: 69–70. Darwin had mentioned George's teeth extraction in a letter to Hooker of 4 February 1861. *Correspondence*, 9: 20, note 3, 21–22.

27. *Correspondence*, 9: 98–99. Darwin spoke in London at the Linnean Society on 16 April. On 19 April, Emma recorded in her diary: "Ch. poorly in London."

28. To get to Hitcham, Darwin would have to take a train to Charing Cross station in central London, then a train to Stowmarket, then travel six miles by coach.

29. *Correspondence*, 9: 133. Within a year of Henslow's death, Darwin would publish his "Recollections of Professor Henslow." *Collected Papers*, 2: 72–74.

30. *Correspondence*, 9: 155–56.

31. Healey 2001, 163, 165.

32. *Correspondence*, 9: 195–96, 391.

33. *Correspondence*, 9: 269.

34. *Correspondence*, 9: 201, 390.

35. *Correspondence*, 9: 220, 221, 223; Bowlby 1990, 365.

36. *Correspondence*, 10: xvii–xix.

37. *Correspondence*, 10: 139.

38. *Correspondence*, 10: 148. When in London Darwin stayed at the home of his brother Erasmus.

39. *Correspondence*, 10: 80, 405.

40. *Correspondence*, 10: 250.

41. *Correspondence*, 10: 378.

42. *Correspondence,* 10: 270–71, 283.

43. *Correspondence,* 10: xxii–xxiii, 300, 627.

44. *Correspondence,* 10: 330. In his 1862 journal, Darwin had written: "Much time wasted June & July from Leonard's illness." His distress over Leonard was influenced by memories of Charles Waring's death from scarlet fever in 1858 and Annie's death from "bilious fever" in 1851.

45. *Correspondence,* 10: 373.

46. *Correspondence,* 10: 395.

47. *Correspondence,* 10: 419, 421–22.

48. *Correspondence,* 10: 481–82.

49. *Correspondence,* 10: 405.

50. Emma to William Darwin, 12 December 1862, quoted in *Correspondence,* 11: 2, note 2.

51. *Correspondence,* 10: 482, 576.

52. *Correspondence,* 10: 491.

53. *Correspondence,* 10: 525.

54. *Correspondence,* 10: 624.

55. *Correspondence,* 10: 635.

56. *Correspondence,* 10: 641.

57. *Correspondence,* 11: 8.

58. *Correspondence,* 11: 14.

59. *Correspondence,* 10: 417.

60. *Correspondence,* 10: 515.

61. *Correspondence,* 10: 626–27. In July 1863, in reply to a correspondent who had been a hydropathy patient with him and Miss Butler in Ilkley in 1859, and who now asked him about her, he wrote: "Owing to the state of our Family we have not seen anything of Miss Butler for a long time, but she has visited us here once or twice & was as pleasant as usual." *Correspondence,* 11: 544.

62. Huxley 1918, 2: 32–33.

Chapter 11

1. *Correspondence,* 11: 7, 11.

2. *Correspondence,* 11: 95.

3. *Correspondence,* 11: 154–55, note 6.

4. *Correspondence,* 11: 122–23, 134, 171–72, note 8.

5. *Correspondence,* 11: 114.

6. *Correspondence,* 11: 173.

7. *Correspondence,* 11: 200.

8. *Correspondence,* 11: 204.

9. *Correspondence,* 11: 207.

10. *Correspondence,* 11: 218.

11. *Correspondence*, 11: 255.

12. *Correspondence*, 11: 265.

13. *Correspondence*, 11: 293.

14. In a May 1863 letter to their son William, Emma wrote: "Your father remains so very languid & weak . . . that we have almost given up all hopes of his being brisk enough to go to L.H.P [Leith Hill Place]." *Correspondence*, 11: 377.

15. *Correspondence*, 11: 410.

16. *Correspondence*, 11: 421, 438. Emma's diary for 1863 records this illness as follows: "Ch. taken with pain in bowels—no flat" (15 May); "very unwell" (16 May); "Ch very unwell with pain" (17 May); "pain left & sickness appears came on" (19 May); "Ditto" (20 May); "sick in mg." (21 May). This appears to be the only recorded instance where Darwin had the symptom of "pain in bowels," which then subsided after four days.

17. *Correspondence*, 11: 423. In June 1863, a deputation of Malvern inhabitants presented Dr. Gully with an illuminated address, congratulating him and themselves on his recovery from a severe (unspecified) illness. I thank Elizabeth Jenkins, author of *Dr. Gully*, a novel (London, 1972), for telling me of this.

18. *Correspondence*, 11: 438.

19. *Correspondence*, 11: 500–501. "Valetudinarian" refers to a person of weak health who is more or less an invalid and difficult to cure.

20. *Correspondence*, 11: 499.

21. *Correspondence*, 11: 504.

22. *Correspondence*, 11: 599. Potassium carbonate (carbonate of potash) was used as an alkaline remedy for stomach upsets. Paris 1825, 2: 273. John Goodsir (1814–67) made many important observations on the normal and pathological functions of cells at a time when the role of cells in health and disease was not generally appreciated. Jacyna 1983.

23. *Correspondence*, 11: 595–96.

24. *Correspondence*, 11: 603–4.

25. *Correspondence*, 11: 604. George Busk (1807–86) studied at the College of Surgeons and for twenty-five years was surgeon to the hospital ship *Dreadnought.* In 1856 he retired from the practice of surgery and devoted himself solely to scientific work; microscopic studies of the Polyzoa and lower forms of life, and paleontological osteology. He was a close friend of Huxley and Hooker, and in 1864 he was one of the nine eminent Victorian scientists who formed the X Club. Jensen 1970.

26. *Correspondence*, 11: 602. Waterbrash was a condition involving eructation of dilute acid from the stomach that caused a burning sensation at the back of the throat, or "heartburn." *Correspondence*, 11: 603, note 3.

27. *Correspondence*, 11: 620, 624–25. James Smith Ayerst (1824/5–84) was first a surgeon to the Royal Navy and a member of the Royal College of Surgeons of England, and then obtained his medical degree from Saint Andrews in 1856. In 1859 Ayerst, in conjunction with Dr. Gully, opened a hydropathic establishment at Wells House, Malvern Wells. He was described as "a successful homeopathic practitioner . . . a great hygienist

and believed as much in fresh air and sunlight as in water. Eventually he retired on account of ill health. This was some time before Dr. Gully's retirement." Metcalfe 1912, 94. Annie's gravestone was located in the Priory churchyard, Great Malvern.

28. *Correspondence*, 11: 642–43. In her diary Emma recorded that Darwin was sick every day from 20 to 23 September, but that over the succeeding six days his sickness stopped, while he suffered intermittently from flatulence, "head swimming," and "sinking."

29. *Correspondence*, 11: 640.

30. *Correspondence*, 11: 646.

31. *Correspondence*, 11: 654. In her 1863 diary Emma recorded: 4 October: "Ch. very swimming in head all day"; 9 October: "very weak swimming & with legs weak all this fortnight."

32. *Correspondence*, 11: 691. There is no record of what Darwin and Dr. Gully said to each other in their 1863 Malvern meetings.

33. *Correspondence*, 11: 654.

34. *Correspondence*, 11: 643.

35. *Correspondence*, 11: 652.

36. *Correspondence*, 11: 656.

37. *Correspondence*, 11: 675.

38. *Correspondence*, 11: 682. For a discussion of the feelings of Darwin and Hooker on Annie and Maria, see Keynes 2001, 246–60.

39. *Correspondence*, 11: 689.

40. *Correspondence*, 11: 695.

41. Stephen Paul Engleheart (1831/1832–85) was a member of the Royal College of Surgeons of England, 1859; surgeon in Down, 1861–70; medical officer, Second District Bromley Union, 1863–70. *Correspondence*, 11: "Biographical Register." Darwin's daughter Etty recollects that Engleheart cared for Leonard Darwin in his 1863 scarlet fever illness and that "He was always in difficulties being too indulgent with his poorer patients. My father used to lend him money, and when his bill came in my father used to pay half and keep half against the debt, which he called 'sharing the booty.'" *Emma Darwin* (1904), 2: 205, note 1.

42. *Correspondence*, 11: 654.

43. *Correspondence*, 11: 603. William Brinton (1823–67) made a special study of intestinal obstruction and diseases of the alimentary canal. His published books include *Pathology, Symptoms, and Treatment of Ulcer of the Stomach* (1857); *Lectures on the Diseases of the Stomach* (1859, 1864); and *On Food and Its Digestion* (1861). He was physician to Saint Thomas's Hospital (1860–64). *Dictionary of National Biography*; "Biographical Register," in *Correspondence*, 11.

44. *Correspondence*, 11: 654.

45. *Correspondence*, 11: 666, 670, 691. On the therapeutic use of acids, Brinton had written: "Acids are regarded chiefly as tonics; with local effects . . . in furthering gastric

secretion, as well as in aiding the solvent powers of the juice already poured out of the stomach. . . . They are contra-indicated by the great irritability of the stomach . . . such potent remedies should only be given in a small and dilute dose . . . during or immediately after a meal." Brinton 1859, 389.

Brinton strongly believed in the beneficial effects of work for some cases of dyspepsia. He wrote:

> In an enumeration of the causes of dyspepsia, perhaps undue intellectual exertion claims the first place. The influence of such exertion must not however be measured by its intensity; but rather by its rapidity, its duration, nay, even by the faculties it involves. The constructive mental efforts of genius are eminently wholesome . . . because they demand a concord of faculties, a symmetry of mind, and an application of reason and judgment—in short, a moderate and varied exercise of all the mental powers. Conversely, I think dyspepsia may be caused by a deficiency of mental exertion; person accustomed to intellectual toil being rendered amenable to this malady by the loss of labour which habit had made pleasant, and comparatively healthy, to him.
>
> Mental anxiety constitutes a cause of dyspepsia which though allied to the preceding, and often concurrent with it, is a far more efficient agent in producing gastric derangement . . . one which sometimes renders the physician as powerless a ministrant to a dyspeptic stomach, as he would be to a mind diseased in the Shaksperian sense. How closely all the phenomena of digestion are connected with the mental states is a matter of common experience . . . the chemistry of the stomach is subjected to the least material and palpable agents of our life, to that world of thought and emotion which works within every one of us. (Brinton 1859, 370–71)

46. *Correspondence*, 11: 687.

47. *Correspondence*, 12: 31.

48. *Correspondence*, 11: 695.

49. *Correspondence*, 12: 28.

50. *Correspondence*, 12: 31.

51. *Correspondence*, 12: 37, 57.

52. For December 1863 and January and February 1864 Emma's diary records her husband's medications and treatments as follows: 4 December, "began Quinine"; 12 December, "Colchicum"; 15 December, "took quinine at night"; 19 December, "opium dinner time," "opium once in night"; 24 December, "began compress," "took opium comf after"; 28 December, "last dose of brandy at 9 p.m."; 29 December, "blue pill"; 30 December, "left off pepsine"; 31 December, "began [illegible word] compress"; 1 January, "good day billiards"; 2 January, "began Quinine," "blue pill"; 4 January, "began pepsine"; 6 January, "began bismuth"; 13 January, "began bismuth took extra opium"; 21 January, "blue pill"; 11 February, "began compress"; 17 February, "began sulph acid"; 18 February,

"acid twice"; 20 February, "began acid once"; 21 February, "took acid once"; 29 February, "left off acid."

53. *Correspondence*, 12: 31, 41, 59, 91.

54. *Correspondence*, 12: 31.

55. *Correspondence*, 12: 52.

56. *Correspondence*, 12: 60.

57. "I am very glad to hear that the Antiquity [*The Geological Evidence of the Antiquity of Man*] goes on selling so well, but if it gets another edition of 'Origin' I shall not be grateful; for I dread the very thought of that job." Darwin to Lyell, 14 August 1863. *Correspondence*, 11: 590.

58. *Correspondence*, 12: 32.

59. *Correspondence*, 12: 30–31.

60. *Correspondence*, 12: 65.

61. *Correspondence*, 12: 77–78. Sir William Jenner (1815–95) became physician in ordinary to Queen Victoria in 1862, and because of the failing health of Sir James Clark (whom Darwin had consulted in 1837), he soon became responsible for the immediate care of the queen. He then received the highest medical honors and, "at the height of his powers, was the undisputed leader of his profession, and he owed his supremacy to his mastery in two of its departments—those of the practicing consultant and of the clinical teacher." *Dictionary of National Biography; Correspondence*, 12, biographical register.

62. *Correspondence*, 12: 91.

63. The indications of when, in cases of dyspepsia, to give alkalines were disputed. Dr. Frederick W. Headland wrote, "Dr. Pereira recommends alkalis in cases of dyspepsia and pyrosis, where there is an excess of acid secreted by the stomach. Yet this must not always be taken as an indication for their employment." He gives his opinion that it is a "tolerable safe rule" to give alkali in those cases of dyspepsia which are thought to be due to "a gouty cause" or which were "accompanied by a marked lithic diathesia and excess of acid in the urine." Headland 1863, 154. Dr. Brinton wrote:

> The alkalines . . . seem chiefly useful in cases in which the close of the digestive act is attended with much flatulence, regurgitation, and heartburn; where their immediate effects may be attributed to a neutralization of those lactic and acetic acids, which the decomposition of the undigested food can produce. In other cases they . . . bring . . . general results at least as valuable towards the cure of the malady; removing . . . the uric acid sediments associated with some of the more obstinate varieties of the malady; or provoking . . . the secretion of the liver, pancreas, or intestines . . . the administration of alkalines should be limited to the latter part of the act of gastric digestion, and to the succeeding period of rest . . . these remedies should be regarded only as . . . temporary measures; and should not be pursued for a longer period than a few weeks at a time. (Brinton 1859, 388–89)

64. It was believed that "liquids not uncommonly cause indigestion and dilute the gastric juice." Roberts 1874, 654.

Chalk was calcium carbonate, while lime water was often a solution of calcium carbonate. Royle and Headland 1865, 118–19. Emma's diary shows that Darwin began chalk, lime water, and carbonate of magnesia on 22 March. On 14 August Jenner directed that, because of alkaline urine and the danger of urinary stones, Darwin should stop taking chalk, take a "combination" of other antacids (identity not known), and increase taking lime water. *Correspondence*, 12: 305.

Carbonate of ammonia, soon after being ingested, produced unusually pleasant sensations which were described as: "a feeling of warmth at the pit of the stomach, which soon spreads to the rest of the body." It was further observed that "as an excitant of the stomach and upper part of the intestines, [carbonate of ammonia] may be used when from exhaustion or weakness, the functions of these parts are depressed, but it is inferior in these respects to brandy or wine.... Ammonia compounds of this group are therefore among the best anti-spasmodics." Ringer 1869, 110. Darwin mentions using carbonate of ammonia in April. *Correspondence*, 12: 135.

65. Colchicum, from the roots of meadow saffron (*Colicum autumnale*), was used in treating gout and as a diuretic and diaphoretic in fevers. Podophyllin, from the roots of the may apple or American mandrake (*Podophyllum peltatum*), was a strong cathartic and emetic. Its side effects included severe dermatitis and conjunctivitis. Estes 1990, 51, 154–55. Taraxacum, from the roots of the dandelion (*Taraxacum officinale*), was used as a mild tonic, laxative, and diuretic. Royle and Headland 1865, 502–3.

While Emma's diary records that Darwin began using both colchicum and podophyllin on 24 March, there is no record of when he started taking taraxacum. After he had benefited from podophyllin for several months, his use of it was criticized by Dr. Henry Holland, who said that podophyllin was "nothing but a strong drastic" and "not good" for him. He may have reported this criticism to Jenner, who in May wrote him a letter stating that "two or three grains" of *Sodae carbonas exsiccata* [dried sodium carbonate] "rubbed up with the podophyllin sometimes makes it act more kindly." In the same letter, Jenner directed that he continue taking colchicum and taraxacum (the only reference to his use of taraxacum), adding a "little ammonia to each dose" if he felt that the medicines were depressing him. In his letter of 14 August, Jenner advised Darwin to omit colchicum and continue with podophyllin. *Correspondence*, 12: 171–72, notes 1–5.

Emma's diary records that Darwin "began bismuth & c." on 17 August. Bismuth was used in "irritable conditions of the mucus membrane of the stomach." Royle and Headland 1865, 186.

66. *Correspondence*, 12: 135. In his journal, Darwin wrote, "Last sickness April 13th." *Correspondence*, 12: chronology, 493.

67. *Correspondence*, 12: 151. Hooker attended the 21 April meeting of the Royal Society where Jenner was elected a fellow. *Correspondence*, 12: 152, note 13.

68. *Correspondence*, 12: 153. In an 1861 paper on "Dimorphic Condition in Primula," Darwin had defined a homomorphic union as a union between the same forms of a

dimorphic plant and a heteromorphic union as a union between a long-styled form and a short-styled form. *Collected Papers*, 2: 55. Also cited in *Correspondence*, 12: 154, note 7.

69. *Correspondence*, 12: 154–55.

70. *Correspondence*, 12: 157.

71. *Correspondence*, 12: 183.

72. Recorded in his journal. *Correspondence*, 12: 492.

73. *Correspondence*, 12: 257. By "routine work" he meant writing the *Variation of Animals and Plants*.

74. *Correspondence*, 12: 259.

75. *Correspondence*, 12: 257, 285–86, 295–96.

76. *Correspondence*, 12: 298, note 2.

77. *Correspondence*, 12: 297.

78. *Correspondence*, 12: 492.

79. *Correspondence*, 12: 337.

80. *Correspondence*, 12: 325.

81. *Correspondence*, 12: 330.

82. *Correspondence*, 12: 337. Following this, Darwin and Hooker do not appear to have further discussed Maria's death.

83. *Correspondence*, 12: 375. Darwin described his crying in his 1865 medical notes to Dr. John Chapman, *Correspondence*, 13: 482. This seems to be the only occasion that Emma and Darwin used the term *hysteria*.

84. *Correspondence*, 12: 386–88.

85. On 14 August, after making visits to Down in March, April, and May, Jenner had written to Darwin: "I do not think any advantage would be derived from a visit—I have now seen you often enough to judge well of your state as described by letter." *Correspondence*, 12: 305. Since the subsequent extant Darwin-Jenner correspondence consists only of Jenner's letters to Darwin, the contents of Darwin's letters have to be inferred from Jenner's letters and from other sources of information about Darwin.

86. Iron and preparations of iron were used as a tonic, cathartic, diaphoretic, and diuretic. Estes 1990, 82. Emma's diary for 1864 records that Darwin "began iron" on 12 April and "began phosph. Iron" on 21 August and 12 September on orders from Dr. Jenner. On 29 October, he wrote Asa Gray that phosphate of iron "has done me good." *Correspondence*, 12: 387.

87. *Correspondence*, 13: 370–71. Spirit of horseradish (*Raphanus Rusticanus*) was derived from the root of horseradish and used as a tonic, diuretic, and diaphoretic. Estes 1990, 163.

88. A syrup preparation of a drug was made by mixing the drug's raw ingredients in simple sugar syrup or honey. At this time syrup of phosphate of iron was mentioned in *British Pharmacopeia*, 1864, and Royle and Headland 1865, 156.

89. *Correspondence*, 12: 412–13.

90. *Correspondence*, 12: 415.

91. *Correspondence*, 12: 416. This is the last extant letter of Jenner to Darwin, although the two would continue to have professional contacts into 1865.

92. *Correspondence*, 12: 389–90, 394–95.

93. *Correspondence*, 12: 401.

94. *Correspondence*, 12: 405–6. In a letter to Hooker he wrote that "Emma quite agrees with me" that attending the anniversary meeting would probably make him "very ill." *Correspondence*, 12: 419.

95. *Correspondence*, 12: 408.

96. *Correspondence*, 12: 410.

97. *Correspondence*, 12: 425.

98. *Correspondence*, 12: 435.

99. *Correspondence*, 12: 421.

100. *Correspondence*, 12: 424.

101. On 15 December 1864, Darwin wrote to a correspondent, who wished to visit him at Down: "My health is so uncertain that I never know how I shall be & some few days I cannot speak to any one. [While he sometimes could not speak to visitors he could always speak to Emma.] On my best days I dare not talk for more than 10 or 15 minutes, though I can repeat the dose two or three times.... All I can say is that I sh^d be *delighted* to see you for a few minutes, but it would not be worth all the trouble of coming here." *Correspondence*, 12: 471–72. Emma's diary for 1864 records that at the time he was writing this letter, he was ill for two consecutive days: 15 December, "Hor[ace] sickness"/"C. bad night"; 16 December, "C. unwell in bed." It seems likely that Darwin's illness, which closely followed Horace's vomiting, was caused by his disturbed feelings over this vomiting.

Chapter 12

1. *Correspondence*, 13: 17. Except for Emma's diary entries for 15 and 16 December 1864, there is no record of the days when Darwin had to spend time in bed. Darwin would start consulting Dr. Henry Bence Jones in July 1865.

2. *Correspondence*, 13: 19–20. Hooker had obtained a medical degree from Glasgow University and was sometimes referred to as "Dr. Hooker." He had also expressed skepticism about the validity of "suppressed gout" as a medical diagnosis in a 2 July 1862 letter to Darwin. *Correspondence*, 10: 295. For a discussion of the concept of "suppressed gout," see chapter 16.

3. *Correspondence*, 13: 35.

4. *Correspondence*, 13: 47–48. Emma's 1865 diary records "sick" for 24 and 25 January, which probably refers to her husband, and on 27 January "C. sick."

5. *Correspondence*, 13: 48.

6. *Correspondence*, 13: 56. Emma's 1865 diary records "C. very languid for 3 days past sick," on 7 February, and that he was "better" the next day. Darwin's anticipation of the

sun's cooling was influenced by William Thomson's 1862 essay, "On the Age of the Sun's Heat."

7. Darwin to Alfred Wallace, 28 May [1864], *Correspondence*, 12: 216. How Darwin developed his theory of sexual selection is discussed by Desmond and Moore in their introduction to the 2004 Penguin edition of Darwin, *The Descent of Man, and Selection in Relation to Sex.*

8. *Correspondence*, 12: 108.

9. *Correspondence*, 12: 111, 132. Dr. Alfred Baring Garrod (1819–1907) was an eminent physician and expert on gout and gouty complaints.

10. The vomiting was chronicled by Emma in her diary. Her only reference to treatments is a 29 April entry, "took blue pill," which may refer to her husband.

11. *Correspondence*, 12: 138, note 6. Darwin's account book shows he paid Jenner £10 10s on 3 May, which was the price for a visit to Down. There is no record of Jenner's thoughts about Darwin's illness on 3 May.

12. *Correspondence*, 13: 137.

13. *Correspondence*, 13: 141–42.

14. *Correspondence*, 13: 146–47.

15. Poynter 1950.

16. Chapman 1864, 5–6.

17. *Correspondence*, 13: 147.

18. The two occasions when illness was prolonged were July 1848–March 1849 and February 1863–April 1864 (chapters 6 and 11). The symptoms of the illness of July 1848–March 1849 included vomiting, shivering, black spots before eyes, and fear of impending death. The onset of Darwin's vomiting in February 1863 was preceded by his having feelings of "faintness." The only time he appears to have had vomiting and "hysterical crying" was in October 1864. He had symptoms of "rocking" in 1864, 1865, 1866, 1871, 1874, and 1875. In January 1865 Darwin wrote that reading "makes my head whiz more than anything else."

19. In the health diary for 1849, on 14 August Darwin recorded "retching up with acid & clots of blood," and on 15 August "bad sickness with acid & slime." In the diary, he then reported acid with vomiting on 11 December 1850; 7, 27 January, and 15, 23 December 1853; 10, 21, November 1854; and 5 January 1855.

20. Darwin's illness was diagnosed as "suppressed gout" by Henry Holland in 1849 and perhaps also by William Brinton and William Jenner in 1863–64. Darwin believed that his father, Dr. Robert Darwin, had gout. His grandfather, Dr. Erasmus Darwin, had gout and believed that his father-in-law, Josiah L. Wedgwood, had died from gout. In 1863–64, Brinton and Jenner each told Darwin that he had "no organic mischief" and that he would recover from his illness.

21. Previous to this Darwin had occasional episodes of lumbago.

22. For a history of Darwin's use of alcohol, see chapter 15. Chalk, magnesia, and other antacids were prescribed for Darwin by Dr. Jenner in March 1864, and at first these checked his vomiting. However, under Jenner's direction he stopped using antacids in

November 1864. Darwin last visited Malvern from September to October 1863 and was then evaluated by Dr. Gully as "not strong enough to bear" hydropathy.

23. The passages "I feel nearly sure. . . . Does not throw up the food" are in Emma's handwriting. Emma first reported in an 1863 letter to Hooker that Darwin had digested food before vomiting, and several months later he reported that same observation to Hooker.

24. The previous transcription of these notes, in Colp 1977, 83–84, contains a number of errors. The present transcription is from *Correspondence* 13: appendix 4, note on Darwin's health," 479–84.

25. *Correspondence,* 13: 167.

26. *Correspondence,* 13: 179–80.

27. *Correspondence,* 13: 194.

28. *Correspondence,* 13: 195.

29. Dr. Chapman finished reading *On the Origin of Species* on 21 February 1860—three months after it had been published——and then wrote in his diary, "It impresses me as one of the most important books of this century, and is likely to effect an immense mental revolution. The sagacity, knowledge and candour displayed in the work are unusually great and wonderful." Haight 1940, 237.

30. *Correspondence,* 13: 167; Olby 1963, 250–63.

31. *Correspondence,* 13: 150–52.

32. Huxley's letter has not survived.

33. *Correspondence,* 13: 196–97.

34. *Correspondence,* 13: 202–4.

35. Emma's diary records that after August 1865 her husband only had "rocking" on 7 February 1866 and 18 August 1871. Darwin reported having "rocking" in letters to Hooker on 4 October [1871], 4 March [1874], and 25 February [1875]. In his March 1874 letter he wrote: "my head has been bad enough of late with rocking, pricking of fingers' end & other nasty symptoms." Darwin to Hooker, 4 March [1874]. This appears to be the only record that "rocking" was a symptom that involved Darwin's head.

36. *Correspondence,* 13: 194–95.

37. *Correspondence,* 13: 168. The plagiarism dispute between Lyell and Lubbock is discussed in appendix 5, "The Lyell-Lubbock Dispute," *Correspondence,* 13: 485–94.

38. *Correspondence,* 13: 209.

39. These contacts of Darwin and Lubbock are mentioned in *Correspondence,* 3: 276–77; 5: 154, 161–62, 189, 253–54, 257–58.

40. Hutchins 1914, 1: 41–42, 48–50, 67, 148.

41. *Correspondence,* 13: 245.

42. *Correspondence,* 13: 279.

43. *Correspondence,* 13: 259, note 6.

44. Coley 1973.

45. *Correspondence,* 13: 223.

46. *Correspondence*, 13: 246.

47. *Correspondence,* 13: 260.

48. Emma's diary.

49. *Correspondence*, 13: 328, 477.

50. *Correspondence*, 14: 3–5. Including all of the notes to this letter on pages 4–5.

51. In his May 1865 notes for Dr. Chapman, Darwin may have described a diminution in the occurrence of his headaches by writing, "Head symptoms ??"

52. The entry in Emma's diary for 8 December 1865 reads "left off sugar." This appears to be the only time that Darwin observed the beneficial effects of taking coffee without sugar. In December 1853 he had briefly recorded the effects of coffee on his sleep in his health diary without reaching any definite conclusions.

53. "Horror about acid" refers to the effects of regurgitating acid from the stomach into the mouth, which Darwin thought corroded his teeth.

54. Darwin had taken iron and phosphate of iron in 1864. It is not known when and why he started to take oxide of iron.

55. Darwin had taken muriatic [hydrochloric] acid frequently, but this may have been the first time he took it with cayenne and ginger. A recipe for a remedy consisting of "Oxley's essence of Ginger" and tincture of cayenne in brandy was given by Darwin in a letter to his son George on 22 January 1873. Cayenne was derived from the species of *Capsicum* and used for the treatment of gout and flatulence. Ginger was valued for its beneficial effects on the stomach.

56. *Correspondence*, 14: 52. "Pottas-ammonia" probably refers to a chalk-potash and ammonia preparation for treating acidity, similar to some of the preparations used by Dr. Jenner in treating Darwin in 1864. This "model diet" has been lost.

57. Darwin to Fox, 6 Feb. [1867], *Correspondence*, 15: 70.

58. *Emma Darwin* (1904), 2: 210.

59. *Correspondence*, 14: 21, 337, 340.

60. Coley 1973, 50. In February 1867 Darwin wrote Fox: "Poor Bence Jones has been for months at death's door, & was quite given up; but has rallied in surprising manner from inflammation of Lungs & heart-disease." *Correspondence*, 15: 70.

61. Henry Bence Jones to Emma Darwin, 1 October [1867], *Correspondence*, 15: 382–83. In her diary for 1867 Emma wrote that Darwin was "very unwell" on 21 September, and "bad" on 27 September. In his journal for 18–24 September 1867, Darwin wrote "poorly all time." *Correspondence*, 15: 522.

62. Henry Bence Jones to Darwin, 2 August 1870, DAR 168: 79. This is the last of Dr. Bence Jones's extant letters to Darwin. He retired in early 1873 and died in April. Coley 1973, 50.

63. Darwin to Huxley, 23 July [1868], College Archives, Imperial College, London; Darwin to Fox, 21 October [1868], Christ College Library, Cambridge.

64. Darwin to Hooker, 17 [July 1868], DAR 94: 78–79.

65. William Allingham (1824–89) is today noted for his poems about Ireland and

for his diary, which revealed "something of Boswell's sharp eye and ear for detail" and gave "many detailed accounts of famous Victorian men and women." This was the only occasion on which he saw Darwin. Warner 1975, 11, 66–78.

66. At this time Hooker was president of the British Association for the Advancement of Science, and he was working on an address that he would make at the Association meeting in August 1868 in Norwich.

67. Allingham 1967, 184.

68. *Emma Darwin* (1904), 2: 226, 228; Darwin to Hooker, 13 November [1869], *More Letters*, 1: 316.

69. Darwin to St. George Mivart, [1872], 01–08, DAR 96: 141–42; *Autobiography*, 126.

70. *Emma Darwin* (1904), 2: 245–46.

71. In her diary for 11 July 1871, Emma wrote: "Ch. v[ery] unwell no vomiting & shock."

72. Henrietta Litchfield to Francis Darwin, 18 March 1887, DAR 112: A79–A82.

73. Litchfield 1910, 124–25.

74. "Reminiscences," *L&L*, 1: 105.

75. Darwin to Hooker, 4 August [1872], DAR 94: 225–26. In 1863 Hooker had expressed his hate for Owen in a letter to Darwin: "I can hate & respect; I cannot hate & despise—& I do on my conscience think that I despise Owen's mind and conduct too single mindedly to care one atom for his individuality—I look on him now as a poor miserable devil of a scotched viper, turning & poisoning with a bite what he can neither strangle nor gorge." *Correspondence*, 11: 169–70.

Chapter 13

1. Darwin to Fox, 29 Oct [1872], Christ's College Library, Cambridge, England; Darwin to Asa Gray, 22 Oct [1872], Gray Herbarium, Harvard University.

2. *Emma Darwin* (1904), 2: 258.

3. Emma's diary, 12–22 December 1872; Darwin's journal.

4. Darwin to Hooker, 12 Sept [1873], DAR 95: 274–276. The date when this episode occurred is given in Emma's diary.

5. Sir Andrew Clark, Bart., M.D. (1826–93). For obituaries on Clark see *Lancet*, 11 November 1893, and *British Medical Journal*, 11 November 1893. Emma recorded in her diary that Dr. Clark came to Down on 30 August 1873.

6. *Emma Darwin* (1904), 2: 266.

7. Andrew Clark to Darwin, 3 Sept 1873, DAR 161: 50.

8. Darwin to Hooker, 12 Sept [1873], DAR 95: 274–76.

9. Darwin to Huxley 5 Dec [1873], College Archives, Imperial College, London. Huxley claimed to have benefited from a "special diet" prescribed by Dr. Clark. Huxley 1913, 1: 402.

10. Darwin to Andrew Clark 10 Jan [1874], Library of the American Philosophical

Society, Philadelphia. In this letter Darwin writes that he has just come to London and that Dr. Clark should please call and see him.

11. This was a diary from 1874 to 1882 containing notations by Darwin about sums of money, the progress of his manuscripts, and trips from and back to Down. There are occasional references to Darwin's health and to Dr. Clark and the latter's treatments.

12. Dr. Clark prescribed what were called "Clark's pills," which contained strychnine or quinine and strychnine. Winslow 1971, 34.

13. Darwin to Hooker, 4 March [1874], DAR 95: 313–16.

14. Darwin to [M. T. Masters] 10 July [1875], Smithsonian Institution, Washington, D.C., Dibner Collection.

15. Darwin to Hooker, 14 April [1875], *Life and Letters*, 2: 381; Darwin to Wallace, 17 June 1876 (Marchant 1916, 237–40). Darwin writes to Hooker of his work in organizing leading scientific men so that, while vivisection will be regulated, serious physiological investigation will be permitted. He thanks Wallace for defending him against Mivart's 1874–75 attacks and writes of the "pain" that these attacks have caused him.

16. Darwin to Hooker [2 March 1878], DAR 95: 453–54; Desmond and Moore 1991, 631–32.

17. Henrietta Litchfield to Francis Darwin, 18 March 1887, DAR 112: A79–A82.

18. *More Letters,* 1: 375.

19. *Autobiography,* 115.

20. "Reminiscences," *L&L,* 1: 121.

21. *Life and Letters,* 2: 356.

22. *Autobiography,* 138.

23. *Emma Darwin* (1904), 2: 216.

24. Keynes 2001, 281–82.

25. *Life and Letters,* 2: 377–78.

26. *Report of the Royal Commission on the Practice of Subjecting Live Animals to Experiments for Scientific Purposes* 1876, 233–34.

27. G. Darwin, "Recollections."

28. "Reminiscences," *L&L,* 1: 101.

29. "Reminiscences," *L&L,* 1: 90.

30. Laura Forster, "Recollections of Charles Darwin," January 1883, DAR 112, A31–A37.

31. *Life and Letters,* 2: 375. Darwin had experienced similar "failings" when during his reading of manuscript papers at meetings of the Geological Society he felt "as if my body was gone, & only my head left." *Correspondence,* 6: 344.

32. "Reminiscences," *L&L,* 1: 106.

33. "Reminiscences," *L&L,* 1: 105. *Emma Darwin* (1904), 2: 269, 284, 301.

34. Darwin to J. W. Judd, 27 June 1878, *More Letters,* 1: 375.

35. Darwin to [J. M. Herbert], 25 December [1880]; de Beer 1968, 74.

36. Nash 1921, 28.

37. De Candolle, translated and quoted in Bettany 1887, 148.

38. *Emma Darwin* (1904), 2: 332.

39. Henrietta Litchfield to Francis Darwin, 18 March 1887, DAR 112, A79–A82.

40. Schwartz 1995.

41. *Autobiography*, 130.

42. Desmond and Moore 1991, 615–16, 618, 621.

43. Darwin to Huxley, 4 February [1880]; *Autobiography*, 187.

44. Henrietta Litchfield to Francis Darwin, 18 March 1887, DAR 142, A79–A82.

45. "Reminiscences," *L&L,* 1: 94–95.

46. *Insectivorous Plants* (1875), *The Effects of Cross and Self Fertilisation in the Vegetable Kingdom* (1876), *The Different Forms of Flowers on Plants of the Same Species* (1877), and *The Power of Movements in Plants*, assisted by Francis Darwin (1880). When he was writing his book on *Insectivorous Plants*, Darwin told Hooker: "You ask about my book, & all that I can say is that I am ready to commit suicide: I thought it was decently written, but find so much wants rewriting. . . . I begin to think that every one who publishes a book is a fool." Darwin to Hooker, 10 February [1875], *Life and Letters*, 2: 501.

47. The saying occurs in a novel by Anthony Trollope when a clergyman who is confronting great social adversity is advised by a brickmaker that "there ain't nowt a man can't bear if he'll only be dogged. . . . It's dogged as does it. It ain't thinking about it." Reflecting on this, the clergyman concludes that "the brickmaker's doggedness simply meant self-abnegation; that a man should force himself to endure anything that might be sent upon him, not only without outward grumbling, but also without grumbling inwardly." Trollope 1867, vol. 2, chapter 18, "It's Dogged as Does It." Wallis Nash, a lawyer who befriended the Darwin family and lived near them in Down from 1873 to 1877, recollected how Darwin once said to him: "Trollope, in one of his novels, gives as a maxim of constant use by a bricklayer, 'It's dogged as does it!' and I have often and often thought this is a motto for every scientific observer." Nash 1919, 133.

48. "Reminiscences," *L&L,* 1: 125–26.

49. De Beer 1968, 74.

50. Darwin 1929, 120.

51. "Reminiscences," *L&L,* 1: 108.

52. *Autobiography*, 46, 139.

53. "I am sorry to hear that you are suffering from boils; I have often had fearful crops; I hope that the doctors are right in saying that they are serviceable." Darwin to Wallace, 24 [May 1862], *Correspondence*, 10: 219. I have not been able to find later references to boils in Darwin's *Correspondence*.

54. *Emma Darwin* (1904), 2: 259.

55. *Autobiography*, 27.

56. "Reminiscences," *L&L,* 1: 92.

57. Darwin to Sarah Haliburton, 1 November [1872], *Life and Letters*, 2: 352.

58. *Autobiography*, 97.

59. Darwin to his son George, 13 July [1876]; *Emma Darwin* (1904), 2: 279.

60. *Emma Darwin* (1904), 2: 302.

61. "Reminiscences," *L&L*, 1: 135; *Emma Darwin* (1904), 2: 330.

62. Judd 1910, 118.

63. *Emma Darwin* (1904), 2: 262.

64. Henrietta Litchfield to Francis Darwin, 18 March 1887, DAR 112: A79–A82.

65. *Autobiography*, 96–97.

Chapter 14

1. *Emma Darwin* (1904), 2: 317. It has been suggested that, in view of subsequent events, these fits of dazzling may have been due to a failing circulation. Bowlby 1990, 437.

2. *More Letters,* 2: 433.

3. Marchant 1916, 261.

4. MacNalty 1964, ii.

5. *Life and Letters,* 2: 527–28.

6. *Emma Darwin* (1904), 2: 323.

7. Judd 1910, 158–59; *Life and Letters,* 2: 524.

8. Allan 1967, 236.

9. *Life and Letters,* 2: 522–25; Freeman 1978, 172.

10. *More Letters,* 2: 446.

11. De Beer 1968, 82.

12. Henrietta Litchfield, "Charles Darwin's Death," DAR, 262.23.2. This is an eleven-page manuscript account of the death of her father.

13. Litchfield, "Darwin's Death"; *Emma Darwin* (1904), 2: 325; Atkins 1974, 38.

14. "He felt the *strongest gratitude* to Dr. Clark & wd not hear of anything that might mortify him." Litchfield, "Darwin's Death," emphasis in original. Seventeen days after Clark's visit, Darwin partially expressed his anger by writing Huxley: "Dr. Clark's kindness is unbounded to me, but he is too busy to come here." *Life and Letters,* 2: 529.

15. Litchfield, "Darwin's Death"; Atkins 1974, 38.

16. Sir Thomas Lauder Brunton introduced amyl nitrite to treat angina pectoris in 1867, and it was widely used in the 1880s. He wrote that "amyl nitrite appears to arrest the spasm of the vessels in Angina Pectoris by causing paralysis of the vessels themselves or the peripheral ends of the vasomotor nerves." Brunton 1885, 212.

17. Sir Norman Moore (1847–1922) had been associated with Saint Bartholomew's Hospital, London, since 1872. He would become an eminent clinician and medical writer, teacher, and historian. Since his student days at Cambridge he had shown "a keen interest in natural history." For an obituary on Moore, see *British Medical Journal,* 9 December 1922. Darwin had seen Moore previously and then said he did not have confidence in him. Litchfield, "Darwin's Death"; Atkins 1974, 38.

18. Litchfield, "Darwin's Death."

19. *Emma Darwin* (1904), 2: 329.

20. Laura Forster to Francis Darwin, 15 November 1885, DAR 112: 38–40.

21. *Collected Papers*, 2: 276–80.

22. Mr. Charles H. Allfrey (1839–1912) obtained his medical degree from Edinburgh University in 1861 and became a fellow of the Royal College of Surgeons in 1867. He practiced in partnership with Dr. Heckstall Smith at Saint Mary Cray and took an active part in founding the Chislehurst and Cray Valley Hospital.

23. Litchfield, "Darwin's Death"; Atkins 1974, 38–39. Nux vomica was an extract from the fruit of an East Indian tree, which contained two active alkaloids—strychnine and brucine. It was used as a tonic and stimulant.

24. Litchfield, "Darwin's Death"; Atkins 1974, 39.

25. Dr. Walter Moxon (1836–86) was a noted and brilliant London physician, associated with Guy's Hospital, who in 1881 delivered the Croonian Lectures at the Royal College of Physicians.

26. Litchfield, "Darwin's Death"; Atkins 1974, 39; Francis Darwin to Huxley, Down, Thursday (20 April 1882), Huxley Papers, College Archive, Imperial College, London. In this letter, written the day after Darwin died, Francis Darwin gives a brief account of his father's final illness.

27. Litchfield, "Darwin's Death"; Atkins 1974, 39–40.

28. *British Medical Journal*, 29 April 1882, 628. There does not seem to have been an autopsy.

Chapter 15

1. "Reminiscences," *L&L*, 1: 99–100; *Correspondence*, 1: 72. Snuff was a preparation of powdered tobacco for inhaling through the nostrils. It was used to facilitate the release of phlegm, in treating colds, and as a mental stimulant. Its use could become addictive.

2. Moorehead 1969, 206.

3. *Correspondence*, 2: 150.

4. *Correspondence*, 3: 311.

5. *Correspondence*, 4: 226.

6. *Correspondence*, 4: 235; Innes 1961, 256.

7. *Correspondence*, 5: 540.

8. Atkins 1974, 98.

9. *Correspondence*, 6: 395, note 8.

10. "Reminiscences," ms, 8, 13–14.

11. "Reminiscences," ms, 8.

12. *Correspondence*, 4: 225, 235.

13. *Correspondence*, 3: 311.

14. "Reminiscences," ms, 31.

15. Judd 1909, 379.

16. *Lancet* 2 (1853): 508–12, 532–36.

17. Goodman and Gilman 1955, 620–23.

18. "Reminiscences," ms, 8.

19. *Correspondence*, 1: 330; *Beagle* diary, 184.

20. "Reminiscences," ms, 14–15.

21. "Reminiscences," *L&L*, 1: 99–100.

22. *Autobiography*, 60.

23. "Reminiscences," ms, 96.

24. Grant Duff 1904, 80–81.

25. *Correspondence*, 5: 194.

26. *Correspondence*, 5: 357.

27. *Correspondence*, 7: 215–16, note 6.

28. *Correspondence*, 8: 133.

29. *Correspondence*, 11: 646.

30. *Correspondence*, 13: 482.

31. Atkins 1974, 35.

32. "Reminiscences," ms, 96.

33. "Reminiscences," ms, 10–11.

34. *Autobiography*, 224.

35. King-Hele 1999, 47–48, 220.

36. *Autobiography*, 36.

Chapter 16

1. *Correspondence*, 13: 482.

2. Gully 1846, 99–121.

3. Lane 1882, 3.

4. *Correspondence*, 11: 602–3, note 3.

5. *British Medical Journal*, 1882, 628.

6. *Correspondence*, 4: 209.

7. *Correspondence*, 13: 482–83, note 6.

8. Dr. Andrew Clark to Charles Darwin, 3 September 1873, DAR 161: 151.

9. Holland 1855, 240, 233.

10. Copeland 1858, 1: 1044.

11. Garrod 1863, 263–65.

12. Garrod 1863, 490–91.

13. Coperman 1964, 107.

14. Lane 1882, 3–4.

15. *Correspondence*, 12: 260; *Life and Letters*, 1: 197.

16. Hague 1884, 759.

17. *Life and Letters*, 1: 198.

18. Darwin, *Variation of Animals and Plants under Domestication,* 1868, 2: 7, 77, 404.

19. *Correspondence,* 13: 482.

20. *Correspondence,* 1: 74; 2: 40.

21. King-Hele 1999, 160–61.

22. Dr. Erasmus Darwin to his son, Dr. Robert Darwin, Derby, 5 January [1792], *Autobiography,* 224.

23. *Life and Letters,* 1: 197.

24. Darwin to Adam Sedgwick, 24 August [1859], *Correspondence,* 6: 325.

25. Darwin to Mrs. Haliburton, 1 November [1872], *Life and Letters,* 2: 353.

26. See chapter 18 for a comparison of Darwin's illness with the illnesses of his relations and children.

Chapter 17

1. *Lancet,* 29 April 1882; *Times,* 21 April 1882; Bacon 1882, 9; Miall 1883, 20; *Life and Letters,* 1: 198; Lane 1882, 3–4; Romanes 1882, 14.

2. Huxley 1912, 293.

3. Huxley 1927, 112.

4. F. Smith 1990.

5. Johnston 1901, 158.

6. Nemiah 1975.

7. Johnston 1901, 157.

8. Guggenheim 2000, 1529–30.

9. Gould 1903, 91–94, 102–3.

10. This was the opinion of two ophthalmologists to whom I described Darwin's symptom.

11. "Reminiscences," ms, 93–94, 114–15.

12. Lane 1882, 5.

13. *Life and Letters,* 1: 496–97.

14. "Reminiscences," ms, 7–8; *Correspondence,* 10: 170. He would wear the pince-nez low down on his nose and carry it suspended around his neck on a ribbon.

15. Darwin 1929, 121. Leonard does not specify what he meant by "other forms of auto-poisoning."

16. *Correspondence,* 13: 482.

17. Bulimia is a pathological condition characterized by an alternation of overeating and vomiting, caused by an obsession with weight. In a majority of those bulimics who have been vomiting three times a week for more than four years, the acid content of their vomit produces significant destruction of the enamel of their teeth, resulting in dental cavities, sensitivities, and pain. Wolcott, Yager, and Gordon 1984, 723–25.

18. Health diary, 15–24 June 1852; *Correspondence,* 5: 101.

Chapter 18

1. Keith 1955, 214.

2. Alvarez 1959, 1110.

3. Alvarez 1959, 1111–12.

4. Cook 1996, 59–63; King-Hele 1999, 89–95. Because of the information contained in Dr. Cook's article on Mary Darwin, the possibility that she may have had porphyria (mentioned in Colp 1977, 131–32) can be discounted.

5. Seward 1804, 406–7.

6. King-Hele 1999, 324–30.

7. Robert Darwin's episodes of "gout" are mentioned in *Correspondence*, 1: 74, 98, 356, 361, 423, 493; 2: 40.

8. Sarah Wedgwood to her brother Tom Wedgwood, Gunville, 14 March 1800, Wedgwood Archives, Keele University Library, W/M 60.

9. In 1804 Susannah's brother Josiah Wedgwood II wrote: "My mother remains very well Susan [Susannah] as usual." Josiah Wedgwood II, to his brother Tom Wedgwood, Maer, 19 July 1804, in Litchfield 1903, 175. In 1805 Susannah wrote Josiah: "All are well except myself who am as usual." Susannah to Josiah Wedgwood II [1805], Wedgwood Archives, Keele University Library, W/M 229-32. In 1807 Susannah commented: "Everybody seems young but me." Susannah to Josiah Wedgwood II [June 1807], Wedgwood Archives, W/M 230-32.

10. During her terminal illness Susannah was visited by her two sisters, Catherine and Sarah, who described her clinical condition in letters to Josiah Wedgwood II: Catherine to Josiah, 14 July 1817 (Wedgwood Archives, 19835-27); Sarah to Josiah, 16 July 1817 (Wedgwood Archives, 20400-28).

11. Wedgwood and Wedgwood 1980, 92, 101, 114, 124; King-Hele 1999, 286–87.

12. Healey 2001, 56.

13. Galton 1908, 79, 153; Pearson 1924, 2: 179.

14. *Autobiography*, 42.

15. *Correspondence*, 6: 335.

16. *Correspondence*, 7: 390. Ague is a feverish condition involving alternating stages of feeling hot and cold and sweating.

17. *Correspondence*, 8: 133.

18. Keynes 2001, 206.

19. Alvarez 1959, 1112.

20. *Correspondence*, 5: 9; Keynes 2001, 199–211, 225–26.

21. Raverat 1952, 146–47.

22. Keynes 2001, 219–20.

23. *Correspondence*, 5: 542–43; 7: 116; 8: 215, 435; 9: 195–96.

24. Raverat 1952, 123.

25. Raverat 1952, 189–91.

26. Keynes 1943, 13.

27. *Correspondence*, 11: 438.

28. Cattermole and Wolfe 1987, 4; Raverat 1952, 204. At this time an appendectomy for gastrointestinal symptoms was a new and unusual therapeutic procedure.

29. F. Darwin 1916, 5: xiv; Pickering 1974, 9; Raverat 1952, 187.

30. Keynes 1943, 13.

31. *Correspondence*, 6: 460; 9: 69; *Life and Letters*, 2: 352–53.

Chapter 19

1. Kempf 1920, 209, 211.

2. Kempf 1920, 250.

3. "To my deep mortification my father once said to me, 'You care for nothing but shooting, dogs, and rat-catching, and you will be a disgrace to yourself and all your family.' But my father, who was the kindest man I ever knew, and whose memory I love with all my heart, must have been angry and somewhat unjust when he used such words.... My father . . . was very properly vehement against my turning an idle sporting man, which then [1827] seemed my probably destination." *Autobiography*, 28, 56.

4. Hubble 1946, 84.

5. Good 1954, 106.

6. Greenacre 1963, 90.

7. Graber and Miles 1988, 98.

8. Rosenberg 1989, 92.

9. Bowlby 1990, 69–70.

10. Bowlby 1990, 71. Support for Bowlby's opinion is contained in the following recollection of Darwin's sister Caroline: "I wish some years ago I had known that Charles thought my Father did not understand or know what ability & power of mind he had—really he was so proud as well as fond of him that I often felt afraid Erasmus might feel mortified & feel undervalued." Caroline Wedgwood to Emma Darwin, 19 November 1887, Wedgwood Archives, W/M 598.

11. Bowlby 1990, 71.

Chapter 20

1. Simpson 1958, 117–22.

2. "Naturalist's Evolution," 1959, 141.

3. Greenacre 1963, 32.

4. Adler 1959.

5. Kohn 1963; Huxley and Kettlewell 1965, 66.

6. Medawar 1967, 61–67; Brussel 1966.

7. Woodruff 1965a, 745–50; 1965b, 1380; 1968, 661–72.

8. Woodruff 1965a, 747–48.

9. Woodruff 1965b.

10. Woodruff 1965a, 749.

11. Adler 1965.

12. Bernstein 1984.

13. Adler 1989.

14. Compensated heat disease probably meant that Darwin would have needed to limit his exercise to his usual daily walks of one to two miles. It does not seem likely that these limitations would have been compatible with the strenuous walks that he was sometimes capable of doing. These included during 1849–55, when he walked three to four miles before breakfast, and then may have taken other long walks during the day, and 1865 when he walked five miles a day. G. Darwin, "Recollections," 21; Emma's diary, 7 October 1865. During his exacerbations of flatulence and vomiting, he was examined by physicians—Jenner, Brinton, and Bence Jones—who assured him that he did not have heart disease.

15. Goldstein 1989, 586–601.

16. Responding to Woodruff's contention that in Chagas' disease stomach symptoms usually occur with heart symptoms, David Adler has drawn attention to a study, "New Light on Chagas' Disease," *Lancet* (1965), 1150–51, which observes that "50% of Chagas' disease cases with esophageal lesions had clinically detectable cardiac damage." Adler 1989, 219, note 8.

17. For an account of how Darwin became ill and developed flatulence in 1840, which is based on the 1840 writings of Darwin and Emma, see chapter 4.

18. Others who believe that Darwin had Chagas' disease include Simpson 1996, Milner 2002; and Sulloway 2003, 36.

Those who do not believe Darwin had Chagas' include Janet Browne and Richard Darwin Keynes. While Browne gives no reasons for her disbelief (Browne 2002, 233), Professor Keynes states that Darwin did not have Chagas' because, after being attacked by *Triatoma infestans* bugs on 26 March 1835, he did not "record any period of the fever that characteristically accompanies the initial [Chagas'] infection." Keynes 2003, 283–84. However, about two weeks after the attack, Darwin wrote in his diary that for eight days he "was not very well & saw nothing & admired nothing." This could have been an acute febrile episode of Chagas' disease.

19. I thank Andie Clare of Icon Films for sending me a video copy of "Diagnosing Darwin."

Chapter 21

1. Colp 1977, 142.

2. Bowlby 1990, 56–57; Kohn 1963, 241, 251.

3. For Allingham's account of Darwin's appearing "yellow," see Allingham 1967, 184. Darwin's account of himself as being "rather sallow" is published in *Life and Letters*, 2: 356. For more on Darwin's complexion, see chapter 22.

4. Tennyson 1897, 2: 57; Hillen 1982, 6: 270–71. Emma's diary for August 1868 makes no mention of any changes in her husband's color. On 21 May 1865, she had written in her diary that he was "pale."

5. Kohn 1963, 252.

6. "Reminiscences," *L&L,* 1: 96–97, 100–101.

7. Stetten 1959, 194–95.

8. Roberts 1967, 160–67.

9. "Reminiscences," *L&L,* 1: 99–100.

10. For a discussion of the theory of Systemic Lactose intolerance as a possible cause for Darwin's craving for sweets, see chapter 30.

11. "Reminiscences," ms, 12.

Chapter 22

1. Kohn 1963, 252.

2. Winslow 1971, 73–74.

3. DuBois and Geiling 1959, 134–35.

4. *Correspondence,* 13: 482.

5. *Correspondence,* 4: 269.

6. *Correspondence,* 6: 384.

7. Winslow 1971, 61–62.

8. Dr. W. D. Foster writes that after studying this photograph in his copy of Lady Barlow's edition of Darwin's autobiography, "I was not able to convince myself of the existence of 'corn-like elevations,' and they are certainly not to be seen on the original photograph at Down." Foster 1972, 591–92.

9. *Emma Darwin* (1904), 2: 22; "Reminiscences," ms, 89; Osborn 1928, 51; Allingham 1967, 184. For a discussion of the clinical meaning of Darwin's appearing to be "yellow," see chapter 21.

10. *Correspondence,* 4: 227; *Life and Letters,* 2: 356.

11. Clark 1917, 478–79; Bettany 1887, 147–48; Ferdinand Cohn, recollections of his visit with Darwin, *Breslauer Zeitung,* 23 April 1882.

12. Osler 1929, 592.

13. Foster 1972, 592.

14. Winslow 1971, 68.

15. "The Late Charles Darwin," *British Medical Journal,* 1882, 628.

16. On 20 April 1853, Darwin reported, in his health diary, that he had a cold, mild fever, and "chest-pain." The nature of this "chest-pain" was not specified, and it seems to have lasted for only one day.

17. Winslow 1971, 66–67.

18. The source that Dr. Winslow gives for the assertion that Darwin "mentioned growing bald at the age of twenty-eight" is a letter that Charles Lyell wrote to Darwin, when Darwin was twenty-eight, in which Lyell said: "Do not flatter yourself that you will be believed till you are growing bald like me, with hard work & vexation at the incredulity of the world." *Correspondence,* 2: 4. When Darwin was about twenty-eight, he

commented that his face was "already beginning to wrinkle," but he said nothing about the state of his hair. *Autobiography*, 234.

19. This portrait of Darwin by George Richmond is reproduced in Wells 1938, 152.

20. For Darwin at forty, see photo no. 36 in Desmond and Moore 1991; at forty-three, a photograph reproduced in *Autobiography*, 111; at forty-four, a portrait reproduced in De Beer 1964, 164.

21. Winslow 1971, 66.

22. Buckston Browne wrote that Darwin's health diary shows that Darwin had "pyorrhea and sore gums," but this is not indicated in the diary. Browne 1943, 14.

23. In February 1861, Darwin wrote Hooker about George's dental problems: "Poor George has [lost] literally [every] tooth in his head, except a few lower incisors decayed: they have all gone suddenly together & been stopped & drawn by Mr. Woodhouse & I fear this points to some deep flaw in his constitution, which has formerly [been] indicated by his intermittent pulse." *Correspondence*, 9: 20. Since Darwin had previously stated that some of his sons had inherited his pulse disorders, he may have been fearful that George had also inherited his sensitivity to teeth erosions.

24. Browne 1943, 14.

25. Winslow 1971, 67.

26. *Correspondence*, 5: 289.

27. *Correspondence*, 6: 249.

28. *Correspondence*, 12: 30.

29. Foster 1965, 477–78.

30. Winslow 1971, 68–69.

31. Winslow 1971, 86, note 21.

32. These physicians published their opinions against the use of mercurials in books that Darwin read: Gully 1846, 77–83; Lane 1857, 36–41.

33. *Correspondence*, 9: 14–20.

34. Emma's diary for 1840 records "bismuth" on 25 September, and "no more bismuth" on 1 October (which may refer to her husband, herself, or to both). In September 1845, Darwin reported: "I have taken my Bismuth regularly . . . it has not done me quite so much good as before." Emma was probably referring to her husband when she wrote in her diary: "began bismuth" on 6 and 13 January, and 17 August 1864; and on 8 July 1865, and made no mention of how long the bismuth was continued.

Darwin took mixtures of hydrochloric and nitric acid in February–April 1857, January–March 1860, and October–December 1863. He continued acids for the first three months of 1864, which Emma recorded as follows in her diary: 17 February, "began sulph. acid"; 21 February "took acid twice"; 2 March "began stronger acid & pills"; 4 March, "left of [sic] pill & acid"; 11 March, "began nitric"; 18 March, "left off nitric."

Under the direction of Dr. Jenner, on 22 March 1864, Darwin began taking a daily combination of alkaline medicines, consisting of carbonate of ammonia, chalk, and magnesia, a combination which checked his severe vomiting. He stopped the chalk on 16 August and stopped the other alkaline medicines on 23 November. Emma's diary recorded "began chalk" on 14 July 1865, and then made no further mention of chalk.

In 1864, also under the direction of Dr. Jenner, Darwin took the following medicines: podophyllin, from 24 March until the end of May; taraxacum at undetermined times; colchicine at undetermined times (and before Jenner on 12 December 1863, and 10 and 11 February 1864); and iron compounds and phosphate of iron from April until September.

Emma's diary records the use of quinine, presumably by her husband, on the following days: 15 December 1863, 2 and 9 January 1864, and 12 July and 28 November 1865.

Darwin reports taking opium for the pains from flatulence in 1846. Emma recorded in her diary that he took opium for his flatulence on 19 and 20 December 1863. On 17 March 1864 she wrote, "Left off opium."

Darwin first began using pepsine in February 1859, for an undetermined period. Emma's diary then records that he took pepsine on the following times: 1862: 7 February, "began pepsine"; 22 February, "½ pepsine"; 23 February, "double pepsine"; 4 March, "left off pepsine"; 7 March, "began pepsine at dinner"; 1864: 30 December, "left off pepsine."

Chapter 23

1. Gruber and Barrett 1974, 44, note 14.

2. See chapter 25.

3. Meteyard 1871, 357.

4. G. Darwin, "Recollections." Darwin stopped raising pigeons after the publication of *On the Origin of Species.* The house, which served as a pigeon aviary, remained standing (but unused) for several decades.

5. Pigeon allergy causes pulmonary fibrosis with symptoms of cough, dyspnea, and (sometimes) fever. This allergy does not cause gastrointestinal or skin symptoms.

Chapter 24

1. Atkins 1974, 70.

2. Pickering 1974, 91.

3. Pickering 1974, 86.

Chapter 25

1. Bowlby 1990, 9.

2. Bowlby 1990, 13.

3. Bowlby 1990, 76.

4. Bowlby 1990, 464.

5. Bowlby 1990, 9.

6. Five publications that discuss the relationship between blood carbon dioxide and the symptoms of panic disorder are Klein 1993, 306–17; Papp, Klein, and Gorman 1993,

1149–57; Gorman, Papp, Coplan et al. 1994, 547–53; Griez and Schruers 1998; and Glass 2000, 573–74.

7. Bowlby 1990, 287.

8. Browne 1995, 21–22.

9. *Autobiography,* 68.

10. Bowlby 1990, 61.

11. Henrietta Litchfield, "Biographical Sketch of Charles Darwin," DAR 262.23.1.

12. *Autobiography,* 22.

13. Sulloway 1991, 29–32.

14. Barloon and Noyes 1997.

15. DSM 4: 1994, 394–403.

16. DSM 4: 396.

17. Barloon and Noyes 1997, 139, 1276–77.

18. Judd 1910, 117–18.

19. *Correspondence,* 4: 50–51, 53, 55; Desmond and Moore 1991, 347–49.

20. Freeman 1984, 43–44.

Chapter 26

1. F. Smith 1992, 291–96, 306; F. Smith 1990, 452–54.

2. F. Smith 1992, 292–94.

3. F. Smith 1992, 291.

4. F. Smith 1992, 295.

5. Keynes 2001, 199–212.

6. F. Smith 1990, 451–52.

7. While a student at Cambridge, Darwin went on "long mountain rambles" and long horseback rides with friends, and on one occasion he made an (apparently) rapid recovery from two "aweful rolls" from a horse. Thomas Butler, "Recollections," 13 September 1882, DAR 112, A10–A12; *Correspondence,* 1: 81–96. Darwin's sensitivity to physical stress mainly occurred after 1842. *Autobiography,* 99.

8. F. Smith 1990, 454.

9. *Autobiography,* 82–83.

10. These neuromuscular effects are first manifested by muscle weakness in the upper extremities. Goodman and Gilman 1985, 1607–8.

11. F. Smith 1990, 455.

12. Wood 1876, 62–69, 63.

13. *Correspondence,* 2: 206–70, 444.

14. F. Smith 1990, 455–56.

15. For determining the kind of barnacle work that Darwin was engaged in for each year of 1850–54, I have consulted the chronology at the end of *Correspondence,* vols. 4 and 5.

16. *Life and Letters,* 1: 318; F. Smith 1990, 456. Francis cites only two widely differ-

ent observations that Darwin made about his health in 1845 and 1849, and he does not compare his father's 1842–54 period of illness with any of the other periods of severe illness. Darwin recollected that it was his 1839–42 period of illness that most impaired his capacity for work. Emma recollected that the "two low water years" for him were 1849 and 1863. Henrietta Litchfield to Francis Darwin, 18 March 1887, DAR 112, A79–A82. I do not believe that there is any way to determine which of the several prolonged illnesses was the most severe.

17. F. Smith 1992, 304–5.

18. Desmond and Moore 1991, 513. After an evening of conversing and dining with his three *Beagle* friends, Darwin became "very ill with violent shaking & vomiting" and could not wish them good-bye the next morning.

19. *Correspondence*, 5: 248–51, 414–15, 508, note 4.

20. F. Smith 1990, 456–57.

21. See chapter 30 for a discussion of the theory of lactose intolerance.

22. F. Smith 1992, 292.

23. F. Smith 1990, 456.

24. *Correspondence*, 4: 29. In a 7 April 1847 letter to Hooker, Darwin described himself as "suffering from four boils & swellings, one of which hardly allows me the use of my right arm & has stopped all my work & damped all my spirits." His "swellings" probably consisted of local cellulites and edema produced by the infection that produced the boils. In a letter to Hooker, written ten days later, he appears to have recovered. *Correspondence*, 4: 35–36.

25. *Life and Letters*, 1: 114; Desmond and Moore 1991, 384; *Correspondence*, 5: 289, notes 5–6; 7: 115–16, note 1, 118–20; 8: 205, note 5; 9: xix; 10: xxii.

Chapter 27

1. King 1994, 47–48, 52–56.

2. *Life and Letters*, 1: 198.

3. Williams and Dluhy 1991, 1729–32.

Chapter 28

1. Young 1997, 83; *Dubois' Lupus Erythematosus*, 410–13. How much Darwin complained about anorexia is uncertain.

2. Young 1997, 83; *Dubois' Lupus Erythematosus*, 290–92.

3. For an account of the role of mental stresses in producing SLE, see *Dubois' Lupus Erythematosus*, 386–88.

4. Young 1997, 84. In September 1831 Darwin complained about his hands in a letter to Susan, being vague about the clinical nature of these complaints. In October 1843 he told his father that he suffered from "dreadful numbness" in his fingers, and in June 1862, he concluded in a letter to Hooker by commenting: "This is a very dull letter, but my

hands are burning as if dipped in hell-fire" (*Correspondence,* 1: 143; 2: 399; 10: 271). For more on Darwin's hands see chapter 31.

5. Young 1997, 83.

6. For most of his *Beagle* land trips he seems to have enjoyed being in sunny weather, although sometimes becoming tired from the heat, and at the end of the voyage he looked back on these trips with a "kind of extreme delight." *Beagle* diary, 39, 154, 158, 159, 202–3, 264, 445.

7. *Correspondence,* 2: 96.

8. *Emma Darwin* (1904), 1: 458; 2: 325.

9. Young 1997, 78, 80, 83, 84; *Dubois' Lupus Erythematosus,* 365–66, 414, 420–21.

10. *Life and Letters,* 1: 90.

11. *Dubois' Lupus Erythematosus,* 343–45.

12. *Dubois' Lupus Erythematosus,* 322–26.

13. For a possible diagnosis of these skin lesions, see chapter 29.

Chapter 29

1. Darwin only rarely mentioned what his dermatitis felt like. In March 1863, he wrote that applying a medical ointment to his eczema was "*certainly* to me very soothing." *Correspondence,* 11: 265. There appears to be no record of his complaining of itchiness, but he may have sometimes experienced this symptom because of the frequent changes that his skin lesions underwent.

2. Sauer 2000, 476.

3. Hanifin and Rajka 1980, 45–46.

4. Sauer 2000, 476.

5. In his May 1865 notes for Dr. Chapman, Darwin wrote: "Eczema—(now constant) lumbago—fundament—rash." *Correspondence,* 13: 482. No further mention is then made of "fundament—rash." Darwin describes other skin symptoms as "erythema" and "eruption."

Chapter 30

1. Campbell and Matthews 2001, 5–27.

2. Emma Darwin's recipe book is kept in the Cambridge University Library, Darwin Papers, *DAR* 214.

3. Campbell and Matthews 2001, 22–26.

4. "Reminiscences," ms, 8.

5. *Correspondence,* 2: 236.

6. Chapters 6 and 10.

7. *Correspondence,* 13: 246.

8. *Correspondence,* 14: 3–4.

9. "Reminiscences," ms, 8.

10. Campbell 2003, 12–13.

11. *Correspondence,* 11: 689.

12. Colvin 1971, 571–72.

Chapter 31

1. Orrego and Quintana 2007, 27, note 16; Colp 1998, 216;
Colp, 2000, 224.

2. Orrego and Quintana 2007, 24.

3. *Life and Letters,* 1: 198.

4. Orrego and Quintana 2007, 24.

5. Colp 1998, 215, 216, note 17.

6. Orrego and Quintana 2007, 26; *Autobiography,* 83, 99. Darwin's illness when he
was at Moor Park is discussed in chapters 8 and 9.

7. Orrego and Quintana 2007, 27.

8. Orrego and Quintana 2007, 25.

9. *Correspondence,* 1: 143. The history of Darwin's paresthesia is given in chapter 1.

10. Health diary, 19 November 1853; 5–9 August 1854; *Correspondence,* 6: 249; 12: 30;
13: 482.

11. Health diary, 14 August 1851, "Poorly Rheumaticks continued"; 15 August 1851,
"Little Rheumatism." "Partly for amusement & partly for change of air we went to London & took a House for a month, but it turned out a great failure, for that dreadful frost
set in when we went, & all our children got unwell & Emma & I had coughs & colds,
& rheumatism nearly all the time." Darwin to Fox, 19 March [1855], *Correspondence,* 5:
289.

Summary

1. *Autobiography,* 68; Herbert, "Recollections."

2. *Autobiography,* 79–80.

3. *Life and Letters,* 1: 193.

4. *Autobiography,* 82.

5. *Autobiography,* 98; chapter 4, notes 1–5, 10, 11, 16–23.

6. *Emma Darwin* (1904), 2: 142.

7. *Correspondence,* 11: 666.

8. *Life and Letters,* 2: 352.

9. *Autobiography,* 106.

10. *Correspondence,* 13: 361.

11. *Correspondence,* 7: 462.

12. *Emma Darwin* (1904), 2: 181.

13. *Autobiography,* 97.

14. *Emma Darwin* (1904), 2: 249.

Appendix. Darwin's Diary of Health

1. " + ," denotes one episode of vomiting.

2. "7 days," written in pencil, refers to days that Darwin was free of vomiting and able to work.

3. On 31 January 1849, Darwin attended a council meeting of the Geological Society in London (*Correspondence*, 4: 385).

4. "9 days," written in pencil, refers to the days of 15–23 February, 1849, when Darwin was free of vomiting and able to work.

5.
stone	lbs	ounces
10	7	12

6. Darwin's "sinking" feeling.

7. "With Flannel Waistcoat is 4 ounces."

8. Five minutes.

9. Evening.

10. On 16 August, 1849, Darwin visited the home of Lord Mahon at Chevening. A visit that was not mentioned in the *Diary*.

11. "Cleansing" may refer to taking an enema.

12. Written in pencil. Refers to Darwin's next weighing of himself being on 10 September 1849.

13. Written in pencil.

14. In her diary for September 1849, Emma recorded that on Tuesday 11 September Darwin went to Birmingham for a meeting of the British Association for the Advancement of Science, and on 12 September she followed him. On Saturday 15 September, they started out for Warwick, but then did not go because Darwin was "unwell." On Sunday 16 September they went to Malvern, and on 17 September returned to Birmingham. On Thursday 20 September they came home to Down. In his manuscript "Journal" Darwin recorded these travels as follows: "Sept 11 to 21. British Assoc. at Birmingham, going to Malvern on that Sunday."

15. "3 double" dashes, written in pencil.

16. Charles and Mary Lyell visited Down 15–18 October. Visit not recorded in *Diary* (*Correspondence*, 4: 385).

17. Written in pencil.

18. Written in pencil.

19. On 2 November 1849 William Fox visited Darwin at Down, although this visit is not mentioned in *Diary*. (*Correspondence*, 4: 385).

20. "T," travelling.

21. On 7 November 1849 Darwin attended a council meeting of the Geological Society (*Correspondence*, 4: 385).

22. This means that in the period of 12 weeks up to Saturday 10 November 1849, for every week Darwin had hydropathy treatments of 5 sweating processes, 2 douches, and 2 dripping sheets.

23. Written in pencil.

24. On 19 December, 1849, Darwin attended a council meeting of the Geological Society (*Correspondence*, 4: 385).

25. "T," travelling.

26. These crossed lines indicate that after 20 December Darwin will begin a new weekly course in hydropathy.

27. In the six-week period from 10 November to 20 December, for every week Darwin had 3 sweating processes, 4 douches, and 2 dripping sheets.

28. Written in pencil.

29. Emma began her confinement on 14 January, and 15 January 1850, Emma gave birth to a son, Leonard Darwin. On this occasion Darwin, for the first time, gave his wife chloroform before the doctor arrived to aid her in delivery (*Correspondence*, 4: 302–3, 311, 385).

30. At this time Darwin wrote Fox: "You ask after water cure.--I go honestly on & had had the douche 36° to 37° for 5 minutes & the shallow bath with water at 39° for 4 minutes this very morning." (*Correspondence*, 4: 303). The double lines may indicate that Darwin will change his hydropathy regimen by again (at times) using a sweating process (SW).

31. The Darwins' son George Howard Darwin born on 9 July, 1845.

32. "Georgey," the Darwins' son George.

33. At this time the Darwins' son William attended a preparatory school at Mitcham in Surrey. Emma's diary records that on Monday 28 January, 1850, "Willy went to school."

34. These notes on the different forms of hydropathy that Darwin used aided him in evaluating the effectiveness of these treatments. At this time he "regularly" reported on the treatments to Dr. Gully, who then gave him instructions (*Correspondence*, 4: 335).

35. Written in pencil.

36. 6 February, 1850, Darwin attended a council meeting of the Geological Society (*Correspondence*, 4: 385).

37. Darwin was nominated for election to the council of the Royal Society at a meeting on 16 November 1849. He attended a meeting of the Council on 7 February 1850, but was not among those who were re-elected at the meeting of 31 October 1850 (Records of the Royal Society).

38. Darwin here describes two successive episodes of vomiting occurring on the same day by first writing " + ," and then by writing "sickness," which was his frequent way of writing vomiting.

39. The parallel lines indicate that Darwin will begin a new regimen of hydropathy.

40. Written in pencil.

41. "16" is written in blue pencil over "15," which was written in black pencil.

42. "T," travelling.

43. On 10 April 1850, Darwin attended a meeting of the Geological Society (*Correspondence*, 4: 385).

44. The line indicates a new regimen of hydropathy.

45. Charles and Mary Lyell visited Down on 28–30 April. Not recorded in *Diary of Health* (*Correspondence*, 4: 385).

46. Written in pencil.

47. The nature of this "excitment" is not known.

48. The line indicates a change in hydropathy.

49. Written in pencil.

50. This was Darwin's third visit to Malvern since his departure in June 1849. It was made for the purpose of being medically evaluated by Dr. Gully (*Correspondence*, 4: 335).

51. Sitz Bath. 19, 20, 21, 22, and 24 June 1850, are the only times that Darwin recorded using Sitz Baths in the *Diary of Health*.

52. Written in pencil.

53. Written in pencil.

54. "T," travels.

55. Leith Hill was the home of Darwin's sister, Mrs. Caroline Wedgwood.

56. Written in pencil.

57. The Darwins' son William Erasmus Darwin, born 27 December, 1839.

58. Written in pencil.

59. Darwin here describes episodes of vomiting in the day, and then at night, by first writing "vomit" and then " + ."

60. Hartfield (a village in East Sussex) usually refers to the home of Sarah Elizabeth Wedgwood, Darwin's maternal aunt. It sometimes also refers to the nearby home of Emma's sister Charlotte, who was married to the Reverend Charles Langton (*Companion*).

61. Ramsgate was a town on the Kent coast, which was a resort for sea-bathing. The Darwins went to Ramsgate to try the effects of sea-bathing on their nine year-old daughter Annie who had begun to be ill (*Annie's Box*, 151–53). The *Diary of Health* shows that on 19, 20, and 21 October Darwin went "swim[ming]" at Ramsgate and did not take any hydropathy.

62. "12 bad days!," added in pencil after the *Diary* had been written in ink.

63. Written in pencil.

64. "Oct. 14 not tired in evening" added in pencil after the *Diary* had been written in ink.

65. Emma's diary for 16 November 1850 reads: "Ch & I went to Mitcham & brought home W[illiam]."

66. Written in pencil.

67. On 18 December 1850, Darwin attended a council meeting of the Geological Society (*Correspondence*, 4: 386).

68. Written in pencil.

69. Tartar Emetic Ointment was an irritant to the skin.

70. Change in hydropathy to "Sh."

71. Written in pencil.

72. "9th began Tartar" written in ink, crossing out in pencil.

73. The last entry on Tartar Emetic Ointment in the *Diary of Health*.

74. Written in pencil.

75. Croton was used as a tonic and in treating dyspepsia.

76. In the week of 24–31 March 1851, Darwin traveled with his sick daughter Annie from Down to London and then to Malvern. After leaving Annie at Malvern for treatment by Dr. Gully, he returned to London, and from there went home to Down (*Annie's Box*, 161–65. *Correspondence*, 5: 535).

77. Written in pencil.

78. Darwin was at Malvern from 17–24 April 1851, and because of his "insufferable" grief over the terminal illness and then death of Annie he did not write any entries about himself in his *Diary of Health* from 15–26 April. During this period he chronicled his grief and states of health in letters to Emma. He recommenced writing the *Diary* two days after he returned to Down from Malvern.

79. Written in pencil.

80. Horace Darwin.

81. Written in pencil.

82. The vertical line from 1 June to 21 June may indicate that during this period Darwin continued to treat himself with "sh" (shallow baths), and that after 21 June he stopped this treatment.

83. The vertical line indicates that the day and night symptoms on 8 and 9 June were the same.

84. Written in pencil.

85. Emma's diary for 1851 records: 22 July, Tuesday, "Rowlands & Armstrongs came"; 23 July, Wednesday, "went." This may refer to Daniel Rowland (1778–1859), antiquarian and philanthropist, born in Shrewsbury, who endowed Shrewsbury with a hospital for women; and William George Armstrong (1810–1900), inventor, who invented guns for the English government.

86. Written in ink. The first time Darwin writes double dashes in ink, instead of pencil. He also first encloses "double dashes" in parentheses.

87. At this time Darwin and his family sojourned at the London home of his brother Erasmus while they saw the Great Exhibition.

88. The horizontal line written on 27 August indicates after this date Darwin will again begin a course of hydropathy.

89. Written in ink.

90. "speudo" probably means "pseudo."

91. Written in ink. In April 1850 Darwin recorded 17 double dashes.

92. These crossed lines indicate that after 7 October Darwin changed his hydropathy regimen to only taking daily "sh," except on 11 October when he was traveling.

93. For more on Darwin's treatments with electrical appliances, see chapter 7, notes 31–33.

94. Written in ink.

95. "SU" means Seldom Up.

96. Bartholomew Sulivan was an officer on the *Beagle*, who then became Darwin's lifelong friend.

97. Written in ink.

98. The vertical lines indicate that the day and night symptoms for 15, 16, and 17 December were the same.

99. On 17 December 1851, Darwin attended a meeting of the Geological Society Club (*Correspondence*, 5: 536).

100. The bottom two lines are written in pencil. On January 1850 Darwin recorded 24 double dashes.

101. The horizontal line indicates that after 14 January Darwin changed his hydropathy regimen.

102. Emma's diary records that on 29 January 1852, Darwin went to London to bring their son William back to Down.

103. Written in ink.

104. These crossed lines indicate that after 29 February Darwin changed his hydropathy regimen.

105. Written in ink.

106. This refers to Darwin's hydropathy treatments from 14 January 1852 to 29 February 1852.

107. On 24 March 1852, Darwin and Emma visited their son William at Rugby School (*Correspondence*, 5: 536).

108. At Shrewsbury Darwin stayed at his family home and visited with his sisters Susan and Catherine (*Correspondence*, 5: 536).

109. Written in ink.

110. From 17–26 April 1852, Hooker and his wife visited Down (*Correspondence*, 5: 536).

111. Written in ink.

112. On 23 May, 1852, Darwin dined at High Elms, the home of his neighbor John William Lubbock (*Correspondence*, 5: 536).

113. Written in ink.

114. In her diary for June 1852 Emma wrote: 2 Wednesday, "Charles went to London sick"; 5 Saturday, "came home pretty well." The reason for Darwin's trip to London is not known.

115. The horizontal line and the crossed lines indicate that after 10 June Darwin had made a change in his hydropathy regimen.

116. The horizontal line on 20 June indicates that on this date Darwin's hydropathy change has stopped.

117. Written in ink.

118. The "Ten Days Treatment" refers to the hydropathy Darwin took on the days between 10 and 20 June.

119. The crossed lines indicate that after 11 July Darwin has begun a new hydropathy regimen.

120. Written in ink.

121. Emma's diary for 1852 records that from 5–9 August Charles and Mary Lyell visited Down, although the visit was not recorded in the *Diary of Health*.

122. The two crossed lines and the extended horizontal line indicate that after 21 August Darwin limited his hydropathy to daily shallow baths.

123. This refers to the weeks of hydropathy treatment from 12 July to 21 August.

124. Written in ink.

125. "Trs" may mean "Transpose"; that Darwin vomited on 6 September instead of 5 September. Emma's diary has no entries for either 5 or 6 September.

126. For Leith Hill, see note 55.

127. Written in ink.

128. Emma's diary for 1852 records that on 15 October "dined at the Normans." This refers to George Warde Norman, who lived at Bromley (*Companion*).

129. Not identified.

130. On 24 October 1852, Darwin wrote Fox: "I have been unusually well of late (no Water Cure) . . ." (*Correspondence*, 5: 100).

131. Emma's diary for 1852 records that on 25 October George Brettingham Sowerby came to prepare the drawings for Darwin's cirripide book.

132. Written in ink. In January 1850 Darwin had 24 double dashes. (Also recorded at end of *Diary* for November 1852).

133. Emma's diary for 1852 records: 8 November, "Ch went to London"; 12 November, "came home," although there is no *Diary* record of this visit. Darwin recollected that he and Hooker watched the funeral of the Duke of Wellington, which took place in London on 17–18 November (*Correspondence*, 5: 194.

134. Written in ink. At the end of the *Diary* for October 1852, Darwin had also mentioned that it was his best month since January 1850.

135. Written in ink.

136. This *Diary* page for January 1853 is written in two kinds of ink. The first two entries for 1 and 2 January and for all of the days of the month of January are written in black ink, which Darwin had used previously. The rest of the *Diary* is written in blue ink, including the last entry on "11 Double Dashes."

137. The vertical line extending from 5–16 January, alongside of which is written "Dr.," shows that Darwin treated himself with dripping sheets during these eleven days in January.

138. On 18 January 1853, Darwin reported to his zoologist friend Waterhouse: "I have just lately had a very bad fortnight, otherwise you w^d. have seen me at the [British] Museum this week" (*Correspondence*, 5: 111–12).

139. The entire *Diary* page for February 1853, including the last entry on "Nine Double Dashes," is written in blue ink.

140. On 1–3 February 1853, Darwin made a trip to London to visit his sisters Susan and Catherine, and brother Erasmus (*Correspondence*, 5: 536).

141. The entire *Diary* page for March 1853, including the last entry on "18 Double dashes," is written in blue ink.

142. There is no other record of Darwin's being in London around the date of 16 March.

143. The *Diary* page for April 1853 is written in two kinds of ink. All of the days of the month, and the entries through 18 April, are written in blue ink. The rest of the entries are written in black ink. From this time on, all of the *Diary* would be written in black ink.

144. Darwin was in London from 4–7 April 1853, and on 6 April attended a meeting of the Geological Society (*Correspondence*, 5: 536).

145. "Swimming" refers to a sensation that Darwin often experienced in his head.

146. For a discussion of the medicinal effects of tea, see Chapter 7, note 34.

147. On 7 May 1853, Darwin attended Lord Rosse's Royal Society party in London, where he talked with Hooker and Charles Bunbury (*Correspondence*, 5: 536).

148. On 1 June 1853, Darwin attended a meeting of the Geological Society (*Correspondence*, 5: 536).

149. The "1" after London probably refers to one fit of flatulence.

150. The Crystal Palace was being rebuilt at Sydenham.

151. Darwin's manuscript "Journal" for 1853 records: "July 14th to Eastbourne: visited Brighton & Hastings. Home Aug. 4th." Darwin and his family stayed at Sea Houses, Eastbourne, from 14 July to 4 August 1853.

152. The Hermitage, near Woking in Surrey, was the home of Harry Allen Wedgwood, Emma's brother. Darwin and his family stayed at the Hermitage from 13 to 17 August, and while there visited Chobham Camp where the English army was engaged in mimic warfare. Darwin "intensely" enjoyed seeing this warfare (*Correspondence*, 5: 539, note 22).

153. On this *Diary* page (as elsewhere in the *Diary*) Darwin sometimes writes "1" as "i."

154. For Crystal Palace, see note 150.

155. The underlining of the "very" is crossed out.

156. The purpose of this London visit is not known. Darwin mentions the visit in a 10 October 1853 letter to the American geologist James Dana (*Correspondence*, 5: 160).

157. The underlining of the "very" is crossed out.

158. The horizontal line indicates that hydropathy, which has been stopped after November 1852, will now begin again after 12 November 1853.

159. Darwin continued to test the effects of tea on his sleep.

160. In these entries for 13, 16, 19, 22, 25, and 28 November 1853, Darwin changed the way he wrote the sweating process. Instead of writing it as "Sw" he respectively wrote it

as: "S.W.," "S.W.," "SW," "SW," "S.W.," and "S.W." The reasons for these changes are not known.

161. Darwin's being "Sick & Heasish" and "<u>Poorly</u>" on 29–30 November, 1853, was caused by his having to attend a public ceremony of the Royal Society on 30 November, where he was awarded the Royal Medal of the Society. The award was for his work on barnacles, and his previous work in geology.

162. "w" means wakeful.

163. The reasons for Darwin's London visits on 1 and 10 December are not known.

164. Darwin's taking coffee or tea on 3–10 and 13 December 1853 was to evaluate how each of these drinks influenced his being wakeful at night. He hoped to be able to sleep better at night so that he would be less tired during the day.

165. In the December entries for 1853 Darwin again changed the way he wrote the sweating process so that he respectively wrote it as: "SW," "SW," "SW," "SW," "SW," "SW," and "SW" from 2–23 December. The reasons for these changes are not known.

166. The horizontal line indicates that hydropathy was stopped after 25 December 1853.

167. Emma's diary for 1854 records: Friday, 6 January, "Mrs Fry's party." This may refer to the wife of James Thomas Fry of Bastan, near the village of Hayes, about four miles northwest of Down. The Post Office directory lists the Frys there from the early 1850s to the early 1870s. In a 25 July 1863 letter to his son William, Darwin reports that "one day" his Down family and relatives "all went to the Frys & had a gorgeous party with about 80 people chiefly from London & dancing on the Lawn & dinner in grand tent, Band, & ices &c &c" (*Correspondence*, 11: 560–62, 562n10).

168. The reasons for Darwin's visit to London are not known.

169. The horizontal line indicates Darwin will try the effects of lemons.

170. On 23 and 24 January 1854, Darwin was evaluating the effects of lemons on his illness.

171. There is no other account of Darwin's 1 February 1854 London trip.

172. The "(Dinner Party)" is not identified.

173. Darwin went to London with Emma, his daughter Etty, and son Leonard (Emma's diary for 23–25 February, 1854).

174. On 23 and 24 January 1854, Darwin was evaluating the effects of lemons on his illness.

175. The Darwins' son Francis became ill on 12 March 1854 when he was at Hartfield. Darwin and Emma then went to Hartfield on 13 March. Darwin returned to Down on 17 March. Emma stayed at Hartfield with Francis, and returned to Down with him on 20 March. (Emma's 1854 diary for 12–20 March).

176. On 23 and 24 January 1854, Darwin was evaluating the effects of lemons on his illness.

177. Not identified.

178. Darwin attended a London meeting of the Linnean Society (*Correspondence*, 5: 537).

179. Emma's dairy for 1854 records: 24 May, "Ch. went to London."

180. On 25 May 1854 Darwin attended a meeting of the Philosophical Club of the Royal Society. At this time he wrote Hooker that his London visits had suited his "stomach admirably" (*Correspondence*, 5: 194, 195n5).

181. On 10 June 1854 Darwin, Emma, and Etty attended the opening of the new Crystal Palace at Sydenham. (Emma's diary for 10 June 1854, *Correspondence*, 5: 194–95, 195n6.)

182. During his 21–23 June 1854 visit to London, Darwin attended a dinner of the Philosophical Club of the Royal Society on 22 June (*Correspondence*, 5: 537).

183. Emma's diary for 1854 records: 12 July, "I very bad"; 13 July, "Ch & I to Hartfield"; 15 July, "Came home."

184. Double dashes under "very" are crossed out.

185. The reasons for Darwin's visit to London are not known.

186. The second dash under "very" is crossed out.

187. "p" means "poor." "S" means "seldom." Darwin uses "S" for seldom in his 1851 *Diary* entries for 6, 12, 21, 22, 23, and 25 November. "E" probably means evacuation, because of the contents of the passage, and Darwin's use of purgatives in his *Diary* entries for 6–8 September 1854.

188. This is the only time in the *Diary* that Darwin uses the term *wretched*. Describing a state of feeling that was worse than "poorly."

189. "(work)" here, and in the following entry on 5 September, refers to the successful actions of a cathartic, that Darwin is taking, which is probably Cordial Aloes.

190. For a discussion of the medical uses of Cordial Aloes, see Chapter 7, note 36.

191. Darwin may have continued to have trouble with his bowels, and tried a different cathartic, because on 22 September 1854, Emma wrote in her diary: "Chalk iron & rhub[arb], to C. did not do good." For a discussion of the Darwin family's use of iron chalk and rhubarb, see Chapter 7, note 36.

192. The dash under "very" is crossed out.

193. Emma's diary for 1854 records that from 9–14 October, she, her husband, and all of their children except for Horace went to Leith Hill.

194. Emma's dairy for 1854 records that on 23 October she and Darwin visited London.

195. Emma's 1854 diary recorded that on 26 October the Lyells and Hookers were at Down for a dinner party.

196. Emma's 1854 diary records that on 28 October the Lyells left Down.

197. On 2 November 1854, Darwin was elected a member of the Council of the Royal Society (*Correspondence*, 5: 537).

198. Emma's diary shows that from 2–4 November 1854, she and her husband visited London.

199. Instead of using Aloes in the form of a "Cordial," Darwin now uses it in the form of "liquid Tincture."

200. "1 w." means 1 drop of the liquid tincture of Aloes works.

201. "(4 ?)" refers to the questionable effectiveness of 4 drops of liquid tincture of Aloes.

202. The second dash under "very" is crossed out.

203. On 30 November–1 December 1854, Darwin was in London for the anniversary meeting of the Royal Society (*Correspondence*, 5: 537).

204. The Darwins' two sons Leonard and Francis were ill from 14–29 December 1854, with what Darwin described as "Fever & Inflammation" (*Correspondence*, 5: 253). Emma wrote in her 1854 diary that Leonard and Francis came home "unwell" from Sarah Wedgwood's on 13 and 15 December respectively. On 22 December she wrote that Francis had a "fit," and on 31 December that he "got up."

205. On 1 January 1855, Darwin wrote his relative Francis Galton that he and Emma were "looking out . . . for a House in London for a month" (*Correspondence*, 5: 253).

206. On 10 January he wrote Lyell: "We are going to take a House in London for 4 weeks, if we can get one, which seems exceedingly doubtful" (*Correspondence*, 5: 255).

207. On 14 January he wrote Lyell: "(I hope we have succeeded in a House, after infinite trouble, but am not sure, in York Place, Baker St)." (*Correspondence*, 5: 256).

208. On Monday, 15 January, he reported to his Down neighbor John Lubbock: "I have taken a House (28 York Place Baker St.) for a month & we all move on Thursday morning" (*Correspondence*, 5: 258).

209. A week after moving into his Baker Street house, on 25 January 1855, Darwin attended a Council meeting of the Royal Society, and a meeting of the Philosophical Club. However, during his sojourn in London his children became unwell, and he and Emma had (what he described as) "cough, & colds, & rheumatism nearly all the time" (*Correspondence*, 5: 289, 537).

Bibliography

Adler, D. 1989. "Darwin's Illness." *Israel Journal of Medical Science* 25 (4): 218–21.

Adler, Saul. 1959. "Darwin's Illness." *Nature* 184 (10 October): 1102–3.

———. 1965. "Darwin's Illness." *British Medical Journal* 8 (May): 1249–50.

Allan, Mea. 1967. *The Hookers of Kew, 1785–1911*. London: Joseph.

Allingham, William. 1967. *William Allingham's Diary*. Fontwell, Sussex: Centaur Press.

Alvarez, W. C. 1959. "The Nature of Charles Darwin's Lifelong Ill-Health." *New England Journal of Medicine* 261: 1110–12.

Atkins, Hedley. 1974. *Down, the Home of the Darwins*. London: Royal College of Surgeons.

Bacon, G. W. 1882. *The Life of Charles Darwin, with British Opinion on Evolution*. London: G. W. Bacon.

Barloon, Thomas J., and Russell Noyes Jr. 1997. "Charles Darwin and Panic Disorder." *Journal of the American Medical Association* 277: 138–42.

Baur, Susan. 1988. *Hypochondria: Woeful Imaginings*. Berkeley: University of California Press.

Bernstein, Ralph. 1984. "Darwin's Illness: Chagas' Disease Resurgens." *Journal of the Royal Society of Medicine* 77: 608–9.

Bettany, G. T. 1887. *Life of Charles Darwin*. London: W. Scott.

Bowlby, John. 1990. *Charles Darwin: A New Life*. London: Hutchinson.

Brace, Emma, ed. 1894. *The Life of Charles Loring Brace, Chiefly Told in His Own Letters*. New York: C. Scribner's.

Brinton, William. 1859. *The Disease of the Stomach*. London: J. Churchill.

Browne, Buckston. 1943. "Darwin's Health." *Nature*.

Browne, Janet. 1995. *Charles Darwin: Voyaging*. New York: Knopf

———. 2002. *Charles Darwin: The Power of Place*. New York: Knopf.

Brunton, T. Lauder. 1885. *A Textbook of Pharmacology, Therapeutics and Materia Medica*. London: Macmillan.

Brussel, James. 1966. "The Nature of the Naturalist's Unnatural Illness: A Study of Charles Robert Darwin." *Psychiatric Quarterly Supplement*, part 2, 1–17.

Calvin, William. 1998. *Down House: The Home of Charles Darwin*. Seattle: privately published.

Campbell, A. K. 2003. "What Darwin Missed." In *Astrophysics and Space Science* 285: 1–5.

Campbell, A. K., and S. B. Matthews. 2001. *Lactose Intolerance and the MATHS Syndrome: What Are They and How Can I Cope?* Wales: Welston Press.

Cattermole, M. J. G., and A. F. Wolfe. 1987. *Horace Darwin's Shop: A History of the Cambridge Scientific Instrument Company, 1878–1968*. Bristol and Boston: Adam Hilger.

Chapman, J. 1864. *Functional Diseases of the Stomach. Part I. Seasickness: Its Nature and Treatment*. London: Trübner.

Clark, James. 1846. *The Sanative Influence of Climate*. 4th ed. London: J. Murray.

Clark, John S. 1917. *The Life and Letters of John Fiske*. Boston: Houghton Mifflin.

Coley, N. G. 1973. "Henry Bence-Jones, M.D., F.R.S. (1813–1873)." *Notes and Records of the Royal Society of London* 28: 31–56.

Colp, R. 1977. *To Be an Invalid: The Illness of Charles Darwin*. Chicago: University of Chicago Press.

———. 1980. "'I Was Born a Naturalist': Charles Darwin's 1838 Notes about Himself." *Journal of the History of Medicine and Allied Sciences* 35: 8–39.

———. 1981. "Charles Darwin, Dr. Edward Lane, and the 'Singular Trial' of *Robinson v. Robinson and Lane*." *Journal of the History of Medicine and Allied Sciences* 36: 205–13.

———. 1985. "Notes on Charles Darwin's *Autobiography*." *Journal of the History of Biology* 18: 357–401.

———. 1986. "'Confessing a Murder': Darwin's First Revelations about Transmutation." *Isis* 77: 9–32.

———. 1987. "Charles Darwin's 'Insufferable Grief.'" *Free Associations* 9: 9–32.

———. 1998. "*To Be an Invalid*, Redux." *Journal of the History of Biology* 31: 211–40.

———. 2000. "More on Darwin's Illness." *History of Science* 38: 221–36.

Colvin, Christina, ed. 1971. *Maria Edgeworth: Letters from England, 1813–1844*. Oxford: Clarendon Press.

Colwell, Hector A. 1922. *An Essay on the History of Electrotherapy and Diagnosis*. London: W. Heinemann.

Coperman, W. S. C. 1964. *A Short History of the Gout and the Rheumatic Diseases*. Berkeley: University of California Press.

Cook, G. C. 1996. "Mary Darwin's Illness." *Notes and Records of the Royal Society of London* 50 (1): 59–63.

Copeland, James. 1858. *A Dictionary of Practical Medicine*. 3 vols. London: Longman, Brown, Green, Longmans and Roberts.

Darwin, Charles. 1839. *Journal of Researches into the Geology and Natural History of the Countries Visited by H.M.S. Beagle*. London: Henry Colburn.

———. 1845. *Journal of Researches into the Natural History and Geology of the Various Countries Visited during the Voyage of H.M.S. Beagle*. London: John Murray.

———. 1859. *On the Origin of Species by Means of Natural Selection, or the Preservation of Favoured Races in the Struggle for Life*. London: John Murray.

———. 1868. *The Variation of Animals and Plants under Domestication*. 2 vols. London: John Murray.

———. 1946. *Charles Darwin and the Voyage of the* Beagle. Edited by Nora Barlow. New York: Philosophical Library.

———. 1958. *Autobiography of Charles Darwin, 1809–1882. With the Original Omissions Restored.* Edited by Nora Barlow. London: Collins.

———. 1975. *Charles Darwin's Natural Selection: Being the Second Part of His Big Species Book Written from 1856 to 1858.* Edited from manuscript by Robert C. Stauffer. Cambridge: Cambridge University Press.

———. 1977. *Collected Papers of Charles Darwin.* Edited by Paul Barrett. 2 vols. Chicago: University of Chicago Press.

———. 1985. *Correspondence of Charles Darwin.* Edited by Frederick Burkhardt et al. 15 vols. Cambridge: Cambridge University Press.

———. 1987. *Charles Darwin's Notebooks, 1836–1844.* Edited by Paul H. Barrett, Peter J. Gautrey, Sandra Herbert, David Kohn, and Sydney Smith. Ithaca, N.Y.: British Museum (Natural History) and Cornell University Press.

———. 1988. *Charles Darwin's Beagle Diary.* Edited by Richard Darwin Keynes. Cambridge: Cambridge University Press.

Darwin, Erasmus. 1794 and 1796. *Zoonomia; or, The Laws of Organic Life.* 2 vols. London: J. Johnson.

———. 1798. *A Plan for the Conduct of Female Education: In Boarding Schools, Private Families, and Public Seminaries.* Philadelphia: John Ormrod.

Darwin, Francis. 1912. "FitzRoy and Darwin, 1831–1836." *Nature* 88: 547–48.

———. 1916. "Memoir of Sir George Darwin." In vol. 5 of Sir George Howard Darwin, *Scientific Papers.* Cambridge: Cambridge University Press.

———. 1882–87. "Reminiscences of My Father's Everyday Life." In *Life and Letters,* 1: 87–136.

———, ed. 1888. *The Life and Letters of Charles Darwin, Including an Autobiographical Chapter.* 2 vols. New York: D. Appleton.

Darwin, Francis, and A. C. Seward, eds. 1903. *More Letters of Charles Darwin.* 2 vols. New York: D. Appleton.

Darwin, Leonard. 1929. "Memories of Down House." *Nineteenth Century and After, 106,* 118–23.

De Beer, Gavin. 1964. *Charles Darwin: Evolution by Natural Selection.* Garden City, N.Y.: Doubleday.

———. 1968. "The Darwin Letters at Shrewsbury School." *Notes and Records of the Royal Society of London.*

Desmond, Adrian, and James Moore. 1991. *Darwin.* London: Michael Joseph.

DuBois, K. P., and E. M. K. Geiling. 1959. *Textbook of Toxicology.* New York: Oxford University Press.

Duncan, Andrew, Jr. 1826. *The Edinburgh New Dispensatory.* Edinburgh.

Estes, J. Worth. 1990. *Dictionary of Protopharmacology: Therapeutic Practices, 1700–1850.* Canton, Mass: Science History.

FitzRoy, Robert. 1839. *Narrative of the Surveying Voyages of His Majesty's Ships* Adventure and Beagle, *between the Years 1826 and 1836.* London: H. Colburn.

Fletcher, Ifan K. 1951. *Splendid Occasions in English History, 1520–1947*. London: Cassell.

Forrest, D. W. 1974. *Francis Galton: The Life and Work of a Victorian Genius*. New York: Taplinger.

Fortescue, John. 1930. *History of the British Army*. London: Macmillan.

Foster, W. D. 1965. "A Contribution to the Problem of Darwin's Ill Health." *Bulletin of the History of Medicine* 39. 477–78.

———. 1972. Review of Darwin's *Victorian Malady: Evidence for Its Medically Induced Origin*, by John H. Winslow. *Isis* 63 (December 1972): 591–92.

Freeman, Richard B. 1978. *Charles Darwin: A Companion*. Folkestone, Kent: William Dawson & Sons; Hamden, Conn: Archon Books, Shoestring Press.

———. 1984. *Darwin Pedigrees*. London: privately printed.

Galton, Francis. 1908. *Memories of My Life*. London: Methuen.

Garrod, Alfred Baring. 1863. *The Nature and Treatment of Gout and Rheumatic Gout*. 2nd ed. London: Walton and Maberly.

Geikie, Sir Archibald. 1895. *Memoir of Sir Andrew Crombie Ramsay*. London: Macmillan.

Glass, R. M. 2000. "Panic Disorder. It's Real and It's Treatable." *Journal of the American Medical Association* 283: 573–74.

Glickman, R. M. 1997. "Inflammatory Bowel Diseases: Ulcerative Colitis and Crohn's Disease." In *Harrison's Principles of Internal Medicine*, 12th ed., 1268–81. New York: McGraw-Hill.

Goldstein, J. H. 1989. "Darwin, Chagas,' Mind, and Body." *Perspectives in Biology and Medicine* 32(4): 586–601.

Good, R. 1954. "The Life of the Shawl." *Lancet*.

Goodman, Louis, and Alfred Gilman. 1955. *The Pharmacological Basis of Therapeutics*. New York: Macmillan.

———. 1985. *The Pharmacological Basis of Therapeutics*. 7th ed. New York: Macmillan.

Gould, G. M. 1903. "Charles Darwin." In *Biographic Clinics*. Philadelphia.

Graber, R. G., and L. P. Miles. 1988. "In Defense of Darwin's Father." *History of Sciences*, 28.

Grant Duff, Mountstuart E. 1904. *Notes from a Diary, 1892–1895*. London: J. Murray.

Greenacre, P. 1963. *The Quest for the Father: A Study of the Darwin-Butler Controversy, as a Contribution to the Understanding of the Creative Individual*. New York: International Universities Press.

Griez, E., and K. Schruers. 1998. "Experimental Pathophysiology of Panic." *Journal of Psychosomatic Research* 45: 493–503.

Gruber, Howard E., and Paul H. Barrett. 1974. *Darwin on Man*. New York: Dutton.

Guggenheim, F. G. 2000. "Somatoform Disorders." In Sadock and Sadock, eds., *Kaplan and Sadock's Comprehensive Textbook of Psychiatry*, ed. Benjamin J. Sadock and Virginia A. Sadock. 7th ed. Philadelphia: Lippincott.

Gully, James Manby, MD. 1846. *The Water Cure in Chronic Disease: An Exposition of the Causes, Progress, and Termination of Various Chronic Diseases of the Digestive Organs,*

Lungs, Nerves, Limbs, and Skin; and of their Treatment by Water and Other Hygienic Means. London: Churchill; New York: Wiley & Putnam.

Hague, J. 1884. "A Reminiscence of Mr. Darwin." *Harper's New Monthly Magazine,* October, 759–63.

Haight, Gordon S. 1940. *George Eliot and John Chapman, with Chapman's Diaries.* New Haven: Yale University Press.

Haller, John S., Jr. 1975. "The Use and Abuse of Tartar Emetic in the Nineteenth-Century Materia Medica." *Bulletin of the History of Medicine* 49: 235–57.

Hanifin, J. M., and G. Rajka. 1980. "Diagnostic Features of Atopic Dermatitis." Acta Dermatol Venereol (Stockholm) 92: 44–47.

Headland, Frederick W. 1852. *Essay on the Action of Medicines in the System.* London: J. Churchill.

———. 1863. *On the Action of Medicines in the System.* 4th American ed. Philadelphia: Lindsay and Blakiston.

Healey, Edna. 2001. *Emma Darwin: The Inspirational Wife of a Genius.* London: Headline.

Herbert, Sandra. 2005. *Charles Darwin, Geologist.* Ithaca, N.Y.: Cornell University Press.

Higginson, Thomas Wentworth. 1900. *Cheerful Yesterdays.* Boston: Houghton Mifflin.

Hillen, A., ed. 1982. *The Letters of Henry Wadsworth Longfellow.* Vol. 6. Cambridge: Harvard University Press.

Holland, Henry. 1840. *Medical Notes and Reflections.* 2nd ed. London.

———. 1855. *Medical Notes and Reflections.* London.

Hooker, Sir Joseph. 1899. "Reminiscences of Darwin." *Nature,* 22 June, 187–88.

Hubble, D. 1946. "The Evolution of Charles Darwin." *Horizon, 14.*

Hutchins, Horace G. 1914. *The Life of Sir John Lubbock, Lord Avebury.* Vol. 1. London: Macmillan.

Huxley, Julian, and H. B. D. Kettewell. 1965. *Charles Darwin and His World.* New York: Studio Book, Viking Press.

Huxley, Leonard. 1912. *Darwiniana.* New York: D. Appleton.

———. 1913. *Life and Letters of Thomas Henry Huxley.* 2 vols. New York: D. Appleton.

———. 1918. *Life and Letters of Sir Joseph Dalton Hooker.* 2 vols. London: J. Murray.

———. 1927. *Charles Darwin.* New York: Greenberg.

Huxley, Thomas. 1912. *Darwiniana: Essays.* New York: D. Appleton.

Innes, John Brodie. 1961. Recollections of Darwin by the Reverend John (Brodie) Innes. In "The Darwin-Innes Letters," ed. Robert M. Stecher. *Annals of Science* 17.

Jacyna, L. S. 1983. "John Goodsir and the Making of Cellular Reality." *Journal of the History of Biology* 16: 75–99.

Jensen, J. V. 1970. "The X-Club: Fraternity of Victorian Scientists." *British Journal for the History of Science* 5: 63–72.

Johnston, W. W. 1901. "The Ill-Health of Charles Darwin. Its Nature and Its Relation to His Work." *American Anthropologist* (n.s.) 3: 157.

Judd, John W. 1909. "Darwin and Geology." In *Darwin and Modern Science,* ed. A. C. Seward. Cambridge: Cambridge University Press.

———. 1910. *The Coming of Evolution.* Cambridge: Cambridge University Press.

Keith, Arthur. 1955. *Darwin Revalued.* London: Watts.

Kempf, Edward J. 1920. *Psychopathology.* St. Louis: C. V. Mosby.

Keynes, M. 1943. *Leonard Darwin, 1850–1943.* Cambridge: Privately printed at the Cambridge University Press.

Keynes, Randal. 2001. *Annie's Box: Charles Darwin, His Daughter, and Human Evolution.* London: Fourth Estate.

———. 2004. "The Sand-walk." In *Thinking Path,* ed. Shirley Chubb, 15–21. Shrewsbury Museum Services: Shrewsbury.

Keynes, Richard Darwin. 2003. *Fossils, Finches, and Fuegians.* New York: Oxford University Press.

King, Betsy. 1994. *The Owl and the Lark (Charles Darwin): A Medical Detective Story.* Penrith, Cumbria, England: Spar House Press. Ms. King is "the Owl" who stays up late in the night and sleeps during the morning. Darwin is "the Lark," who feels at his best in the morning and becomes tired in the evening, although often having difficulty in going to sleep. Ms. King believes that these differences in night and day activities are caused by differences in the hypoadrenocortical state.

King-Hele, Desmond. 1999. *Erasmus Darwin: A Life of Unequaled Achievement.* London: Giles de Mare.

Klein, D. F. 1993. "False Suffocation Alarms, Spontaneous Panics, and Related Conditions: An Integrative Hypothesis." *Archives of General Psychiatry* 50.

Kohn, Lawrence A. 1963. "Charles Darwin's Chronic Ill Health." *Bulletin of the History of Medicine* 37: 239–56.

Lane, Edward Wickstead. 1857. *Hydropathy; or, The Natural System of Medical Treatment: An Explanatory Essay.* London.

———. 1882. *Letter Read by Dr. B. W. Richardson F.R.S. at His Lecture on Chas. Darwin F.R.S. in St. George's Hall Langham Place, October 22nd, 1882 by Richard Lane.* Dr. Lane begins his *Letter* by writing Dr. Richardson that "in accordance with your request, I gladly send you a few reminiscences of the late Mr. Darwin, derived from an intimate acquaintance with him during a period of several years." The *Letter* takes the form of a pamphlet of 7 pages, without the name of a publisher or date of publication.

Lewis, John. 1909. "A Visit to Darwin's Village: Reminiscences of Some of His Humble Friends." *Evening News,* February 12, 4.

Licht, Sidney, ed. 1967. *Therapeutic Electricity and Ultraviolet Radiation.* 2nd ed. New Haven: E. Licht.

Litchfield, Henrietta, ed. 1904. *Emma Darwin, Wife of Charles Darwin: A Century of Family Letters.* 2 vols. Cambridge: Cambridge University Press.

———. 1910. *Richard Buckley Litchfield: A Memoir Written for His Friends.* Cambridge: privately printed at the Cambridge University Press

———. 1915. *Emma Darwin: A Century of Family Letters, 1792–1896.* 2 vols. London: John Murray.

———. n.d. "Biographical Sketch of Charles Darwin." DAR 262.23.1.

Litchfield, Richard Buckley. 1903. *Tom Wedgwood, the First Photographer.* London: Duckworth.

MacNalty, A. S. 1964. "The Ill Health of Charles Darwin." *Nursing Mirror, 4.*

Marchant, James, ed. 1916. *Alfred Russel Wallace: Letters and Reminiscences.* New York: Cassel.

Mayr, Ernst. 1992. *The Growth of Biological Thought.* Cambridge: Harvard University Press.

Medawar, P. B. 1967. *The Art of the Soluble.* London: Methuen.

Metcalfe, Richard. 1912. *The Rise and Progress of Hydropathy in England and Scotland.* London: Simpkin, Marshall, Hamilton, Kent.

Meteyard, Eliza. 1871. *A Group of Englishmen.* London: Longmans, Green.

Miall, L. C. 1883. *The Life and Work of Charles Darwin.* Leeds.

Milne, D. 1847. *On the Parallel Roads of Lochaber; with remarks on the changes of relative levels of sea and land in Scotland, and on the detrital deposits in that country.* Edinburgh: privately printed.

Milner, R. 2002. "Putting Darwin in His Place." *Scientific American* 287 (4): 103–4.

Mitchell, J. E. 1991. "Dental Complications of Bulimia Nervosa." *Journal of the New Jersey Dental Association.*

Moody, J. W. T. 1971. "The Reading of the Darwin and Wallace Papers: An Historical 'Non-event.'" *J. Soc. Bibliography of Natural History* 5 (6): 471–76.

Moorehead, Alan. 1969. *Darwin and the Beagle.* New York: Harper and Row.

Nash, L. A. 1921. "Some Memories of Charles Darwin." *Overland Monthly 77.*

Nash, Wallis. 1919. *A Lawyer's Life on Two Continents.* Boston: R. G. Badger.

"Naturalist's Evolution." 1959. *MD,* September.

Nemiah, J. C. 1975. "Neurasthenic Neurosis." In *Comprehensive Textbook of Psychiatry,* 2nd ed., eds. Alfred M. Freedman, Harold I. Kaplan, and Benjamin J. Sadock, 264–67. Baltimore: Williams and Wilkins.

Olby, R. C. 1963. "Charles Darwin's Manuscript of Pangenesis." *British Journal for the History of Science.*

Orrego, F., and C. Quintana. 2007. "Darwin's Illness: A Final Diagnosis." *Notes and Records of the Royal Society of London* 61: 23–29.

Osborn, Henry Fairfield. 1928. "Charles Darwin." In *Impressions of Great Naturalists.* New York: Charles Scribner's Sons.

Osler, William, ed. 1929. *Bibliotheca Osleriana.* Oxford: Clarendon Press.

Papp, L. A., D. F. Klein, and J. M. Gorman. 1993. "Carbon Dioxide Hypersensitivity, Hyperventilation, and Panic Disorder." *American Journal of Psychiatry* 150: 1149–57.

Paris, John Ayrton. 1825. *Pharmacologia.* 2 vols. New York: E. Duyckinck.

Pearson, Karl. 1914, 1924, 1930. *The Life, Letters, and Labours of Francis Galton.* 3 vols. Cambridge: Cambridge University Press.

Pickering, George. 1974. *Creative Malady.* London: Allen and Unwin.

Pike, E. Royston. 1974. *Human Documents of the Victorian Golden Age, 1850–1875.* London: Allen and Unwin.

Porter, Dorothy, and Roy Porter. 1989. *Patient's Progress: Doctors and Doctoring in Eighteenth-Century England.* Stanford: Stanford University Press.

Porter, Duncan M. 1983. "More Darwin Beagle Notes Resurface." *Archives of Natural History* 11: 315–16.

Poynter, F. N. D. 1950. "John Chapman (1821–1894): Publisher, Physician and Medical Reformer." *Journal of the History of Medicine.* Winter, 1–22.

Raverat, Gwen. 1952. *Period Piece: A Cambridge Childhood.* London: Farber and Faber.

Report of the Royal Commission on the Practice of Subjecting Live Animals to Experiments for Scientific Purposes: with Minutes of Evidence and Appendix. London: Her Majesty's Stationery Office, 1876.

Richardson, Benjamin Ward. 1901. *Disciples of Aesculapius.* New York: Dutton.

Ringer, Sydney. 1869. *A Handbook of Therapeutics.* London: H. K. Lewis.

Roberts, Frederick Thomas. 1874. *A Handbook of the Theory and Practice of Medicine.* Philadelphia: Lindsay and Blakiston.

Roberts, H. 1967. "Reflections on Darwin's Illness." *Geriatrics* 160–67.

Romanes, George J. 1882. "Life and Character." In *Charles Darwin: Memorial Notices,* reprinted from *Nature.* London: Macmillan.

Rosenberg, D. 1989. "Mr. Darwin Collects Himself." In *Nineteenth-Century Lives: Essays Presented to Jerome Hamilton Buckley,* ed. Laurence Lockridge, John Maynard, and Donald Stone. New York: Cambridge University Press.

Rowbottom, Margaret, and Charles Susskind. 1984. *Electricity and Medicine: History of Their Interaction.* San Francisco: San Francisco Press.

Royle, J. Forbes, and Frederick W. Headland. 1865. *A Manual of Materia Medica and Therapeutics.* 4th ed. London: John Churchill and Sons..

Rudwick, M. 1974. "Darwin and Glen Roy: A 'Great Failure' in Scientific Method?" *Studies in History and Philosophy of Science* 5: 97–185.

Sauer, Gordon, C. 2000. "Charles Darwin Consults a Dermatologist." *International Journal of Dermatology* 474–78.

Schwartz, J. S. 1995. "George John Romanes's Defence of Darwinism: The Correspondence of Charles Darwin and His Chief Disciple." *Journal of the History of Biology* 28 (2): 281–316.

Schweber, S. S. 1977. "The Origin of the *Origin* Revisited." *Journal of the History of Biology* 10: 229–316.

Secord, James A. 2000. *Victorian Sensation: The Extraordinary Publication, Reception, and Secret Authorship of "Vestiges of the Natural History of Creation."* Chicago: University of Chicago Press.

Seward, Anna. 1804. *Memoirs of the Life of Dr. Darwin*. Philadelphia: W. Poyntell.

Sheppard, Francis. 1971. *London, 1808–1870: The Infernal Wen*. London: Secker and Warburg.

Simpson, G. G. 1958. "Charles Darwin in Search of Himself." *Scientific American* 199: 117–22.

Simpson, Larry. 1996. "From Molecular Evolution to Biomedical Research: The Case of Charles Darwin and Chagas' Disease." In Charles R. Marshall and J. William Schopf, eds., *Evolution and the Molecular Revolution*. Sudbury, Mass.: Jones and Bartlett.

Smith, Fabienne. 1990. "Charles Darwin's Ill Health." *Journal of the History of Biology* 23: 443–59.

———. 1992. "Charles Darwin's Health Problems: The Allergy Hypothesis." *Journal of the History of Biology* 25: 285–306.

Smith, K. G. V., ed. 1987. "Darwin's Insects: Charles Darwin's Entomological Notes." *Bulletin of the British Museum Natural History* 14: 1–143.

"Snuff and Its Adulteration." 1853. *Lancet*, 2.

Southey, Charles Cuthbert, ed. 1855. *The Life and Correspondence of Robert Southey*. New York: Harper.

Stetten, D. 1959. "Gout." *Perspectives in Biology and Medicine*, Winter, 194–95.

Stott, Rebecca. 2003. *Darwin and the Barnacle*. London: Faber and Faber.

Sulloway, Frank J. 1991. "Darwinian Psychobiography." *New York Review of Books*, October 10, 29–32.

———. 2003. "Darwin and His Doppelgänger." *New York Review of Books*, 18 December, 36.

Tennyson, Hallam. 1897. *Alfred Lord Tennyson: A Memoir by His Son*. 2 vols. New York: Macmillan.

Thomson, William. 1862. "On the Age of the Sun's Heat." *Macmillan's Magazine*, 5 March, 288–93.

Topham, Jon. 1997. "Charles Darwin of Woking? Emma Darwin's Recollections of House-Hunting." *Darwin College Magazine*, March, 50–54.

Trollope, A. 1867. *The Last Chronicle of Barset*. 2 vols. London: Smith, Elder.

Wallace, Daniel J., and Bevra Hannahs Hahn, eds. 1993. *Dubois' Lupus Erythematosus*. 4th ed. Philadelphia: Lea and Febiger.

Ward, Thomas H. 1926. *History of the Athenaeum, 1824–1925*. London: privately published.

Warner, Alan. 1975. *William Allingham*. Lewisburg, Pa: Bucknell University Press.

Wedgwood, Barbara, and Hensleigh Wedgwood. 1980. *The Wedgwood Circle, 1730–1807*. Don Mills, Ont.: Collier Macmillan.

Wells, Geoffrey. 1938. *Charles Darwin: A Portrait*. New Haven: Yale University Press.

Williams, G. H., and R. G. Dluhy. 1991. "Diseases of the Adrenal Cortex." In *Harrison's Principles of Internal Medicine*, 1713–35. 12th ed. New York: McGraw-Hill, Health Profession Division.

Wilson, Leonard G., ed. 1970. *Sir Charles Lyell's Scientific Journals on the Species Question.* New Haven: Yale University Press.

———. 1977. "The Puzzling Illness of Charles Darwin." *Journal of the History of Medicine and Allied Sciences, 32.*

———, ed. 1978. "Fevers and Science in Early Nineteenth-Century Medicine." *Journal of the History of Medicine and Allied Sciences* 33: 286–407.

Winslow, John H. 1971. *Darwin's Victorian Malady.* Philadelphia: American Philosophical Society.

Wolcott, R. B., J. Yager, and G. Gordon. 1984. "Dental Sequelae to the Binge-Purge Syndrome (Bulimia): Report of Cases." *Journal of the American Dental Association* 109: 723–25.

Wood, E. S. 1876. "Illuminating Gas in Its Relation to Health." *Public Health Papers Rep.* 3.

Woodham-Smith, Cecil. 1972. *Queen Victoria.* New York: Knopf.

Woodruff, A. W. 1965a. "Darwin's Health in Relation to His Voyage to South America." *British Medical Journal* 1: 745–50.

———. 1965b. "Darwin's Illness." *British Medical Journal* 1: 1380.

———. 1968. "The Impact of Darwin's Voyage to South America on His Work and Health." *Bulletin of the New York Academy of Medicine* 44: 661–72.

Young, D. A. B. 1997. "Darwin's Illness and Systemic Lupus Erythematosus." *Notes and Records of the Royal Society of London* 51 (1): 77–86.

Index

Ralph Colp Jr., M.D., is assistant professor of psychiatry at Columbia University and senior attending psychiatrist at St. Luke's Roosevelt Hospital in New York City.